T0215494

Advanced Survival
Models

Chapman & Hall/CRC Biostatistics Series

Series Editors
Shein-Chung Chow, Duke University School of Medicine, USA
Byron Jones, Novartis Pharma AG, Switzerland
Jen-pei Liu, National Taiwan University, Taiwan
Karl E. Peace, Georgia Southern University, USA
Bruce W. Turnbull, Cornell University, USA

Recently Published Titles

Mathematical and Statistical Skills in the Biopharmaceutical Industry: A Pragmatic Approach
Arkadiy Pitman, Oleksandr Sverdlov, L. Bruce Pearce

Bayesian Applications in Pharmaceutical Development
Mani Lakshminarayanan, Fanni Natanegara

Innovative Statistics in Regulatory Science
Shein-Chung Chow

Geospatial Health Data: Modeling and Visualization with R-INLA and Shiny
Paula Moraga

Artificial Intelligence for Drug Development, Precision Medicine, and Healthcare
Mark Chang

Bayesian Methods in Pharmaceutical Research
Emmanuel Lesaffre, Gianluca Baio, Bruno Boulanger

Biomarker Analysis in Clinical Trials with R
Nusrat Rabbee

Interface between Regulation and Statistics in Drug Development
Demissie Alemayehu, Birol Emir, Michael Gaffney

Innovative Methods for Rare Disease Drug Development
Shein-Chung Chow

Medical Risk Prediction Models: With Ties to Machine Learning
Thomas A Gerds, Michael W. Kattan

Real-World Evidence in Drug Development and Evaluation
Harry Yang, Binbing Yu

Cure Models: Methods, Applications, and Implementation
Yingwei Peng, Binbing Yu

Bayesian Analysis of Infectious Diseases
COVID-19 and Beyond
Lyle D. Broemeling

Statistical Meta-Analysis using R and Stata, Second Edition
Ding-Geng (Din) Chen and Karl E. Peace

Advanced Survival Models
Catherine Legrand

Structural Equation Modeling for Health and Medicine
Douglas Gunzler, Adam Perzynski and Adam C. Carle

For more information about this series, please visit: https://www.routledge.com/
Chapman--Hall-CRC-Biostatistics-Series/book-series/CHBIOSTATIS

Advanced Survival Models

Catherine Legrand

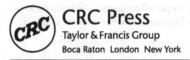

CRC Press
Taylor & Francis Group
Boca Raton London New York

CRC Press is an imprint of the
Taylor & Francis Group, an **informa** business

A CHAPMAN & HALL BOOK

First edition published 2021
by CRC Press
6000 Broken Sound Parkway NW, Suite 300, Boca Raton, FL 33487-2742

and by CRC Press
2 Park Square, Milton Park, Abingdon, Oxon, OX14 4RN

ISBN: 978-0-367-14967-3 (hbk)
ISBN: 978-0-367-71536-6 (pbk)
ISBN: 978-0-429-05416-7 (ebk)

Typeset in Computer Modern font
by KnowledgeWorks Global Ltd

To Adèle and Hugo.

Contents

Preface

What is often referred to as "survival data analysis" is actually a very broad field of statistics, encompassing a large variety of methods used in various fields of application. The analysis of "time-to-event" data has exploded over the last decades resulting in numerous new developments and a multitude of publications and textbooks on the subject. While the main goal is to analyze a response variable of the form "time from a given origin to the occurrence of a well defined event", the main specificity of time-to-event data is the presence of censoring. This pertains to the fact that at the time of analyzing the data, the time of interest will not be fully observed for all individuals, and this will actually precludes the use of most standard statistical analyzes techniques developed for continuous variables.

Time-to-event data are common in medical research, the basic example being time to death which led to the denomination "survival analysis". However, we can think of plenty of other examples: time to progression of a cancer, time to HIV sero-conversion for AIDS patients, time to organ rejection for transplanted patients, time to occurrence of influenza in a vaccination study, ... Note that the event of interest does not necessary have to be negative and we could also consider for example time to first pregnancy in female suffering from fertility problems, time to hospital discharge for covid-19 hospitalized patients, time to the disappearance of a given symptoms, ... As mentioned before, survival data analysis find its place in many other fields and examples are numerous: time to the breakdown of a machine in engineering, time to the first cigarette in epidemiology, time to the first child in sociology, time to finding a solution to a problem for a child in psychology, time to completion of a PHD in educational science, ... This book will mainly focus on applications from the medical research as these two fields are closely related. It is indeed recognized that several methodological research questions in the field of survival analysis are (partly) induced by progress made in medicine. This is for example the case of the cure model, originally proposed to take into account the possibility of cure in cancer patients or of the joint models whose rise over the last 20 years is certainly to put in conjunction with the development of personalized based medicine. However, all the techniques considered in this books also have applications in many other fields, and may actually have been developed in parallel in economy, engineering, demography, ...

There exist numerous very good books on "classical methods" for survival data, and by classical I mean assuming independent observations, one single event of interest that would be observed for all observations if follow-up would be long enough, no competing risks,and considering only covariates measured at baseline. Several of these books include one or two chapters dedicated more specific issues such as correlated observations, multiple types of event, presence of a "cure fraction", multiple outcomes, or handling of a longitudinal prognostic marker. Also, most of these topics have also been more specifically addressed in dedicated textbooks. However, to my knowledge there was no book addressing all of these issues with a practical perspective. Since, I missed such a book for my course on "Advanced Survival Models" in the master program in biostatistics at the Université catholique de Louvain (Belgium), my idea in writing this book was to fill this gap.

This book therefore aims to gather in a single reference some more advanced survival models, such as frailty models (in case of unobserved heterogeneity or clustered data), cure models (when a fraction of the population will not experience the event of interest), competing risk models (in case of different types of event), and joint survival models for a time-to-event endpoint and a longitudinal outcome. Main focus is on the understanding of the methods and models and of the appropriate estimation techniques (with sufficient methodological details to grasp a sound understanding of these techniques while avoiding too advanced methodological developments). A key point will also be their implementation and the interpretation of the output of such models. This book is therefore illustrated with numerous real-life examples as well as some real-life data analyzed in R and SAS. All the datasets analyzed in this book are either available in referenced R packages or can be freely available for download from to complete . Main part of R and SAS code to re-produce the analyzes presented in this book can also be downloaded from the same place. Note that these codes have been written with the objective to illustrate the methodologies presented in this book and experts R/SAS programmers may find several ways to optimize these codes.

After a first general introductory chapter which also serves to introduce the datasets that will be further analyzed in the next chapters, Chapter 2 aims to sum-up the main ideas of survival data analysis, while focusing primarily on the concepts required for a good understanding of the following chapters. Chapter 3 deals with the frailty models; introducing the idea of univariate and multivariate (clustered) survival data, and pursuing with a discussion of several parametric and semi-parametric frailty models. Chapter 4 introduces cure models, describing the context and motivation for such models, and then describing the two main families of cure models, namely mixture cure models and promotion time (cure) models. Chapter 5 describes the methods for competing risks, starting from the different possible research questions one may envisage when facing competing risks (combined analysis, marginal analysis, or competing risk analysis) and introducing the various quantities of interest and how they differ (e.g., cause-specific and sub-distribution hazard) as well as corresponding estimation and modeling approaches. Finally, Chapter 6 will provide a broad overview of joint modeling of a survival endpoint and a longitudinal marker, both via the shared random effect approach and via the latent-classes approach. The idea and advantages of joint models will be presented, followed by a general presentation of the main estimation techniques for each approach. Throughout the book, I concentrate on right censored data (extensions to left and interval censoring will be referenced when available), and on frequentist methods, although Bayesian references will also be mentioned.

This book is mainly dedicated to applied statisticians in the pharmaceuticals industry and in medical research institutes but also to be used to accompany a graduate course on survival data analysis in a (bio-)statistics program. While the book is mainly illustrated with examples from the medical field, it should also be accessible for applied statisticians in other fields of application. I hope this book could also be a good introductory reference for methodological researchers interested in discovering (some) of the main extensions of classical survival analysis. Of course, if the objective is to perform advanced research on a specific topic addressed in this book, then more in-depth references will be necessary and I've try to provide at the end of each chapter some interesting further references. These lists of further references are not to be considered as exhaustive but rather as a starting point to dig further into the subject. This comment also applies to the overview provided at the end of each chapter on available software. I have mainly considered R and SAS but even for these two software the packages, functions and macro mentioned certainly do not represent an exhaustive list.

When writing this book I have assumed that the reader has already some basic knowledge of statistical data analysis and inference, and in particular already a good background on standard maximum likelihood theory and standard regression models for a continuous or survival endpoint. This comes of course with minimum prerequisites in mathematics (matrix algebra, concept of limit, derivatives and integrals, ...). I also assume basic familiarity with the use of R and/or SAS in particular with regards to data import and manipulation.

I am very grateful to all who will take the time to read this book. I hope you will find in it, depending on what you are looking for, answers to your questions, further lines of research or simply some interest in reading it. Writing this book was a first experience for me, and I'm sure that there are things that I should have done differently, or that you will still find some typos, errors or ambiguities despite all my efforts. If this is the case, please do not hesitate to let me know about these (catherine.legrand@uclouvain.be).

Acknowledgment for use of data

The example datasets that accompany this book are either already available from existing R packages (colon cancer data, diabetic retinopathy data, advanced ovarian cancer) or can be freely downloaded from complete . Researchers who download and analyze these data accept the following conditions:

1. The research shall be scientifically sound and peer reviewed before publication

2. The source of data shall be acknowledge in all presentations and publications, including a reference to publication(s) by the investigator or group of investigators who generated the data

3. The results of the analyses shall be made available to the research community and not used for commercial purposes

4. The confidentiality of individual patient data shall be protected

The author acknowledges that the rectal cancer data (AERO98) [99] were provided for re-analysis by the International Drug Development Institute (IDDI) with permission from the Sponsor of the trial, the European Association for Research in Oncology (AERO). The children ALL data (EORTC 58951) [104] and the melanoma data (EORTC 18891) [109] were provided for re-analysis by the European Organisation for Research and Treatment of Cancer (EORTC). The contents of this book and methods used are solely the responsibility of the author and do not necessarily represent the official views of IDDI or the EORTC.

Acknowledgment

I could not go ahead without a very warm thank you to my two former PhD promoters, Prof. Paul Janssen and Prof. Luc Duchateau, who transmitted me their passion for statistical research on survival data analysis. I also would like to thank my former EORTC colleagues with whom I learned at the beginning of my career what it really means to analyze survival data in the quest to improve the treatment of cancer patients. A special thought also to all my PhD students with whom I have been working on several of the topics addressed in this book, I'm very proud of them, of the work we did together and of their current career.

I would also like to thank the anonymous reviewers of the book proposal for their very valuable feedback and suggestions. Some made me suffer, but all were very useful. Also, Rob Calver and Vaishali Singh at Chapman and Hall/CRC deserve all my gratitude for their support and their infinite patience.

Last but not least, I would like to thank my colleagues, friends, and family for their support while I was writing this book, some of them have even promised me to read it! I'm particularly grateful to Caroline for her endless encouragements and of course to my husband Marc for always believing I could do it! I will end by apologizing to my children, Adèle and Hugo, the two best children ever, for all the time spent working on this book and in particular during these very peculiar lockdown weeks we had to face this year.

Catherine Legrand
July 2020

List of Figures

List of Tables

Author

Catherine Legrand is Professor in Statistics and Biostatistics at the Institute of Statistics, Biostatistics, and Actuarial Sciences (ISBA-LIDAM) of the Université Catholique de Louvain (UCLouvain, Belgium). She obtained a Master Degree in Mathematics from the Université Libre de Bruxelles (ULB, Belgium) in 1998. She worked for 7 years at the European Organization for Research and Treatment of Cancer (EORTC, Brussels) and became the primary statistician of the EORTC Lung Cancer Group. She was also a member of the EORTC Treatment Outcome Research Group, the Elderly Task Force, and coordinator of the EORTC Independent Data Monitoring Committee. In parallel, she completed a PhD in 2005 at the Center for Statistics, Hasselt University, in the field of survival analysis (frailty models). Early 2006, she started working as biometrician at Merck Sharp & Dohme (MSD) where she was involved in the design and analysis of clinical trials in respiratory diseases. In September 2007, she joined the
Université Catholique de Louvain (UCLouvain). Her area of research includes survival data analysis, design and analysis of clinical trials and analysis of medical data. Along with these professional experiences, she co-authored more than 80 papers in peer-reviewed clinical and statistical journals.

Symbols

Symbol Description

$I(.)$ Indicatrice function, equal 1 if the argument is true and zero otherwise

$sgn(.)$ Sign function, equal -1 if the argument is negative and +1 otherwise

T Non-negative continuous random variable representing the real time to the event of interest.

$F(.)$ Distribution function

$f(.)$ Density function

$S(.)$ Survival function

$h(.)$ Hazard function

$H(.)$ Cumulative hazard function

C Non-negative continuous random variable representing the time to censoring.

Y Non-negative continuous random variable representing the observed time (time to censoring or to the event of interest whichever comes first), $Y = min(T, C)$.

δ Censoring indicator, with value 1 if the real time to event is observed and 0 otherwise

$G(.)$ Distribution function of the time to censoring variable C, $\delta = I(T \leq C)$

$g(.)$ Density function of the time to censoring variable C

n Number of observations in a sample

y_i Observed time to event or censoring for the ith observation

$y_{(i)}$ i^{th} ordered distinct event time

$d_{(i)}$ Number of observed events at the ith ordered distinct event time

$\mathfrak{R}(y_{(i)})$ Risk set at $y_{(i)}$

$R(y_{(i)})$ Size of the risk set at $y_{(i)}$

$\mathfrak{R}^\star(y_{(i)})$ Extended risk set at $y_{(i)}$

$R^\star(y_{(i)})$ Size of the extended risk set at $y_{(i)}$

$z_{\alpha/2}$ $\alpha/2$ percentile of the standard normal distribution

$\mathbf{X}$ Vector of covariates, with $\mathbf{X}^t = (X_1, \ldots, X_p)$

$\mathbf{x}_i$ Observed vector of covariates for the ith individual, with $\mathbf{x}_i^t = (x_{i1}, \ldots, x_{ip})$

$\mathbf{U}$ Frailty (random variable)

$f_{\mathbf{U}(.)}$ Frailty density

$\mathscr{L}(.)$ Laplace transform

$\mathscr{L}^{(q)}(.)$ q^{th} derivative of the Laplace transform

B Cure status: $B = 1$ for a susceptible (uncured) observation and $B = 0$ for a cure observation

$S_u(.)$ Survival function of the uncured observations; $S_u(t) = S(t \mid B = 1)$

E	Event type in a competing risks setting; $E = 1, ..., K$	$h_k(.)$	Sub-distribution hazard function
$F_k(.)$	Cause specific cumulative incidence function or sub-distribution function; $F_k(t) = P(T \leq t, E = k)$	$\lambda_k(.)$	Cause-specific hazard function

1

Introduction

1.1 Survival data analysis

Survival data or more generally speaking "time-to-event" data considers the time from a given origin to the occurrence of an event of interest, for example the time from the diagnosis of a certain disease to the death of the patient. While it is common to speak about *survival time*, the event considered is not necessarily death and we could, for example, be interested in the time to cancer relapse in an oncology study, the time to rejection of the transplanted organ in a transplantation study, the time to pain relief post surgery in an analgesic studies, or the time to the first pregnancy. Obviously, survival data are not restricted to medicine, and one can also think of time to first employment after graduation, time to the first claim for an insurance policy, time to break down of an engine, ... As can be seen from these examples, the event of interest can be either negative (death, rejection, break down, ...) or positive (pain relief, first employment, ...). While the term *survival analysis* is commonly used in the biomedical area, the terms of *duration analysis* and *reliability analysis* are more common in human sciences and engineering.

Survival data have two main distinguishing features. First, the time-to-event, often denoted T, is obviously a positive continuous random variable. A second typical feature of survival data is that they may be subject to censoring and truncation, which leads to incomplete data. Censoring means that for certain individuals under study, the time-to-event of interest is not known precisely. For example, a patient may still be alive at the time of the last follow-up visit in a clinical study. In that case, we know that the real survival time is longer than the observed survival time and the survival time is said to be right-censored at the date of the last information available. Although right-censoring is usually considered to be the more common form of censoring, one also speaks about left censoring and interval-censoring, and these concepts will be shortly wrapped up in Section 1.2.1, together with truncation. While for censored observations, "some" information is available, truncation occurs when a part of the relevant subject's observations will not at all appear in the data. Unless specified otherwise, we will concentrate in this book on right-censoring and provide further references for left- and interval-censoring and/or truncation whenever available.

Time-to-event or survival data analysis has been the subject of numerous textbooks, amongst which are [13, 78, 91, 181, 186, 372]. For a more applied perspective, we can also mention [8, 193] and [260] amongst many others, or [249, 282] who focus on the design and analysis of clinical trials with a time-to-event endpoint. These books mainly consider what can be called *classical* or *standard survival data*. Such data are characterized by a single event of interest (e.g. death from any cause). Furthermore, one assumes that this event would be observed for all experimental units if the follow-up would be long enough. One assumes further that all experimental units are independent and that the population is homogeneous given the observed covariates.

These classical survival data analysis techniques encompass estimation, hypothesis tests, and regression models. Such regression models are useful to analyse simultaneously the impact of several factors on the time-to-event under investigation. For example, in the context of a clinical trial, such regression models are often used to estimate the treatment effect on time to death while adjusting for important prognostic factors such as the stage of disease at randomization. These models are particularly useful in the context of observational studies where one has to adjust for confounding factors. The Cox proportional hazards model is certainly the most popular regression model for time-to-event data and is covered in a wide range of references.

While these methods are applicable in a wide series of practical situations, these assumptions are not always realistic. For example, observations may be correlated, or the population may be heterogeneous due to some unobserved factors, or observations may be subject to more than one type of events, or on the contrary some observations may be *non-susceptible* or *cured* for the event of interest. These features have led to the development of more *advanced survival models* which will be the topic of this book.

In the late seventies, Vaupel [397] introduced the idea that the population may not be homogeneous, even when accounting for known prognostic factors, and formalized this idea through the introduction of a *univariate frailty*, that is, a latent variable acting multiplicatively on the risk of event of each individual. This allows the "more frail" individuals to experience the event quicker and the "less frail" individuals to experience the event later, even if the factors explaining the presence of more and less frail individuals have not been measured. This idea has been further developed to take into account correlation between clustered observations. The idea is that observations within the same cluster share some unobserved risks factors that make them "more alike" in terms of fragility than observations from different clusters, leading to the concept of *multivariate frailty*. A cluster may be a single individual on which repeated measurements are taken. For example, in the analysis of time to repeated asthma attacks in young children, we can obviously expect time to successive asthma attack within a same child to be more correlated than time to asthma attacks in different children. However, clustered data can also occur when several observations are grouped together, sharing some "features" together. A common example is the analysis of twins (e.g., time to death in twins), or paired organs (e.g., time to blindness of each of the two eyes) where both components or a pair share the same genetic material and environmental factors. But the cluster can also be of various sizes, like students grouped in a class or school or patients grouped in hospitals with the individuals from a same cluster being expected to be more correlated than individuals from different clusters. One popular way (but not the only one as we will see) to analyse such data is using a (shared) frailty model. Frailty models are presented in one or more dedicated chapters of most of the general references mentioned above [13, 78, 181, 186, 260, 372], as well as in few dedicated textbooks [107, 93, 152, 406]. Frailty models will be discussed in Chapter 3 of this book, considering both the univariate and multivariate settings.

A classical assumption in survival analysis is that if the follow-up would be long enough, all observations under study would experience the event of interest. In other words, one assumes that all observations are at risk for the event of interest. There are, however, several applications in different fields for which this assumption is not realistic. Some typical examples are time to recurrence after treatment for a curable disease (some patients are cured and will therefore not experience recurrence of the disease) or time to a second pregnancy after a first child (some women will never have a second child for various reasons). In these situations, the population is said to include a fraction of *non-susceptible* or *cured* observations. As a consequence, we will see that, at the level of the population, the traditional cumulative distribution function is not proper anymore (i.e., does not tend to 1 when time tends to infinity), and appropriate modeling techniques have to be used to account for this. The first developments on *cure models* have been presented in the book of Maller and Zhou [244] and despite the fact that cure models have been the subject of a lot of attention in the literature over the last two decades, this remains to the best of our knowledge, the only book available on the subject. We will present in Chapter 4, the main two families of cure models, and discuss when and how to apply them in practice.

Another specific feature of survival data occurs when each individual under study is at risk of several types of events, which is further complicated by the fact that the occurrence of one type of event can preclude the occurrence of the other type(s) of event or at least modify the risk of these other event type(s) to occur. This situation is usually refer to as the presence of *competing risks*. The most popular example is probably the case of cause-specific death. Assume we follow patients suffering from a given disease, e.g. AIDS, and our interest lies in the time to AIDS-related deaths. Obviously patients suffering from AIDS may still die from another cause (cardiovascular death, car accident, ...) and such a death would prevent us from observing the time of AIDS-related death for this patient. Other examples are the time to progression for patients suffering from a cancer (with death as a competing event) or time to in-hospital infection for hospitalized patients (with death or discharge as a competing event). While an intuitive way to address this situation is to censor individuals experiencing a competing event, it will in most cases not be an appropriate way to analyse such data and specific techniques have been developed. Competing risk analysis is presented in some general reference books on survival data [78, 91, 181, 193, 260, 372] and is also the subject of some dedicated book such as [93, 132, 300] . Chapter 5 will be devoted to techniques for the analysis of survival data in the presence of competing risks.

Finally, we will consider a situation where we want to analyse information on a survival endpoint (e.g. time to death) and a longitudinal (continuous) outcome. This will typically occur if we are interested in studying the impact of biomarker measured at repeated time-points on the survival of the patients. A common example is the follow-up of the PSA level in prostate cancer patients as a predictor of a recurrence of the disease. A first idea could be to include this latter information as a time-dependent covariate in survival model. We would, however, see that, in many situations, considering a *joint modeling approach* may be a better option. Both outcomes are then modeled separately and joined together by some structure. The nature of the structure joining the two models will lead to two main broad classes of joint models, namely random effect joint model and latent classes joint model. The first approach is detailed in [114, 320], as well as in [393] with this last reference a special focus being on the question of dynamic prediction in the context of survival data. We will present these two classes of joint models in Chapter 6 and discuss their competitiveness over time-dependent variables.

Each chapter (except Chapter 6) will be illustrated with some real-life data, which are either publicly available data or data provided by IDDI and by the EORTC. A brief presentation of these datasets is included at the end of this chapter (see Section 1.3). We will come back to these examples in the next chapters to illustrate the techniques discussed as well as their implementation in R [371] and in SAS [174].

This book assumes that the reader is familiar with the main classical concepts of survival data analysis, and their implementation in R and SAS. A short summary of the main basic concepts required for the understanding of this book is presented in this chapter, which is also an opportunity to introduce the notations that will be used thoroughout the book. However, we advise a reader not familiar with survival data analysis to start with a more introductory textbook, such as [193, 260], or [78].

1.2   Basic concepts

1.2.1   Censoring and truncation

In its basic formulation, survival data analysis deals with the analysis of the time from an origin until the occurrence of an event of interest. This time can therefore be represented by a positive random variable, and, if observed

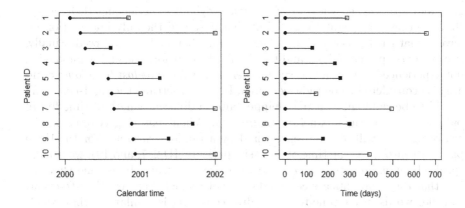

FIGURE 1.1
Graphical representation of the time-to-event of 10 patients in an hypothetical clinical trial in the calendar time scale (*left panel*) and in the individual-trial time scale (*right panel*). Dark circles represent the entry of the patient in the trial, dark squares the death of the patients, and empty square the censoring of the patient.

for everyone, standard statistical analysis methods for continuous (positive) random variable could be used. However, a specificity of survival data is that usually for part of the observations in the study, this duration time is not fully observed. This will for example occur if not all the individuals have experienced the event of interest at the time of the analysis. In such a case, the observation is said to be right-censored at the last observation time and we know that the real event time is actually larger than this censoring time.

A classical example is to consider patients entered in a clinical trial. Patients are typically recruited at different times during what is called the *recruitment period*. This recruitment period is then followed by a *follow-up period* at the end of which data are analyzed. The left panel of Figure 1.1 represents 10 hypothetical patients from such a trial, for which the recruitment period spans from January 1st 2000 until December 31st 2000, with a follow up period until December 31st 2001, time at which the analysis was performed. Note that a more classical representation of these patients is on the *patient trial time scale* rather than on a *calendar time scale*, therefore putting the origin of the time clock at the time of recruitment of each patient, as shown on the right panel of Figure 1.1.

Obviously the patients entered earlier can potentially be followed up for a longer time than the patients entered later in the trial. In this example, a dark square represents the death of the patient and we can see that five patients' (patients ID 3, 4, 5, 8, and 9) died before the end of the study. For these patients, their complete time-to-event is known. Three patients (patients' ID 2, 7, and 10) reached the end of the trial without experiencing their death, they are therefore (right-)censored at that date and the only information we have is that their survival time is longer than what we have observed. Finally, two patients (patients' ID 1 and 6) left the study before the end while having not experienced the event yet, such patients are said to be *lost to follow up* and are also considered to be right-censored. In such a setting, the right-censoring is said to be random, as it may happen after a different length of time for all patients (see the right panel of Figure 1.1). When censoring is *random*, the censoring time will also be represented by a random variable. For the three patients censored at the time of analysis (patients' ID 2, 7, and 10), we usually speak about *administrative censoring* and we can generally assume that the fact that these patients are censored does not impact their real time-to-event. In other words, their time-to-event after censoring is similar to what would have been observed if they would not have been censored. The censoring and event time are then said to be non-informative or independent, which are very important assumptions for most standard survival analysis techniques. On the other hand, this assumption is already more discussable in the case of the two patients who are lost-to-follow up (patients' ID 1 and 6) as it actually depends on the reason of this drop-out. It is indeed not unusual that patients who feel very bad prefer to leave the study to spend their last months peacefully at home. In that case, the fact that the patient drops out brings some information on his event-time. It is then less reasonable to assume that their real event-times are similar to what it would have been if they would not have dropped out.

The assumption of non-informative and independent censoring are actually not identical, independent censoring being a stronger assumption than non-informative censoring; we refer the reader to [202] for a very interesting, although quite technical, discussion on independent and uninformative censoring. Broadly speaking, independent censoring relates to the fact that the random variables representing the real time to the event and the censoring time are independent (usually given the covariates if present), while we speak about uninformative censoring when the distribution of the censoring random variable does not depend on parameters appearing in the survival distribution. The assumption of non-informative and independent censoring become doubtful (if not unacceptable) as soon a subject withdraws from the study for reasons linked to the expected event of interest. In that case, the individuals that remain in the study can not be anymore considered to be representative of the individuals who have left the study and all standard methods will fail to provide correct inference. Unfortunately, the data at hand usually does not allow us to test these assumptions.

Other types of right-censoring exist but are less frequent, at least in biomedical application, and are often called Type I and Type II censoring.

In Type I censoring, the censoring time is pre-specified for all observations under study. A classic example is an animal experiment in which all animals enter the study at a given time (e.g., on the first day of the month) and are all followed up for the same duration (e.g., 30 days), with not possibility of drop-out. So all the animals who did not experience the event of interest are censored with the same censoring time (here 30 days) and this censoring is not random anymore. In Type II censoring, all observations enter the study at the same time (e.g., on the first day of the month) and they are all followed-up until a pre-specified number or proportion of them (e.g., 70%) have experienced the event of interest, and at that time, all the remaining observations are censored. So, again all censored observations are censored at the same time (here the largest event time among the first 70% events). An example of a study with 10 observations with Type I censoring after one month (left panel) and Type II censoring after 70% of events (right panel) is shown on Figure 1.2. These two censoring scheme are far less common in biomedical studies, first due to the difficulty of recruiting all patients at the same time, but also because it is not permitted to force human beings to remain under study until the end, and the right to withdraw from a study at any time is one of the fundamental pillars of ethical clinical research.

A peculiarity of administrative and Type I censoring that will become useful in Chapter 5 is that in these case, the hypothetical censoring time is actually known for all individuals in the study, even those who actually experience the event before being censored and are not followed-up further. This is obviously not the case with random (and Type II) censoring.

Besides right-censoring, one also has to mention left-censoring and interval-censoring. For a left-censored observation, the event of interest has already occur at the first observation time. For example, if we consider the time from birth to the first dental decay some children will already have their first dental decay before they see the dentist for the first time, in such a case we know that the event occur before the age of the first dentist visit and the real time to first dental decay is therefore smaller than the observed (left-)censoring time. Usually left-censoring can be avoided at the time of designing the study. Interval-censoring happens if the event is only known to have occur in between two known dates; taking the same example as before, the exact date of the appearance of the first dental decay will most certainly not be known, and will only be known to have occurred between two successive dentist visits. Interval censoring is actually the more general type of censoring, as one can see right and left censoring as a special case, by considering for right censored data that the event occurs in an interval whose lower bound is the time of right censoring and the upper bound is infinity and for left censored data and interval with zero as the lower bound and the time of left censoring as upper-bound. While interval censoring is actually often present in practice, it is often ignored considering the time the event is observed the first time as the event time. Depending on the context, ignoring interval-censoring may in some case leads to biased results and wrong conclusions. We refer the reader

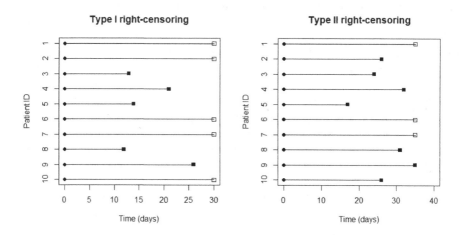

FIGURE 1.2
Graphical representation of the event time of 10 observations in two hypothetical studies, one with Type I censoring at 30 days (*left panel*) and one with Type II censoring at 70% of the event (*right panel*). Dark circle represents the entry of the patient in the trial, dark square represents the death of the patients, and empty square represent the censoring of the patient.

to dedicated textbooks for a thoughtful treatment of interval censored data [42, 64, 366].

Censoring therefore occurs when for part of the individuals in the study, the time to the event of interest is only known to be within a certain interval. In the case of right censoring only a lower bound of the interval is known while for left censoring only an upper bound of the interval is known. In the case of interval censoring, the event is known to occur within a lower and an upper bound. All kind of censoring may occur in the same dataset, as would probably be the case in the example above on time to first dental decay. For example, consider the time to first teeth decay in 10 children as represented on Figure 1.3. Assume that for practical reasons our study takes place among children from age 2 to 7, and that only one dentist visit per year is foreseen. In that case, we see that child ID 3 (who actually got his first teeth decay before the beginning of our study) is left censored (we only know that the real time-to-event is smaller than 2 years) and child ID 2 (who actually got his first teeth decay after the end of the study) is right-censored (we only know that the real time-to-event is longer than 7 years). All the other children are interval-censored; for example for child ID 6, 7, and 8, we only know that the event took place between 3 and 4 years old. Note that in a real study, the time interval between consecutive studies are usually not

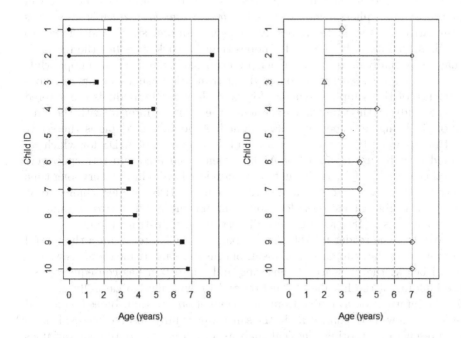

FIGURE 1.3
Graphical representation of time to first teeth decay for 10 hypothetical children. *Left:* Real time-to-event. Dark squares represent the age of first teeth decay. *Right:* Observed time-to-event. Vertical lines represent time of dentist visit in this study (every year from age 2 to 7); empty circles represent right censored observations, empty diamonds represent interval-censored observations, and empty triangles represent left-censored observations.

so regular, and this can be taken into account in the analysis of time-interval data.

Another typical feature of survival data is truncation. While for censoring some observations are incomplete, for truncation the issue is that some observations are actually not present in our dataset. Truncation is therefore linked to a problem of biased sampling. Left truncation often occurs when the individuals of interest must first meet a particular condition before they can be entered in the study and followed-up for the event of interest. A classical example is a study about time to spontaneous abortion in pregnant women; obviously women need to be aware of their pregnancy before entering the study and women experiencing spontaneous abortion within the first weeks of pregnancy will most probably not even realize that they were pregnant and will therefore not enter the study. So, only the women for whom spontaneous abortion occur after they have been aware that they were pregnant will have a chance to enter in the study, and all short time to spontaneous abortion will be missed. This phenomenon is linked to *length time bias* which is sometimes summarized by the quote "popes lives longer than rock stars", indeed time to death is "significantly" longer for popes than for rock stars but the reason is that you actually need to have reach an advanced age to become a pope while you can be a rock start very young! Right truncation usually occurs as a consequence of the sampling scheme, for example when individuals are entered in the study at the time they experience the event of interest with the time of origin being retrospectively ascertained. A popular example is the study of time between HIV seroconversion and development of AIDS for which we would actually use a sample of AIDS patients and ascertain retrospectively the time of HIV infection. In that case, individuals who have a very long time between HIV seroconversion and development of AIDS have less chance to be sampled. Right truncation is less common, and more difficult to account for the analysis, see [186] for a general discussion on right-truncation.

We refer the reader to [186], and in particular Chapter 3, for a thoughtful discussion on the different mechanisms of censoring and truncation. As we will detail below, the presence of censoring and truncation has consequences on the building of the likelihood function and we will have to carefully account for the information available from each type of observation. Indeed, censored observation will not contribute in the same way as fully observed cases. Due to the presence of censoring, classical analysis techniques for continuous variables can therefore not be used. If present, truncation should ideally also be taken into accounted in the building of the likelihood function. Most of the time, only right-censoring is taken into account when analyzing the data, and a major part of the survival data analysis literature focus on right censoring. Note that the different right-censoring mechanisms actually lead to the same survival likelihood function, and can therefore be handled by the same survival analysis techniques [107]. This book will mainly focus on right-censored data, but whenever available, we will provide references for extension to other censoring and truncation schemes of the methods presented .

1.2.2   Basic functions

Let denote T the non-negative continuous random variable representing the real time to the event of interest. In statistics, it is common to use the distribution function $F(t) = P(T \leq t)$ and the density function

$$f(t) = \lim_{\Delta t \to 0} \frac{1}{\Delta t} P(t \leq T \leq t + \Delta t)$$

to characterize the distribution of the variable T. However, in survival data analysis, it is more common to work with the *survival function* which represent the probability that a randomly selected individual will survive beyond time

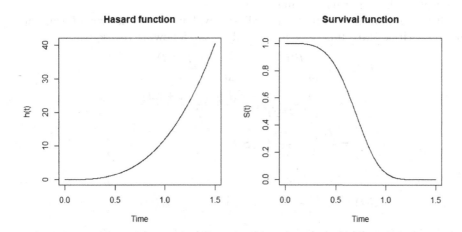

FIGURE 1.4
Example of a hazard function and corresponding survival function.

t and is therefore given by

$$S(t) = 1 - F(t) = P(T > t). \tag{1.1}$$

It is a decreasing function defined in $[0, 1]$, with value 1 at $t = 0$ and value 0 at $t = \infty$. By definition,

$$f(t) = \frac{d}{dt}F(t) = -\frac{d}{dt}S(t).$$

and the density function can thus be thought of as the (instantaneous) unconditional probability of experience the event at time t.

Two other functions are also very popular to characterize the distribution of event times, namely the *hazard function* and the *cumulative hazard function*. The hazard function is also known as the instantaneous conditional risk of event, and is given by

$$h(t) \quad = \quad \lim_{\Delta t \to 0} \frac{P(t \leq T < t + \Delta t \mid T \geq t)}{\Delta t}. \tag{1.2}$$

It is a non-negative function, but not necessarily monotone. Note that $h(t)$ is not a probability and can take value larger than 1. See for example, the hazard function depicted on Figure 1.4 with its corresponding survival function.

In addition to the survival function and the hazard function, a third important characterization of the event times distribution is the cumulative hazard function, which is an increasing function over the interval $[0, +\infty]$ and is defined as

$$H(t) = \int_0^\infty h(u)du.$$

The cumulative hazard at time t can be interpreted as the expected number of events to be observed by time t.

It is well known that, in "standard" survival analysis (one type of event of interest) these three functions are linked by the following relationships:

$$h(t) = \lim_{\Delta t \to 0} \frac{P(t \leq T < t + \Delta t \mid T \geq t)}{\Delta t}$$

$$= \frac{1}{P(T \geq t)} \lim_{\Delta t \to 0} \frac{P(t \leq T < t + \Delta t)}{\Delta t}$$

$$= \frac{f(t)}{S(t)} = \frac{-d}{dt} \log S(t)$$

and

$$S(t) = \exp\left(-\int_0^t h(u)du\right) = \exp(-H(t)). \tag{1.3}$$

So, knowing one of these functions suffices to characterize the event times distribution and to determine the other functions. Given a survival function $S(t)$, its complement give the cumulative distribution function $F(t)$, and the density function $f(t)$ can be obtained by differentiating the negative of the survival function with respect to t. The hazard function $h(t)$ can be obtained as the ratio of the density and the survival function and on the other hand, given a hazard function $h(t)$ one can obtain the survival function $S(t)$ by exponentiating the negative of the integral of the hazard function (which is the cumulative hazard function $H(t)$). Looking back at the example on Figure 1.4, we indeed see that when the hazard is low, the slope of the survival function is small while a steepest decrease is seen when the hazard increases.

For people not familiar with event times data, it is interesting to note that given the intrinsic time component, we may actually distinguish an *instantaneous* and a *cumulative* quantification of the event times distribution [132]. Indeed, the hazard is obviously an *instantaneous* description of the data; it quantifies, at each time-point, the fraction of individuals that develops the event of interest at that time amongst the ones that are still at risk of an event at that time. It is therefore sometimes also referred to as a *rate* and is linked to the concept of *incidence* in epidemiology. The hazard function is also sometimes called the *instantaneous death rate*, the *intensity function* or the *force of mortality*. On the other hand, the (cumulative) distribution function (so the complement of the survival function) is a cumulative measure, based at time t on the fraction of individuals who have experienced the event up to that time amongst all those that were at risk at the beginning of the observation period. As a consequence, it can never decrease when the time span increases. Other common names for this cumulative distribution function are the *cumulative incidence*, the *cumulative risk* or the *actuarial risk* function.

One can define the *mean survival* time as

$$\mu = E(T) = \int_0^\infty u f(u)du = \int_0^\infty S(u)du$$

However, due to censoring, this mean survival time can not really be used in practice. An alternative is then to use the τ-*restricted mean survival time* (RMST) [339, 391, 432], which corresponds to the area under the survival curve before a landmark time τ, and can be interpreted as the mean life before this landmark

$$\mu_\tau = E[min(T, \tau)] = \int_0^\tau S(u)du$$

It is however not to be confused with the mean survival conditional on events occurring before that landmark τ. As an example, the 5 years restricted mean survival time of children in developed countries is close to 5 while the mean survival time conditional on death before 5 is close to zero, as most infant deaths in developed countries actually occur very early in life (mainly due to death of premature babies and to the sudden infant death syndromes).

From the RMST, we can easily derive the number of (years of) life lost before time τ:

$$YL(0, \tau) = \tau - \int_0^\tau S(t)dt$$

which has been proposed in (oncology) clinical trial [378] as an alternative to the hazards ratio in situation of non-proportional hazards (see Section 2.5.1 in Chapter 2).

Another alternative is to define the *median survival time* which is defined as the time t_M such that,

$$S(t_M) = 0.5.$$

It corresponds therefore to the time after which half of the individuals have experienced the event of interest. As we will see, in practice due to censoring this median survival time may not have been reached at the time of the analysis, and other percentile can be considered.

The percentage event-free survival at a given time-point is also often used to summarize event times distribution. It simply corresponds to the value of $S(.)$ at a given time t. We can then define for example the 1 year survival or the 2 years progression-free survival.

1.3 Examples

1.3.1 Colon cancer data

The `colon` dataset contains data on patients recruited in a clinical trial conducted in colon cancer patients by the North Central Cancer Treatment Group in the US. The design of this clinical trial has been described in detail in [216] while the main clinical results where published in [255, 256]. The main objective of this randomized controlled trial was to assess the effectiveness of two adjuvant therapy regimens (Levamisole alone and Levamisole in combination with 5-Fluorouracil) in stage III (Dukes stage C) colon cancer patients.

Eligible patients who had curative-intent resection of stage III colon cancer one to five weeks prior to randomization were randomized to either observation only, Levamisole alone, or a combination of Levamisole and 5-Fluorouracil. The randomization was stratified for time interval since surgery, depth of invasion of the primary tumor, and number of lymph nodes with metastases. After a specific schedule for initiation of the treatment, Levamisole was administered every two weeks for one year, while in the combination arm 5-Fluorouracil was maintained weekly for 48 weeks. The main endpoints of this trial were overall survival (time to death) and time to recurrence. A total of 971 patients were randomized, however 42 (4.3%) were a posteriori assessed as ineligible and are not included in this dataset. Among the remaining 929 eligible patients, 315 were in the observation only arm (Obs), 310 in the Levamisole alone arm (Lev), and 304 in the Levamisole and 5-Fluorouracil arm (Lev-5FU). At the time of publication of the study results by [255, 256], the median follow-up time was 6.5 years and the combination of Levamisole and 5-Fluorouracil showed a significant advantage both in terms of time to recurrence (p-value < 0.0001) and overall survival (p-value $= 0.0007$). Furthermore, this combination was found to be associated with acceptable toxicity and became the new standard treatment for these patients.

This dataset is available in the R package `survival` and is shortly described in Chapter 8 of [372, 374]. For each patient, the `colon` dataset contains information on the patient identifier the treatment arm (Obs, Lev, Lev-5FU), and a series of baseline characteristics. In addition, the time-to-event, censoring status as well as the event type are also available. The available variables are listed in Table 1.5. To access the data, one first has to load the `survival` package:

```
> library(survival)
```

and the first line of the datasets can then be displayed using the `head()` command:

```
> head(colon)
  id study     rx sex age obstruct perfor adhere nodes status
1  1     1 Lev+5FU   1  43        0      0      0     5      1
2  1     1 Lev+5FU   1  43        0      0      0     5      1
3  2     1 Lev+5FU   1  63        0      0      0     1      0
4  2     1 Lev+5FU   1  63        0      0      0     1      0
5  3     1     Obs   0  71        0      0      1     7      1
6  3     1     Obs   0  71        0      0      1     7      1
  differ extent surg node4 time etype
1      2      3    0     1 1521     2
2      2      3    0     1  968     1
3      2      3    0     0 3087     2
4      2      3    0     0 3087     1
5      2      2    0     1  963     2
6      2      2    0     1  542     1
```

Variable	Control $n(\%)$	Lev $n(\%)$	Lev+5FU $n(\%)$	Total $n(\%)$
Gender				
Male	149 (47.3%)	133 (42.9%)	163 (53.6%)	445 (47.9%)
Female	166 (52.7%)	177 (57.1%)	141 (46.4%)	484 (52.1%)
Obstruction of the colon by the tumor				
No	252 (80.0%)	247 (79.7%)	250 (82.2%)	749 (80.6%)
Yes	63 (20.0%)	63 (20.3%)	54 (17.8%)	180 (19.4%)
Perforation of the colon				
No	306 (97.1%)	300 (96.8%)	296 (97.4%)	902 (97.1%)
Yes	9 (2.9%)	10 (3.2%)	8 (2.6%)	27 (2.9%)
Adherence to nearby organs				
No	268 (85.1%)	261 (84.2%)	265 (87.2%)	794 (85.5%)
Yes	47 (14.9%)	49 (15.8%)	39 (12.8%)	135 (14.5%)
Differentiation of the tumor				
Well	27 (8.6%)	37 (11.9%)	29 (9.5%)	93 (10.0%)
Moderate	229 (72.7%)	219 (70.6%)	215 (70.7%)	663 (71.4%)
Poor	52 (16.5%)	44 (14.2%)	54 (17.8%)	150 (16.1%)
Missing	07 (2.2%)	10 (3.2%)	6 (2.0%)	23 (2.5%)
Extent of local spread				
Submucosa	8 (2.5%)	3 (1.0%)	10 (3.3%)	21 (2.3%)
Muscle	38 (12.1%)	36 (11.6%)	32 (10.5%)	106 (11.4%)
Serosa	249 (79.0%)	259 (83.5%)	251 (82.6%)	759 (81.7%)
Contig. struc.	20 (6.3%)	12 (3.9%)	11 (3.6%)	43 (4.6%)
Time from surgery to registration				
Short	224 (71.1%)	230 (74.2%)	228 (75.0%)	682 (73.4%)
Long	91 (28.9%)	80 (25.8%)	76 (25.0%)	247 (26.6%)
More than 4 positive nodes				
No	228 (72.4%)	221 (71.3%)	225 (74.0%)	674 (72.6%)
Yes	87 (27.6%)	89 (28.7%)	79 (26.0%)	255 (27.4%)
Age (years)				
Mean (Range)	60 (18–85)	60 (27–83)	60 (26–81)	60 (18–85)

TABLE 1.1
Colon cancer data: Baseline characteristics

As we can see, an important characteristic of this dataset is that it actually contains two rows per patient, one for each type of event considered (death and recurrence). One can however easily derive one dataset per type of event:

```
colon.OS <- colon[etype==1,]
colon.TR <- colon[etype==2,]
```

Baseline characteristics of the patients per treatment arm are summarized in Table 1.1 and are well balanced between the three treatment arms.

We will use these data to illustrate standard survival techniques in Section 2.6 of Chapter 2.

1.3.2   Rectal cancer data

Colorectal cancer is one of the most frequent cancer in most Western countries and is usually acknowledged as the second cause of cancer death. Among these colorectal cancers, about one third are cancers of the rectum. The French R98 Intergroup trial for patients with resected stage II–III rectal cancer has been conducted in the first half of the 2000's and patients were followed-up until the final analysis in 2013, with a median follow up of 13 years [99]. This trial aimed to assess the efficacy of the addition of irinotecan to a postoperative 5FU/LV regimen. Before initiation, each center had to opt for one of two 5FU-LV regimens for the control arm (Mayo Clinic regimen or LV5-FU2 regimen) and all analyses were stratified according to this choice.

The primary endpoint for this trial was disease-free survival (DFS), defined as time from randomization until the first event of recurrent disease (persistent or progressive disease or second primary colon cancer) or death from any reasons. Secondary endpoints included overall survival, time to loco-regional relapse and time to distant relapse. This trial was aiming at a 80% power to detect an increase in median disease-free survival from 50% to 61% and should have recruited 600 patients to base the analysis on 270 DFS events. The trial was launched by the Association Européenne de recherche en Oncologie (AERO) and quickly became an Integroup trial with three other French Groups joining, leading to a total of 66 participating centers. However despite these efforts, the trial recruited only 357 patients from March 1999 to December 2005 and was then closed for slow recruitment following the recommendations of an Independent Data Monitoring Committee.

The final analysis of this trial was performed in 2013 based on a total of 173 events and a median follow-up of 13 years. A total of 178 patients were randomized to the control group (61 in the Mayo Clinical Regimen sub-arm and 117 in the LV5FU2 sub-arm) and 179 patients in the experimental group (LV5FU2 + irinotecan). Results for DFS and OS were both in favor of LV5FU2 + irinotecan although they did not reach significance (p-value = 0.154 and p-value = 0.433 respectively).

The list of the main variables for this dataset is presented in Table 1.6 and relates to the patient identification, treatment, outcome, and some important baseline characteristics. The main characteristics of the patients by treatment group and strata are summarized in Table 1.2. These data were provided for re-analysis by the International Drug Development Institute (IDDI) with permission from the Sponsor of the trial, the European Association for Research in Oncology (AERO).

These data are used in Section 2.6.3 of Chapter 2 to illustrate how to apply the main classical survival analysis techniques with the SAS software. In this trial, the patients were entered by a total of 66 French centers from different groups. In Section 3.7 of Chapter 3 we will see how we can investigate the heterogeneity in outcome between centers, and whether this heterogeneity can be partly explained by the choice made for the 5FU-LV regimens.

| Variable | Control (5FU/LV) | | Exp. (5FU/LV + Irinotecan) | | Total |
| | MC Reg | LV5-FU | MC Reg | LV5-FU | |
	$n(\%)$	$n(\%)$	$n(\%)$	$n(\%)$	$n(\%)$
Gender					
Male	37 (60.7%)	84 (71.8%)	41 (73.2%)	79 (64.2%)	241 (67.5%)
Female	24 (39.3%)	33 (28.2%)	15 (26.8%)	44 (35.8%)	116 (32.5%)
Localization of cancer					.
Low-rectum	36 (59.0%)	59 (50.4%)	29 (51.8%)	65 (52.8%)	189 (52.9%)
High-rectum	25 (41.0%)	58 (49.6%)	27 (48.2%)	58 (47.2%)	168 (47.1%)
Number of involved nodes					
0	26 (42.6%)	31 (26.5%)	23 (41.1%)	33 (26.8%)	113 (31.7%)
1–3	23 (37.7%)	63 (52.8%)	21 (37.5%)	65 (52.8%)	172 (48.2%)
>3	12 (19.7%)	23 (19.7%)	12 (21.4%)	25 (20.3%)	72 (20.2%)
Preoperative chemotherapy					
No	15 (24.6%)	41 (35.0%)	11 (19.6%)	45 (36.6%)	112 (31.4%)
Yes	46 (75.4%)	76 (65.0%)	45 (80.4%)	78 (63.4%)	245 (68.6%)
Sphincter conservation					
No	16 (26.2%)	20 (17.1%)	16 (28.6%)	21 (17.1%)	73 (20.4%)
Yes	45 (73.8%)	97 (82.9%)	40 (71.4%)	102 (82.9%)	284 (79.6%)
Time from surgery					
0–4 wks	30 (49.2%)	48 (41.0%)	28 (50.0%)	51 (41.5%)	157 (44.0%)
>4 wks	31 (50.8%)	69 (59.0%)	28 (50.0%)	72 (58.5%)	200 (56.0%)
Age (years)					
Mean (Range)	65 (41–82)	63 (33–80)	60.5 (32–72)	61 (39–80)	62 (32–82)

TABLE 1.2
Rectal cancer data: Baseline characteristics

1.3.3 Diabetic retinopathy data

Diabetic retinopathy is a complication associated with diabetes mellitus and is caused by damage to the blood vessels of the retina. It can lead to mild to severe vision problems, and eventually to blindness. It is associated with any type 1 or type 2 diabetes and people with long history of diabetes and poor blood sugar level control are at higher risk. Diabetic retinopathy is a major cause of blindness in people below the age of 60.

The retinopathy dataset contains a random sample of the 1742 patients included in the Diabetic Retinopathy Study (DRS) run in the seventies with the objective to investigate the efficacy of photocoagulation (laser) treatment on visual loss. In this trial, one eye per patient was randomly allocated to the experimental treatment while the other eye received no treatment, and served as control. For each eye, the outcome of interest was the time from initiation of treatment to the time when visual acuity dropped below 5/200 two visits in a row.

This subset of the original dataset available in the survival R package and contains 197 patients, which represents 50% of the patients with "high-risk" diabetic retinopathy included in the original study. This dataset has been used first by [171] to illustrate their work on the modeling of bivariate survival data, and is briefly discussed and analyzed as an illustrative example in some books on survival data analysis [152, 218, 372].

Data on each of the two eyes (one being treated with laser treatment and the other one used as a control) are available for the 197 patients. The dataset is therefore composed of 394 observations (two per patient) and contains information about the treatment (which eye was treated, laser type used for the treated eye), and few baseline characteristics at the level of the patient (age at diagnosis of diabetes, type of diabetes). These characteristics are obviously common to the two eyes of a same patient. In addition, we also have information on the value of a risk score measured at the level of the eye; note that only patients with risk score equal or above 6 in at least one eye are included in this subset of the original data. A summary of these variables is provided in Table 1.7.

In addition, we have for each eye the time to loss of vision or last follow-up and the censoring indicator (equal to 0 for a censored observation and a 1 for an event, i.e. loss of vision for this eye). Patients were censored in case of death, dropout, or end of the study. Note that we can have patients with two censored observations, and then equal follow-up time for both eyes (patients still not blind at the end of the study, or patients who die or left the study before experiencing the event), patients with one censored observed and one uncensored observation (patients for whom only one eye got blind before the end of the follow-up), and patients with two uncensored observations. One should also note that given the nature of the outcome of interest there is a built-in lag time of approximately 6 months, as at least 2 visits are required to evaluate the endpoint and visits were planned every 3 months. Therefore, the survival times in this dataset are in fact the actual time to vision loss (in months) minus the minimum possible time-to-event (6.5 months).

To access the data, one first has to load the **survival** package and the first few lines of the dataset are given below:

```
>  library(survival)
>  head(retinopathy)
   id laser    eye age     type trt futime status risk
1   5 argon  left  28     adult  1  46.23      0    9
2   5 argon  left  28     adult  0  46.23      0    9
3  14 argon right  12 juvenile  1  42.50      0    8
4  14 argon right  12 juvenile  0  31.30      1    6
5  16 xenon right   9 juvenile  1  42.27      0   11
6  16 xenon right   9 juvenile  0  42.27      0   11
```

As can be seen we indeed have two lines per patient. Among the 197 patients included in this dataset, 108 (54.8%) had their left eye treated while the remaining 89 patients (45.2%) had their right eye treated. The type of laser used was xenon in 100 (50.8%) treated eyes and argon for the other 97 (49.2%) treated eyes. Mean age at diagnosis was 21 years old with a median of 15 y.o. (min-max: 1–58 y.o.) and 114 patients (57.9%) were diagnosed with juvenile diabetes (i.e. diagnosed before the age of 20 y.o.). Risk score distribution was similar between the treated and control eyes, with a majority of eyes having

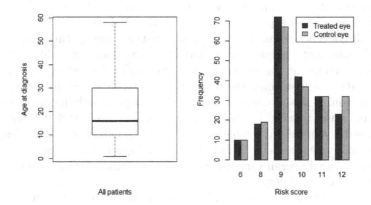

FIGURE 1.5
Diabetic retinopathy data: Distribution of age at diagnosis of diabetes (*left*)
and risk score per eye (*right*).

a score of 9. Descriptive graphs for age at diagnosis and risk score per eye are
provided in Figure 1.5.

The particularity of these data is that we are face with what is often
called *bivariate survival data* as we have two observations per individual, one
for each eye. These data are therefore clustered, with clusters of size 2, and
the observations on the two eyes of a same patient obviously share much more
in common than eyes from different patients. They are therefore expected to
be more correlated than the observations on different patients. As we will
discuss in Chapter 3, appropriate models are required to take into account
this clustered structure of the data. These data will be used to illustrate the
use of frailty models in Section 3.7 of Chapter 3.

1.3.4   Children ALL data

The EORTC CLG 58951 trial is a randomized phase III clinical trial in children and adolescents (under 18 years of age) with previously untreated acute
lymphoblastic leukemia (ALL). The treatment of these patients involved different steps and was based on a so-called Berlin-Frankfurt-Munster (BFM)-
like protocol. The design of this trial is relatively complex as it embeds three
main randomization, each with is own objectives. The first randomization
takes place in the induction phase of the treatment and aim to compare dexamethasone to prednisolone amongst all recruited patients ($n = 1947$) [104].
The patients with a non-high risk profile ($n = 1552$) where then randomized
at the end of the induction phase between prolonged or standard asparaginase treatment during the consolidation and late intensification phase [259].

Finally, the third randomization aimed to compare corticosteroids pulses versus vincristine during maintenance in the continuation therapy of $n = 411$ consecutive average risk patients included in the trial [96].

We will concentrate on the first randomization, aiming thus to compare dexamethasone and prednisolone as induction treatment in childhood ALL. The primary endpoint was event-free survival (EFS) defined as the time between the date of first complete remission to relapse or death in first complete remission. It was planned to analyse this endpoint only for patients who started induction therapy (according to protocol or not), and this endpoint was assigned a value of 0 if the patient did start the induction therapy but did not enter complete remission or died during the induction therapy. Secondary endpoints included overall survival (i.e. time from randomization up to death from any cause) and safety.

A total of 358 events were required to have a 90% power to detect a 5-year EFS rate increase from 80% in the prednisolone arm to 85.5% in the dexamethasone arm (HR = 0.70), with a two-sided 5% alpha level logrank test. A total of 1947 patients were randomized, 972 to the dexamethasone arm and 975 to the prednisolone arm, of which respectively, 971 and 970 started the induction therapy.

The results, as reported in the main publication of this trial [104], are based on a median follow-up of 6.9 years and a total of 346 events (287 relapses, 35 death without relapse, and 24 patients without complete remission). Main results are displayed in Table 1.3. Although, this trial did not succeed to demonstrate a higher efficacy of dexamethasone over prednisolone neither for event-free survival (p-value = 0.73) nor for overall survival (p-value = 0.42), it is interesting to see that the outcome of these patients is actually very good, with more than 80% of the patients being still alive and event-free after 8 years.

Indeed, while ALL is the most frequent malignant disease in childhood, the outcome for these patients is generally very good, with overall survival percentage at 5 years well above 80%. The rate of success in the treatment of childhood ALL has increased steadily since the 1970s and it is nowadays well recognized that a majority of these patients will not die from their disease and can be considered as *cure* [259]. We will therefore come back to this example in Section 4.5 of Chapter 4 on Cure models to demonstrate how take into account such a (large) fraction of cure patient when analyzing these data, and in particular we will be interested in disentangling the effect of treatment and of some known prognostic factors on the short and long term.

The dataset we consider here only concerns the 1941 patients who have started induction therapy, and contains a subset of all available variables. These variables are displayed in Table 1.8 and the dataset contains one line per patient. The main baseline characteristics for these 1941 patients are summarized in Table 1.4 and were adequately balanced between treatment arms. The outcome results for these patients were basically the same as those presented in Table 1.3. These were provided for re-analysis by the European Organisation for Research and Treatment of Cancer (EORTC). The results

Outcome	Dexamethasone	Prednisolone
Event-free survival		
N	971	970
8-yrs EFS (s.e.)	81.5%(1.2%)	81.2%(1.0%)
HR (95% CI), p-value	0.96 [0.78 ; 1.19], p=0.73	
Overall survival		
N	972	975
8-yrs OS (s.e.)	87.2%(1.2%)	89.0%(1.1%)
HR (95% CI), p-value	1.12 [0.85 ; 1.46], p=0.42	

TABLE 1.3
Children ALL data: Main published results of the EORTC CLG 58951 trial
[104]

presented in this book and methods used are solely the responsibility of the
author, and do not necessarily represent the official views of the EORTC.

1.3.5 Melanoma data

This dataset contains observations for the patients randomized to the control group of the EORTC 18991 trial [109]. The objective of this randomized
phase III clinical trials was to compare adjuvant treatment with Pegylated
Interferon Alfa-2b (PEG-IFN-α-2b) versus observation in patients with resected stage III Melanoma. A total of 1256 patients were randomized between
October 2000 and August 2003 by 99 centers in 17 countries. The primary
endpoint of this trial was recurrence-free survival (RFS), defined as time from
randomization until any local or regional recurrence, distant metastasis or
death from any cause. Secondary endpoints were distant metastasis-free survival (DMFS), defined as time from randomization until distant metastasis or
death of any cause and overall survival (OS). Based on the main results of
this trial, obtained after a median follow-up of 3.8 years, PEG-IFN-α-2b was
approved in 2011 by the US Food and Drug administration for the adjuvant
treatment of stage III resected melanoma patients [109].

Long-term results were analyzed and published in 2013 after patients have
been followed-up for a median time of 7.6 years [110]. In this analysis, the
advantage of adjuvant PEG-IFN-α-2b was still observed for the primary endpoint recurrence-free survival, but was now marginally not statistically significant (p-value = 0.055). No significant improvement could be demonstrated
at that time for the secondary endpoint distant-metastasis-free survival and
overall survival.

It is well known that stage III melanoma patients are an heterogeneous
group of patients, with sentinel nodes staging, the presence of ulceration, and
the presence of more than one positive lymph node as important prognostic
factors [111]. We will concentrate on the impact of these factors on OS for the
patients randomized in the control arm of this trial ($n = 629$). Among these

Variable	Prednisolone ($n = 970$) $n(\%)$	Dexamethasone ($n = 971$) $n(\%)$	Total ($n = 1941$) $n(\%)$
Gender			
Boy	533 (54.9%)	533 (54.9%)	1066 (54.9%)
Girl	437 (45.1%)	438 (45.1%)	875 (45.1%)
Age (years)			
<1y	3 (0.3%)	2 (0.2%)	5 (0.3%)
1-<2y	65 (6.7%)	81 (8.3%)	146 (7.5%)
2-<6y	448 (46.2%)	464 (47.8%)	912 (47.0%)
6-<10y	214 (22.1%)	187 (19.3%)	401 (20.7%)
>10y	240 (24.7%)	237 (24.4%)	477 (24.6%)
NCI risk group			
Standard risk	597 (61.5%)	586 (60.4%)	1183 (60.9%)
High risk	373 (38.5%)	385 (39.6%)	758 (39.1%)
EORTC Group			
Very low risk (VLR)	124 (12.8%)	126 (13.0%)	250 (12.9%)
Average risk (AR) 1	564 (58.1%)	556 (57.3%)	1120 (57.7%)
Average risk (AR) 2	155 (16.0%)	144 (14.8%)	299 (15.4%)
Very high risk (VHR) initial	126 (13.0%)	144 (14.8%)	270 (13.9%)
Unknown/missing	1 (0.1%)	1 (0.1%)	2 (0.1%)
Immunophenotype			
B-lineage	822 (84.7%)	825 (85.0%)	1674 (84.9%)
T-lineage	148 (15.3%)	145 (14.9%)	293 (15.1%)
AUL	0 (0.0%)	1 (0.1%)	1 (0.1%)
White Blood Cell Count ($\times 10^9/L$)			
<10	490 (50.5%)	507 (52.2%)	997 (51.4%)
$10 - < 25$	183 (18.9%)	165 (17.0%)	348 (17.9%)
$25 - < 100$	198 (20.4%)	193 (19.9%)	391 (20.1%)
>100	99 (10.2%)	106 (10.9%)	205 (10.6%)

TABLE 1.4
Children ALL data: Main baseline characteristics (AUL: acute undifferentiated leukemia)

629 patients, 272 (43.2%) were reported at randomization with microscopic nodal disease (N1 – microscopic involvement) and 357 (56.8%) with clinically palpable nodes (N2 – palpable). Also, ulceration was present for 181 (28.8%) patients, absent for 338 (53.7%) and reported as unknown for the remaining 110 (17.5%) patients. Finally, 344 (54.7%) patients were reported to have only one positive nodes, 279 (44.4%) more than one, and 6 (0.9%) with zero or an unknown number of positive lymph nodes.

We will see in Chapter 4 that after such a long follow-up, only respectively 63.4%, 59.6%, and 53.4% of the patients have experienced the event of interest for RFS, DMFS, and OS and it is actually reasonable to assume the remaining patients as "cured" form the disease. We are therefore interested in analyzing these data while taking this cure fraction into account, and in particular to investigate whether nodal stage, ulceration, and the presence of more than one positive lymph node are prognostic for the occurrence of the event of interest, for the timing of occurrence of this event or both (see Section 4.5 of Chapter 4).

A summary of the variables we will consider is provided in Table 1.9, and the first few lines of the dataset are given below. We can see for example that patient number 3 got a distant metastases after 349 days but was still alive at the end of the followup after 3750 days. On the other hand, patient number 10 was diagnosed with a relapse 196 days after randomization, with distant metastases 1198 days after randomization, and finally died 2670 days after randomization.

```
> head(Melan.na)
  seqid        rndstage ulceration2c nb_lymphnodes osstat ostime
1     3 N2(palpable)            No             1     No   3750
2     6 N2(palpable)            No             2    Yes    665
3     8     N1(micro)           No             3    Yes   2269
4     9 N2(palpable)            No            15    Yes    263
5    10     N1(micro)          Yes             1    Yes   2670
6    12     N1(micro)          Yes             1    Yes    595
  rftime rfstat dmstime dmsstat          Stade
1    349  Event     349   Event Stade IIIB-C
2     29  Event     274   Event Stade IIIB-C
3   2261  Event    2261   Event    Stade IIIA
4      5  Event     169   Event Stade IIIB-C
5    196  Event    1198   Event Stade IIIB-C
6    595  Event     595   Event Stade IIIB-C
```

These were provided for re-analysis by the EORTC. The results presented in this book and methods used are solely the responsibility of the author and do not necessarily represent the official views of the EORTC.

1.3.6 Advanced ovarian cancer data

This dataset combines the data from four double-blind randomized clinical trials in advanced ovarian cancer. The objective of each of these trials was to assess the efficacy of cyclophosphamide plus cisplatin (CP) versus cyclophosphamide plus adriamycin plus cisplatin (CAP) for these patients. The dataset contains information about progression free survival (time to progression or death, whichever come first) and overall survival (time to death of any cause).

A version of this dataset, containing limited information in terms of variables, is available in the `frailtypack` R package. It contains information about progression free survival (PFS) defined as time from randomization to progression or death, whichever come first, overall survival (OS) define as the time from randomization to death of any cause, and information on the center in which the patient was treated and the treatment group (CP versus CAP), see Table 1.10 for information on the variables available in the dataset. This dataset has already been used to investigate whether PFS could be used as a surrogate marker for OS [356].

The first lines of this datasets are:

```
> head(dataOvarian)
patienID trialID trt timeS        statusS  timeT     statusT
1        1       2   0 0.105158    1        0.185714  1
2        2       2   0 0.895238    1        1.408730  1
3        3       2   0 0.078968    1        0.126190  1
4        4       2   1 1.739285    0        1.739285  0
5        5       2   0 0.091269    1        0.127381  1
6        6       2   1 0.169841    1        0.225396  1
```

A total of 1192 patients are included in this dataset, 606 in the CA group and 586 in the CAP group. These patients were treated in a total of 50 centers, between 2 and 274 patients in each center (mean of 23.84 and median of 11.5 patients per center). A total of 977 patients (82.0%) experienced at least one event, of which 777 experienced a progression of disease (PD) as first event and the remaining 200 patients died before experiencing a progression.

If we are interested in time to progression for these patients, death before progression will act as "competing risks" since it will prevent us from observing the time to progression for these patients. A naive approach consists in censoring these patients at the time of death, however we will see in Chapter 5 on competing risks analysis that this is often not appropriate. These data will be used to illustrate basic concepts of competing risks analysis in Section 5.6 of Chapter 5.

1.4 Scope of this book

As we will describe in Chapter 2, "classical analysis" techniques include parametric and non-parametric estimation of the survival function and its characteristics, as well as hypothesis testing, with the most popular test being the non-parametric logrank test, and a lot of work has been devoted to the modeling of the impact of covariates either on the hazard function, such as in the proportional hazards (PH) model or directly on the (log) time, such as in the accelerated failure time model (AFT). The (Cox) PH model is most certainly the most popular one, however it should not be used without any thought as it relies on the strong PH assumption. The AFT model is often presented as an alternative to the PH model, but other alternatives have also been proposed such as the proportional odds model. We will show that all these models can be fitted parametrically (assuming a parametric distribution of the event times) or semi-parametrically, leaving the distribution of the event time unspecified up to the covariate coefficients.

While these methods are applicable in a wide series of practical situations, "classical" survival analysis methods do not adequately apply to all situations and several extensions of these methods have been proposed to address specific issues.

Variable	Description	Value
id	Identification number of a patient	Integer number
study	Study identifier	1
rx	Treatment	**Obs:** Control ($n = 315$)
		Lev: Levamisole alone ($n = 310$)
		Lev+5FU: Combination of Levamisole and 5-Fluorouracil ($n = 304$)
time	time-to-event	Time from randomization to event
status	Censoring status	0 = Censored observation
		1 = Event
etype	Event type	1 = Death
		0 = Recurrence
age	Age	Age in years
sex	Gender	1 = Male, 2 = Female
obstruct	Obstruction of the colon by the tumor	0 = No, 1 = Yes
perfor	Perforation of the colon	0 = No, 1 = Yes
adhere	Adherence to nearby organs	0 = No, 1 = Yes
differ	Differentiation of the tumor	1 = Well, 2 = Moderate, 3 = Poor
extent	Extent of local spread	1 = Submucosa, 2 = Muscle, 3 = Serosa, 4 = Contiguous structure
surg	Time from surgery to registration	0 = Short, 1 = Long
node4	More than 4 positive nodes	0 = No, 1 = Yes

TABLE 1.5

Colon cancer data: List of variables available in colon dataset of the `survival` R package

Variable	Description	Value
patient	Identification number of a patient	Integer number
centre	Identification of the patient's center	Integer number
treat	Treatment indicator	0 = 5FU/LV ($n = 178$)
		1 = 5FU/LV + CPT-11 ($n = 179$)
Strat	Strata indicator	1 = Mayo Clinic regimen
		2 = LV5-FU2 regimen
dfsm	Observed DFS time	Time from randomization to
		first event or last follow-up
censd	DFS Event indicator	0 = Censored observation
		1 = Event
osm	Observed OS time	Time from randomization to
		death or last follow-up
cens	OS Event indicator	0 = Censored observation
		1 = Event
Age	Age	Age in years
gender	Gender	0 = Male, 1 = Female
loccancer2	Localization of cancer	0 = Low-rectum, 1 = High-rectum
ganglenv3	Number of involved nodes	0, 1 = 1 − 3, 2 => 3 nodes involved
radpreop2	Preoperative radiotherapy	0 = No, 1 = Yes
sphincons2	Sphincter conservation	0 = No, 1 = Yes
tchir2	Time from surgery	0 = 0-4 weeks, 1 = > 4 weeks

TABLE 1.6
Rectal cancer data (R98 trial): List of main variables

Variable	Description	Value
id	Identification number of a patient	Integer number
laser	Type of laser used for treatment	"argon" or "xenon"
eye	Treated eye	"left" or "right"
trt	Treatment indicator	0 = control eye
		1 = treated eye
futime	Observed time	Time from randomization to
		loss of vision or last follow-up
status	Event indicator	0 = censored observation
		1 = event (loss of vision for the eye)
risk	Risk score for the eye	Integer number between 6 and 12

TABLE 1.7
Diabetic retinopathy data: Variables available in the dataset from survival

Variable	Description	Value
seqid	Identification number of a patient	Integer number
trt1n	Allocated treatment	1=Dexa; 2=Pred
sex	Gender	1=Boy; 2=Girl
age	Age (days)	Integer number
ageg	Age group	1=[0 -1year[; 2=[1 2 years[; 3=[2 - 6 years[; 4=[6 - 10 years[; 5=[10 years- [
nci	NCI risk group	1="Standard risk"; 2= "High risk"
rg4c	EORTC Group	1=VLR; 2=AR1; 3=AR2; 4=VHR initial
nci	Immunophenotype	1=B-Lineage; 2=T-Lineage; 2=AUL
wbc	White Blood Cell Count ($\times 10^9/L$)	Integer number
wbcc	White Blood Cell Count ($\times 10^9/L$)	1=¡10; 2=10-¡25; 3=25¡100;4=¿100
respre2c	Response to pre-phase (blasts/μL)	1=¡ 1000; 2=≥ 1000
survt	Follow-up time	Time from randomization to death or last follow-up
ssurv	OS Event indicator	1=Alive; 2=Dead
efs	EFS time	Time from first complete remission (after induction or consolidation) until relapse or death in remission or last follow-up
sefs	EFS Event indicator	1=No event; 2=Event
dmstime	DMFS time	Time from randomization to distant metastasis or death from any cause or last follow-up
dmsstat	DMFS Event indicator	1=No event; 2=Event

TABLE 1.8
Children ALL data: List of main variables

Variable	Description	Value
seqid	Identification number of a patient	Integer number
rndstage	Stage of disease (*)	"N1 (micro)" or "N2 (palpable)"
ulceration2c	Ulceration of primary (**)	"No" or "Yes" or "Unk"
Stage	Combined stage	"Stage IIIA" or "Stage IIIB-C"
ostime	Follow-up time	Time from randomization to death or last follow-up
osstat	OS Event indicator	"No" (censored) or "Yes" (event)
rftime	RFS time	Time from randomization to any local or regional recurrence or distant metastasis or death from any cause or last follow-up
rfstat	RFS Event indicator	"No event" (censored) or "Event"
dmstime	DMFS time	Time from randomization to distant metastasis or death from any cause or last follow-up
dmsstat	DMFS Event indicator	"No event" (censored) or "Event"

TABLE 1.9

Melanoma data: List of main variables (*) as reported at randomization, (**) as reported on the CRF

Variable	Description	Value
patienID	Identification number of a patient	Integer number from 1 to 1192
trialID	Identification number of the center in which the patient was treated	Integer number from 1 to 50
trt	Treatment indicator	0 = Cyclophosphamide plus cisplatin (CP)
		1 = Cyclophosphamide plus adriamycin plus cisplatin (CAP)
timeS	Progression-free Survival (PFS)	Time from randomization to progression or death whichever come first
statusS	PFS indicator	0 = Censored observation
		1 = Event (progression or death)
timeT	Overall survival (OS)	Time from randomization to death
statusT	PFS indicator	0 = Censored observation
		1 = Event (death)

TABLE 1.10

Advanced ovarian cancer data: Variables available in the dataset from frailtypack

The assumption of independent observations can be violated, for example, when considering *clustered data* or *repeated events*. This will occur, for example, if we consider paired organs in which case the cluster size will be fixed to two (e.g. in the diabetic retinopathy data, see Section 1.3.3) or when considering patients treated in different hospitals in a clinical trial. The (shared) frailty models have been introduced to cope with this situation. The main idea is to introduce a random effect in a PH model to capture all the unobserved characteristics shared by the observations of the same cluster. This model is actually an extension of the univariate frailty models, originally proposed to cope with over-dispersion in survival data. The frailty model will be the subject of Chapter 3.

"Classical" survival analysis methods assume that if followed-up is long enough all observations will experience the event of interest. However, this is not always necessarily the case. For example, in the children ALL data (see Section 1.3.4), we know that a quite important fraction of these children will survive from this cancer, and will therefore not progress and not die due to this cancer. They are many situations in different fields where it is more reasonable to assume the presence of a fraction of *cure* patients in the population of interest, e.g. when studying time to relapse from a cancer, time to second pregnancy, time to start a new job in a study of duration of unemployment,... . As we will discuss in Chapter 4, a difficulty in this situation is that due to censoring, the *cure status* is partially unobserved. Indeed, it is obvious for the individuals for whom we observe the event of interest that they are not cured, but for the individuals who are right-censored, we don't know whether the event will occur or not. It is known that ignoring the presence of this cure fraction in the analysis can lead to wrong conclusions. Also, when such a cure fraction is indeed present, it is often of interest to distinguish the impact of the treatment (or more generally of some factor of exposition) both on the probability to be cure or and on the time-to-event for the "uncured" observations, i.e., those who will experience the event of interest. In Chapter 4, we will present two broad classes of models developed for this type of situation, namely the mixture cure models and the promotion time cure models.

While "classical" survival analysis methods consider that there is only one possible type of event, in many situations the individuals in the study may actually be at risk for different types of events. Furthermore, these different types of events may be competing in the sense that the occurrence of one will prevent the occurrence of another one, or may have strong consequences (e.g. change of treatment) that may dramatically modify the risk of the event of interest. For example, in the advanced ovarian cancer data (see Section 1.3.6), if we are interested in time to loco-regional recurrences, the occurrence of death before progression will prevent us from observing the time to progression. A common approach is then to concentrate on the time to the first event, whatever it is, however this approach might not be satisfactory. An alternative is to define one specific type of event, e.g. loco-regional recurrences, as the event of interest and to consider all the other types of events as *competing risks*, and to analyse the data accordingly. Survival analysis methods and models specific for this context will be presented in Chapter 5.

Finally, we will also discuss possible extensions of "classical" survival analysis methods to consider covariates whose values are not fixed at baseline but do evolve over time. A first idea is to extend classical models to include time-dependent covariates, but such extensions may suffer from some limitations. We discuss the case of time-dependent covariates in Chapter 6, and in particular we will see how joint models allow to model jointly the evolution of a marker and the time to an event of interest.

Reference textbooks on survival analysis (see Section 1.1) often include one or two chapters to address some of these situations, considering most often the case of correlated survival times or the presence of more than one type of event [78, 181, 186, 248, 260, 372]. In this book, each of this subject will be treated in a Chapter. The most common methods will be presented, and references will be provided for further reading on more specific topics. This list of further readings will however not be exhaustive as a wide literature is available. The methods will also be illustrated with the analysis in SAS and R of the data presented in Section 1.3. Other softwares allow to perform survival analysis, such as STATA [77], but will not be illustrated in this book.

We will concentrate mainly on the extensions of survival models in the case of right-censoring. The case of left- and interval-censoring have been less studied, and we will refer the reader to appropriate references when available. We will also focus on frequentist approaches, although Bayesian methods [172] will also be shortly discussed and references will be provided.

2

Classical Survival Analysis

2.1 Introduction

The analysis of survival data usually starts with the estimation of the survival function and related summary quantities. Hypotheses testing for the comparison of the survival functions of two or more sub-populations is often of prime interest. This is typically the case in a randomized clinical trial with a time-to-event outcome, where our interest is to identify whether the experimental treatment leads to a longer time-to-event (assuming that the event is a bad outcome for the patient) for the patients in this treatment arm compared to the standard treatment. This is for example the case in the colon trial presented in Section 1.3.1 of Chapter 1. In addition to the information on the outcome of interest, one often has at our disposal information on one or more predictors, such as the treatment group in the case of a randomized clinical trial but also information on baseline characteristics of the individuals or on some exposure factors or confounding factors. The objective can then be to adjust for such confounding factors and/or to identify variables having an impact on the survival distribution. As mentioned previously, the presence of (right-)censoring prevent us from using standard analysis techniques for continuous outcome such as ANOVA or linear regression, and this chapter provides a short summary of the methods most often encountered in classical survival analysis. For more details, we refer to the textbooks mentioned in Chapter 1 as well as to [8, 77, 260] for the implementation of these techniques respectively in R, SAS, and STATA.

2.2 Likelihood function

In the case of (random) right-censoring, one actually do not observe T for all individuals but rather

$$Y = min(T, C)$$

the observed event time, where C is a non-negative random variable representing to time to censoring. One also observes

$$\delta = I(T \leq C)$$

the censoring indicator, meaning that we know which individual is censored or not. In the following, we will denote respectively by $g(.)$ and $G(.)$ the density and the distribution function of C.

The first objective of survival analysis is to estimate the characteristics of the distribution of the real event time T in the population using only the available information, that is, the observed time and the censoring indicator (Y, δ) for a sample of individuals. In this book, we will consider that the censoring and time-to-event variables are independent random variables. Fleming and Harrington [125] have shown that this assumption is sufficient for the distribution of the event time T to be identifiable from the censored data (Y, δ).

Let's consider a random sample of n individuals and denote for each individual $t_1, \ldots, t_n$ the real time-to-event of interest, and $c_1, \ldots, c_n$ the censoring time-to-event of each individual. The observed data are then composed of couples $(y_i, c_i), i = 1, \ldots, n$ with $y_i = min(t_i, c_i)$ the observed event time and $\delta_i = I(t_i \leq c_i)$ the censoring indicator. Under random right-censoring, and assuming independent observations and independent censoring, the likelihood function is then given by

$$L = \prod_{i=1}^{n} [(1 - G(y_i))f(y_i)]^{\delta_i} [(1 - F(y_i))g(y_i)]^{1-\delta_i} .$$

Furthermore, if we assume uninformative censoring, that is, the censoring process does not depend on the parameters of the survival distribution of the survival process [125], the terms depending on $g(.)$ and $G(.)$ can be dropped from the likelihood to obtain

$$L \propto \prod_{i=1}^{n} (f(y_i))^{\delta_i} (S(y_i))^{1-\delta_i}$$

$$\propto \prod_{i=1}^{n} (h(y_i))^{\delta_i} S(y_i). \tag{2.1}$$

An extension of the likelihood function to the case of other types of censoring and truncation is given for example in [186].

2.3 Estimation of the survival and hazard function

2.3.1 Parametric estimation

Parametric estimation of the survival and hazard function can be obtained by assuming a parametric distribution for T. Event-times are, by definition,

Distribution	$f(t)$	$h(t)$	$S(t)$
Exponential ($\lambda > 0$)	$\lambda \exp(-\lambda t)$	λ	$\exp(-\lambda t)$
Weibull ($\rho, \lambda > 0$)	$\rho \lambda t^{\rho-1} \exp(-\lambda t^\rho)$	$\lambda \rho t^{\rho-1}$	$\exp(-\lambda t^\rho)$
Gompertz ($\gamma, \lambda > 0$)	$\lambda \exp(\gamma t) \exp[-\lambda \gamma^{-1}(\exp(\gamma t) - 1)]$	$\lambda \exp(\gamma t)$	$\exp[-\lambda \gamma^{-1}(\exp(\gamma t) - 1)]$
Rayleigh ($\alpha > 0, \gamma \geq 0$)	$(\alpha + 2\gamma t) \exp[-(\alpha t + \gamma t^2)]$	$\alpha + 2\gamma t$	$\exp[-(\alpha t + \gamma t^2)]$
Loglogistic ($\alpha \in R, \kappa > 0$)	$\frac{\exp(\alpha)\kappa t^{\kappa-1}}{(1+\exp(\alpha)t^\kappa)^2}$	$\frac{\exp(\alpha)\kappa t^{\kappa-1}}{1+\exp(\alpha)t^\kappa}$	$\frac{1}{1+\exp(\alpha)t^\kappa}$
Lognormal ($\mu \in R, \gamma > 0$)	$\frac{1}{t\sqrt{2\pi\gamma}} \exp\left[-\frac{1}{2\gamma}(\log(t) - \mu)^2\right]$	$f(t)/S(t)$	$1 - \Phi\left(\frac{\log(t)-\mu}{\sqrt{\gamma}}\right)$

TABLE 2.1
Most often used parametric distribution (and parameters) and their corresponding density $f(t)$, hazard $h(t)$, and survival $S(t)$ function. The function $\Phi(.)$ is the normal distribution function.

positive and often present a skewed distribution. Therefore usual standard distribution, such as the normal distribution, can not be used. Amongst the non-negative parametric density, the most popular ones in survival analysis are the Exponential, Weibull, or Log-normal distribution. Of course, each choice of a parametric distribution leads to a different expression of the density function and therefore a different shape for the associated survival and the hazard function. The expression for the density, hazard, and survival function for the most commonly used distributions are given in Table 2.1. The exponential distribution leads to a constant hazard function, the Weibull density to a monotonic hazard function, increasing (if $\rho > 1$) or deacreasing (if $0 < \rho < 1$) according to some power function (and with the Exponential as special case when $\rho = 1$), the Gompertz density to a monotonic hazard function increasing (if $\gamma > 1$) exponentially with time, and the Rayleigh density to linear increasing (if $\gamma > 0$) hazard function (with the Exponential as a special case when $\gamma = 0$), see Figure 2.1. The expression of the hazard function for the log-normal distribution is less easy to interpret.

Once we have assumed a particular parametric distribution for T, we can simply plug the corresponding expression for the density and survival function ($f(.)$ and $S(.)$) in the likelihood expression (2.1) and maximize this function to obtain the maximum likelihood estimators (MLEs) of the parameters of the assumed distribution. Using standard mathematical statistics theory, the variance of the MLEs can be estimated by the observed information. Confidence intervals can be obtained from the asymptotic normality of the MLEs. See for example [181] for more details.

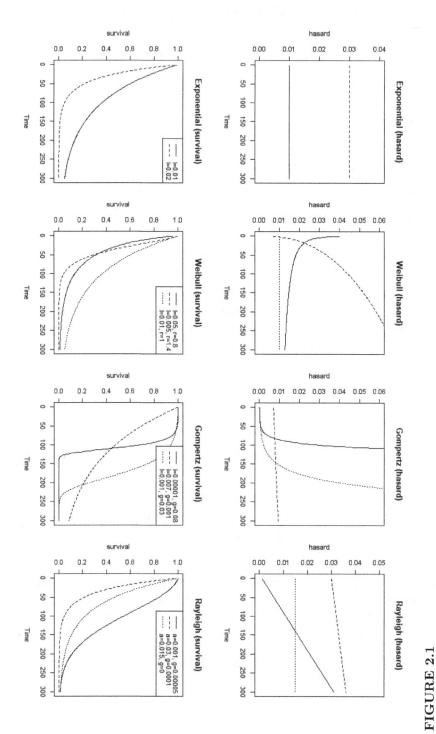

FIGURE 2.1
Survival and hazard function for the Exponential, Weibull Gompertz, and Rayleigh distribution of event times with different parameter value.

2.3.2 Non-parametric estimation

As we have seen in the previous section, parametric estimation is easy to handle but in practice it is often difficult to figure out the appropriate parametric distribution. The (relatively) simple form (often monotonic or unimodal) of the hazard function of most commonly used distribution rarely fits well with the situation we want to study. Also, due to the presence of censoring, inference can be more sensitive to a misspecification of the distribution of the survival times compared to complete data [320]. Non-parametric estimation has therefore became very popular in survival analysis.

In case of no censoring, an obvious *empirical estimator* of the survival function would be

$$\hat{S}^{emp}(t) \quad = \quad \frac{\text{Number of observations with time-to-event} > t}{\text{Number of observations in the data set}}$$
$$= \quad 1 - \hat{F}^{emp}(t)$$

This estimated survival function is assumed to be constant between successive event times, and is therefore a decreasing step function starting at 1 (value of $\hat{S}^{emp}(t)$ before the first event time) and going down to 0 after the last event time.

However, such an estimator can not be applied in the case of censored observation as it actually disregards the information provided by the censored observations. Specific non-parametric estimators of the survival function which allows to take into account the partial information available from the censored observations have therefore been proposed. The two most commonly used non-parametric estimator for right-censored data are the Kaplan-Meier (KM) estimator of the survival function and the Nelson-Aalen (NA) estimator of the cumulative hazard function. Both estimators allow to make inference on the distribution of the real event times T based on the available information (Y_i, δ_i) while making no particular parametric assumption about this distribution.

As is often the case in non-parametric statistics, one actually considers the order in which events and censored observations occur rather than the actual times at which these occur. We therefore need to introduce some new notations. Assume we have n observations with observed times $y_1, \ldots, y_n$ and censoring indicators $\delta_1, \ldots, \delta_n$ corresponding to r distinct event times (obviously $r \leq n$). We will then denote by $y_{(1)}, \ldots, y_{(r)}$ the r ordered distinct event times with $d_{(1)}, \ldots, d_{(r)}$ the corresponding number of events and $R(y_{(1)}), \ldots, R(y_{(r)})$ the size of the risk set at each event time, i.e $R(y_{(j)})$ is the number of observations still event-free and not censored right before $y_{(j)}$. Note that we can also define $y_{(0)} = y_0$ the time origin, at which $R(y_{(0)}) = n$ and with no event in the time interval $[y_0, y_{(1)}]$. We can also define $y_{(r+1)} = \infty$ and $R(y_{(r+1)}) = 0$.

The Kaplan-Meier (KM) estimator is certainly the most popular non-parametric estimator of the survival function for right- censored data [182]. Since we assume that the times to event are independent, the probability for an individual to survive over time t, included in the interval $[y_{(j)}, y_{(j+1)}]$, is actually the product of surviving each interval up to this one, knowing one has survived the previous one. So we can write for t in $[y_{(j)}, y_{(j+1)}]$

$$
\begin{aligned}
S(t) &= P(T > t) \\
&= P(T > y_{(1)} \mid T > y_{(0)}) \times P(T > y_{(2)} \mid T > y_{(1)}) \times \cdots \\
&\times P(T > y_{(j)} \mid T > y_{(j-1)})
\end{aligned}
$$

The idea, as explained for example in [78], is that given the definition of the time-intervals, no one experience the event during the intervals, and if we consider an infinitesimal time interval $[y_{(j)} - \Delta, y_{(j)}]$, the probability to have an event during it can be estimated by $d_{(j)}$, the number of events in this interval divided by $R(y_{(j)})$, the number of individuals still at risk at the beginning of the interval. The probability to survive through that interval is then

$$
1 - \frac{d_{(j)}}{R(y_{(j)})} = \frac{R(y_{(j)}) - d_{(j)}}{R(y_{(j)})}
$$

The Kaplan-Meier (KM) estimator of the survival function is then given by

$$
\begin{aligned}
\hat{S}^{KM}(t) &= \prod_{j:y_{(j)} \leq t} \left(1 - \frac{d_{(j)}}{R(y_{(j)})} \right) \\
&= \prod_{j:y_{(j)} \leq t} \frac{R(y_{(j)}) - d_{(j)}}{R(y_{(j)})}
\end{aligned}
\tag{2.2}
$$

with $\hat{S}^{KM}(t) = 1$ for $t < y_{(1)}$. This estimator is often referred to as the product-limit estimator. It is a decreasing step function, starting at $\hat{S}^{KM}(0) = 1$ and with jumps at each event times. If the largest observed time, say y_n, corresponds to an event, then the KM estimated survival function reaches 0, that is, $\hat{S}^{KM}(y_n) = 0$. On the other hand if this largest observed time is censored, then $\hat{S}^{KM}(t)$ does not reach zero and $S(t)$ can actually not be estimated consistently beyond this time, so for $t > y_n$. The most common solution is to leave $\hat{S}^{KM}(t)$ undefined after this timepoint.

When all data are uncensored, then $R(y_{(j)}) - d_{(j)} = R(y_{(j+1)})$, and (2.2) becomes for $t \in [y_{(k)}, y_{(k+1)}]$

$$
\begin{aligned}
\hat{S}(t) &= \frac{R(y_{(2)})}{R(y_{(1)})} \times \frac{R(y_{(3)})}{R(y_{(2)})} \times \cdots \times \frac{n_{(k+1)}}{R(y_{(k)})} \\
&= \frac{R(y_{(k+1)})}{R(y_{(1)})}
\end{aligned}
$$

Thus, we can easily see for complete data, the Kaplan-Meier estimator reduces to the empirical estimator of the survival function.

The variance of the Kaplan-Meier estimator can be approximated by the so-called Greenwood formula (see for example [78] or [181] for details):

$$\hat{V}\left(\hat{S}^{KM}(t)\right) = (\hat{S}(t))^2 \sum_{j:y_{(j)} \leq t} \frac{d_{(j)}}{R(y_{(j)})(R(y_{(j)}) - d_{(j)})}$$

Furthermore, we have the following asymptotic results

$$\frac{\hat{S}^{KM}(t) - S(t)}{\sqrt{\hat{V}(\hat{S}^{KM}(t))}} \xrightarrow{d} N(0,1)$$

We refer the reader to [13, 125] for a rigorous derivations of this result and of the statistical properties of the Kaplan-Meier estimator. From this asymptotic normality, one can obtain an asymptotic pointwise $100(1 - \alpha)\%$ confidence interval (CI)

$$\hat{S}^{KM}(t) \pm z_{\alpha/2}\sqrt{\hat{V}\left(\hat{S}^{KM}(t)\right)} \tag{2.3}$$

where $z_{\alpha/2}$ is the $\alpha/2$ percentile of the standard normal distribution. However, this CI has the disadvantage that it may contain points outside the $[0,1]$ interval and one often prefers a CI obtained using a log-log transform

$$\hat{S}^{KM}(t)^{\exp\left[\pm z_{\alpha/2}\sqrt{V(\log(-\log \hat{S}^{KM}(t)))}\right]}. \tag{2.4}$$

If we consider again the 10 hypothetical patients represented on Figure 1.1, we actually have 5 distinct event time, see Table 2.2 for the data. The computation of the KM estimator is summarized in Table 2.3 and the result is shown on Figure 2.2. As expected, the KM estimated survival curve starts at one, and we have one step at each event time; since the longest observation (patient 9 with a time of 657 days) is censored, the KM curve does not reach zero. Confidence intervals given by 2.4 are also represented (dotted line), it is important to actually interpret them as pointwise CI and not as confidence bands. An example of the KM estimate of the survival function obtained on real data is presented on Figure 2.7 in Section 2.6.2. Obviously when the number of event times becomes large the number of steps increases and the fact that it is a step function becomes less distinguishable on the picture.

Adjustment of the KM estimator for a categorical covariate is simply done by computing (2.2) in each category defined by the levels of this covariate. The non-parametric KM estimator of the survival function has been extended to account for a continuous covariate [34, 394].

An alternative estimator of the survival function is based on the so-called Nelson-Aalen (NA) estimator of the cumulative hazard function, proposed independently by Nelson [270] and Aalen [2], see also [125] for more details.

Patient	1	2	3	4	5	6	7	8	9	10
Time	390	176	298	493	142	255	230	125	657	286
Event	0	1	1	0	0	1	1	1	0	0

TABLE 2.2
Data of the 10 hypothetical patients presented in Figure 1.1

$t_{(j)}$	$d_{(j)}$	$R(y_{(j)})$	$1 - \dfrac{d_{(j)}}{R(y_{(j)})}$	$\prod \left\{ 1 - \dfrac{d_{(j)}}{R(y_{(j)})} \right\}$
0	10	0	1	1
125	10	1	0.900	0.900
176	8	1	0.875	0.788
230	7	1	0.857	0.675
255	6	1	0.833	0.563
298	4	1	0.750	0.422

TABLE 2.3
Computation of the Kaplan-Meier estimator of the survival function for the
data of the 10 hypothetical patients presented in Figure 1.1

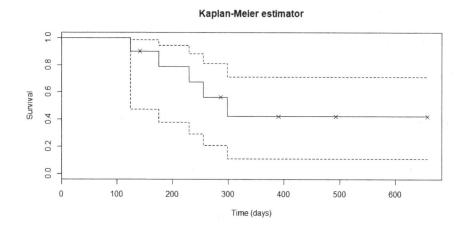

FIGURE 2.2
Kaplan-Meier estimator of the survival function for the data of the 10 hypothetical patients presented in Figure 1.1.

This estimator is given by

$$\hat{H}(t) = \sum_{j:y_{(j)}\leq t} \frac{d_{(j)}}{R(y_{(j)})} \qquad \text{for } t \leq y_{(r)} \qquad (2.5)$$

with

$$\hat{V}\left(\hat{H}(t)\right) = \sum_{j:y_{(j)}\leq t} \frac{d_{(j)}}{(R(y_{(j)}))^2}$$

and the corresponding asymptotic result:

$$\frac{\hat{H}(t) - H(t)}{\sqrt{\hat{V}(\hat{H}(t))}} \xrightarrow{d} N(0,1)$$

From this estimator, one can obtain the following NA estimator of the survival function

$$\hat{S}^{NA}(t) = \exp(-\hat{H}(t)) \qquad (2.6)$$

$$= \exp\left(-\sum_{j:y_{(j)}\leq t} \frac{d_{(j)}}{R(y_{(j)})}\right) \qquad (2.7)$$

$$= \prod_{j:y_{(j)}\leq t} \exp\left(\frac{-d_{(j)}}{R(y_{(j)})}\right) \qquad (2.8)$$

This estimator is also called the Breslow estimator of the survival function [46] and sometimes the Altshuler or Nelson-Altshuler estimator given its roots in [9]. Confidence interval can be obtained as for the KM estimator using a formula similar to the Greenwood's formula.

Interestingly, the Kaplan-Meier estimator of the survival function can actually be seen as a first-order Taylor expansion approximation of the NA estimator. Remind that based on the Taylor expansion, we can write

$$e^{-x} = 1 - x + \frac{x^2}{2!} - \frac{x^3}{3!} + \cdots$$

and that e^{-x} is therefore approximately equal to $1 - x$ when x is small. Applying this result to (2.9), we have

$$\hat{S}^{NA}(t) \approx \prod_{j:y_{(j)}\leq t} (1 - d_{(j)}/R(y_{(j)})) = \hat{S}^{KM}(t) \qquad (2.9)$$

as long as $d_{(j)}$ is small relative to $R(y_{(j)})$ which will usually be the case, except at the latest survival times. The two estimators of the survival functions are consistent and asymptotically equivalent, however in practice we can see

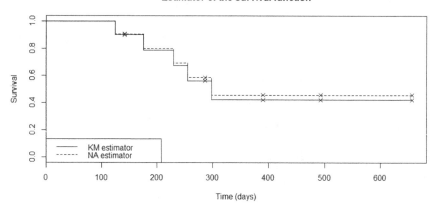

FIGURE 2.3

Kaplan-Meier (*solid line*) and Nelson Aalen (*dotted line*) estimator of the survival function for the data of the 10 hypothetical patients presented in Figure 1.1.

differences and in particular in small samples. Based on (2.9), we have that $e^{-x} \geq 1 - x$ for all values of x. Therefore, at any timepoint, the NA estimator of the survival function will always be greater or equal to the KM estimator. However, in most of the practical cases, both estimates will be very close, except maybe for the longer observed survival times for which both estimates should anyhow be interpreted with care given the little information on which it is based. Note that, as we can see from (2.2) and (2.9) if the largest observed time, say $y_{(n)}$ is a true event, then $\hat{S}^{KM}(y_{(n)}) = 0$ while $\hat{S}^{NA}(y_{(n)}) > 0$. The NA estimator has been shown to perform somewhat better than the KM estimator for small samples. The NA estimator has generally a lower variance but may be biased upwards, however in terms of means square errors these two aspects trade-off with therefore no clear conclusions on which estimator has to be preferred [124]. Nevertheless, the KM estimator has gain more popularity, probably due to its link with the empirical estimator of the survival function when there is no censoring. Figure 2.3 plots both the KM and the NA estimator of the survival function for our 10 hypothetical patients from Figure 1.1, and as mentioned above, the Nelson-Aalen estimator is (slightly) above the KM estimator.

Although non-parametric estimation usually focus on the survival function, one may also be interested in obtaining a non-parametric estimate of the hazard function. From (1.2), a first idea to estimate the hazard function at

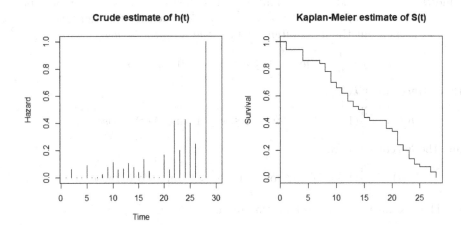

FIGURE 2.4
Crude hazard estimate and corresponding KM estimate for 50 generated survival times.

the ith ordered event time is simply

$$\hat{h}^{crude}(y_{(i)}) = \frac{d_{(i)}}{R(y_{(i)})} \qquad i = 1, \ldots, r \qquad (2.10)$$

so the number of events at time $y_{(j)}$ divided by the number of observations still at risk at that time. Note that at each timepoint, the value of this crude estimator of the hazard corresponds to the size of the jumps of the cumulative hazard function. An example based on 50 randomly generated survival times is shown on Figure 2.4 together with the corresponding KM estimate of the survival function. These data have been generated from a uniform distribution over $[0, 100]$ with the `floor(runif(50,1,30))` command in R (and the option `set.seeds(123)`) and for the sake of illustration, no censoring has been considered. As we can immediately see, such a crude estimate of the hazard function has the disadvantage to be unstable from one time to the next and does not really help in determining the shape of the hazard function.

This crude estimate of the hazard function is rarely used and one will often prefer a *smooth* version. A general expression of a non-parametric smoothed estimator of the hazard function is given by

$$\hat{h}(t) = \frac{1}{b} \sum_{i=1}^{r} K\left(\frac{t - y_{(i)}}{b}\right) \Delta \hat{H}(y_{(i)})$$

where $\hat{H}(t)$ is a non-parametric estimator of the cumulative hazard function and $\Delta \hat{H}(y_{(i)})$ represents the estimated jump of $\hat{H}(t)$ at time $y_{(i)}$. The function

$K(u)$ is a *kernel* or *window* function used to weight the observations within a window around u, and b is a parameter which allows to control the amount of smoothing and is often called the *bandwidth*. Any density function could be used as kernel, but the most often used are the *uniform kernel*,

$$K(u) = \frac{1}{2} \quad \text{for } -1 \leq u \leq 1 \text{ and } 0 \text{ otherwise}$$

the *Epanechnikov kernel*,

$$K(u) = \frac{3}{4}(1 - u^2) \quad \text{for } -1 \leq u \leq 1 \text{ and } 0 \text{ otherwise}$$

and the *biweight kernel*,

$$K(u) = \frac{15}{16}(1 - u^2)^2 \quad \text{for } -1 \leq u \leq 1 \text{ and } 0 \text{ otherwise}$$

The variance of $\hat{h}(t)$ can be estimated by [312]

$$\hat{V}(\hat{h}(t)) = \frac{1}{b^2} \sum_{i=1}^{r} K\left(\frac{t - y_{(i)}}{b}\right)^2 \Delta\hat{V}(\hat{H}(y_{(i)}))$$

with $\Delta\hat{V}(\hat{H}(y_{(i)})) = \hat{V}(\hat{H}(y_{(i)})) - \hat{V}(\hat{H}(y_{(i-1)}))$.

The value of the bandwidth can be fixed a priori, but since the estimated curve of the hazard function will change with the value of the bandwidth, it is advised to choose it appropriately and data-driven method, such as cross-validation, are often preferred. Figure 2.5 plots on the same graph the the crude estimate hazard for the same data as in Figure 2.4 together with smooth kernel estimates obtained with the kernels mentioned above and different choices of the bandwidth. When estimating the hazard function with a kernel, we must be careful about a possible *boundary effect* since the windows computed at the first and last event times will usually contains less data points and we might have some mass points attributed to negative timepoints. Corrections have been developed to address this. We refer the reader to [262, 312] for more technical details, to [260] for a practical perspective, and to [161] for a large simulation study investigating various types of kernel, bandwidth choice methods, and boundary correction.

Finally, let's mention the life-table estimate of the hazard and survival function, also called the actuarial estimate of these functions [78]. These estimators are constructed by dividing the period of observations into m time intervals, for an arbitrary m (usually between 5 and 15) and are based on the assumption that the censoring process is such that the censored survival times occur uniformly throughout the ith interval. So, if we note R_i the number of individuals at risk at the start of interval i, and c_i the number of individuals censored during that interval then based on this assumption the average number of individuals who are at risk during this interval is

$$R_i' = R_i - \frac{c_i}{2}$$

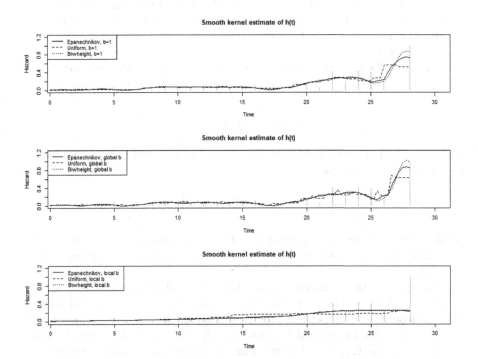

FIGURE 2.5
Smooth kernel estimators of the hazard function for data from Figure 2.4.
The crude estimate in gray, while the black lines are estimates obtained with a
Epanechnikov, uniform or biweight kernel. These kernel estimates are obtained
considering either a fixed bandwidth (*top*), a global bandwidth, with an equal
value for all grid points obtained by minimizing the IMSE (*middle*), and a local
bandwidth, with a potentially different value for each grid point obtained by
minimizing a local MSE (*bottom*).

So, in this interval, the probability of an event can be estimated by d_i/R_i'
where d_i is, as above, the number of events in this interval. So, following the
same reasoning as for the KM estimator, the life-table estimate of the survival
function is based on the product of the conditional probability to survive each
interval, given one has survived the previous ones, and is given by

$$\hat{S}^{LT}(t) = \prod_{i=1}^{k} \left(\frac{R_i' - d_i}{R_i'} \right) \qquad \text{for } t_k' \leq t < t_{k+1}', k = 1, \ldots, m$$

where the t'_k are the boundaries of the m intervals. This estimator is assumed to be constant within each interval, and is thus a decreasing step function. However, in case there is at least one event in the first interval, this estimator will not start at one.

Following the same reasoning and assuming that the death rate is constant during the ith interval, the average time survived in that interval is

$$\frac{d_i}{(R'_i - d_i/2)\Delta_i}$$

where Δ_i is the length of the the ith interval, and an estimate of the hazard function is then given by

$$\hat{h}^{LT}(t) = \frac{d_i}{(R'_i - d_i/2)\Delta_i} \qquad \text{for } t'_k \le t < t'_{k+1}, k = 1, \ldots, m$$

Again, this estimate of the hazard function is assumed to be constant within each time interval, and is therefore a step function, however not necessarily monotone.

The form of the estimated survival and hazard life-table estimator will change according to the choice of the intervals, just as the shape of an histogram depends on the choice of the class intervals [78]. These estimators are rarely used in the biomedical field but may be very useful for example when dealing with registry data. Indeed, a major advantage of these estimators is that they don't require to know the exact time of the events, but only rely on the number of events and the number of censored observations that occur in a series of consecutive periods (e.g. civil year). One should also note that the Kaplan-Meier estimate of the survival function can actually be seen as a particular case of this estimate, for which the time-intervals are design such that only one distinct event time is contained in each interval, and is taken to occur at the start of the interval. Also, the life-table estimate of the hazard function can be seen as a smoothed-estimate with a uniform kernel and arbitrary time-intervals.

2.4   Hypothesis testing

When comparing the survival curves between two groups, it is important to consider overall difference over time

$$H_0 : S_1(t) = S_2(t) \qquad \text{for all } t \le y_{(r)}$$
$$H_1 : S_1(t) \ne S_2(t) \qquad \text{for some } t \le y_{(r)}$$

The most popular test to compare the survival curves between two groups is certainly the logrank test. The idea behind the logrank test is to compare,

	Number with an event at $y_{(i)}$	Number without an event at $y_{(i)}$	Number at risk just before $y_{(i)}$
Group 1	d_{1i}	$R_{1i} - d_{1i}$	R_{1i}
Group 2	d_{2i}	$R_{2i} - d_{2i}$	R_{2i}
Total:	d_i	$R_i - di$	R_i

TABLE 2.4
Notations for the logrank test: number of events and number at risk in each of the two groupes

at each event time, the observed number of events with the expected number of events under the null hypothesis. The information available at each event time $y_{(i)}$ is often represented in a 2×2 contingency table as in Table 2.4.

If we fix the margin in Table 2.4, then all the entries are determined by only one value, let's say d_{1i}. One can show that under the null hypothesis d_{1i} has an hypergeometric distribution from which we can deduce that the expected value of d_{1i} under H_0 is, using the notation of Table 2.4,

$$e_{1i} = E(d_{1i} \mid H_0) = R_{1i} \frac{d_i}{R_i}$$

which therefore represents the expected number of events in group 1 under H_0 (see for example [78] for more details). The idea is then to compare the number of observed and expected events and to combine the information from all event times. The most intuitive way is simply to sum the difference between the observed and expected number of events under H_0 in group 1 at each event times [246]. This leads to the well known logrank U-statistic

$$U_L = \sum_{i=1}^{r} (d_{1i} - e_{1i}) = \sum_{i=1}^{r} \left(d_{1i} - \frac{R_{1i} d_i}{R_i} \right) \tag{2.11}$$

Obviously, this is also equivalent to $\sum_{i=1}^{r} d_{1i} - \sum_{i=1}^{r} e_{1i}$, sometimes abbreviated $O - E$ (for observed minus expected).

Furthermore, one can show that under H_0

$$\frac{U_L}{\sqrt{V(U_L)}} \approx N(0, 1)$$

where

$$V(U^L) = \sum_{i=1}^{r} v_{1i} = \sum_{i=1}^{r} \frac{R_{1i} R_{2i} d_i (R_i - d_i)}{R_i^2 (R_i - 1)}$$

is obtained using the properties of the hypergeometric distribution. And we have

$$\frac{U_L^2}{V(U_L)} \approx \chi_1^2.$$

This logrank test is sometimes also called the Mantel-Haenszel test, the Mantel-Cox test or the Peto-Mantel-Haenszel test. It has been shown that this logrank test have maximal power in case of proportional hazards (i.e., when the ratio of the hazards function in the two groups is constant over time, see Section 2.5.1 for more details).

As can be seen from (2.11), the U_L statistic for the logrank test gives the same weights to the difference between observed and expected number of events at all timepoints. A possible extension is to consider a weighted sum of the differences at each event time $y_{(i)}$. The test statistic then writes

$$U = \sum_{i=1}^{r} w(y_{(i)})(d_{1i} - e_{1i}) = \sum_{i=1}^{r} w(y_{(i)}) \left(d_{1i} - \frac{R_{1i}d_i}{R_i} \right) \qquad (2.12)$$

The variance of this weighted sum can be obtained as above, and we still have

$$\frac{U^2}{V(U)} \approx \chi_1^2.$$

We find back the logrank test if we consider $w(y_{(i)}) = 1$ for all $i = 1, \ldots, r$. Another popular choice for these weights is to consider $w(y_{(i)}) = R(y_{(i)}) = R_i$ for all $i = 1, \ldots, r$ leading to the Wilcoxon test also called the Breslow test. The idea is to give less weight to the difference between observed and expected number of events for the event times where we have less information, i.e. when the risk set becomes small. It will therefore give more emphasis on the deviation from the null hypothesis earlier in time when we have more individuals still at risk, and less emphasis to the deviation from the null occurring later in the tails of the survival functions.

For this Wilcoxon test, we have

$$U_W = \sum_{i=1}^{r} R_i(d_{1i} - e_{1j}) = \sum_{i=1}^{r} (d_{1i}R_i - d_i R_{1i}) \qquad (2.13)$$

and

$$V(U^W) = \sum_{i=1}^{r} R_i^2 v_{1i} = \sum_{i=1}^{r} R_i^2 \frac{R_{1i}R_{2i}d_i(R_i - d_i)}{R_i^2(R_i - 1)}.$$

An example is given in Table 2.5, where we compute the logrank and the Wilcoxon test statistics for 60 hypothetical patients randomized to two treatment groups. The KM estimated survival curves are depicted for these two groupes are displayed in Figure 2.6. There are 21 distinct event times, and based on the computations in Table 2.5, the test statistic for the logrank test is

$$\frac{\sum_{i=1}^{21}(d_{1i} - e_{1i})^2}{\sum_{i=1}^{21} v_{1i}} = \frac{5.11^2}{9.83} = 2.65$$

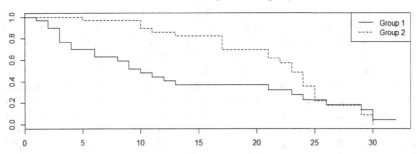

FIGURE 2.6

KM estimated survival curves for 60 hypothetical patients randomized to two treatment groups.

leading to a p-value of $p = 0.103$. On the other hand, the Wilcoxon test lead to a test statistic equal to

$$\frac{\sum_{i=1}^{21}(R_i(d_{1i} - e_{1i}))^2}{\sum_{i=1}^{21}(R_i^2 v_{1i})} = \frac{(378)^2}{14075.52} = 10.15$$

corresponding to a p-value of p-value $= 0.001$. As can be expected from the survival curves, the Wilcoxon test, which give more weight to the earlier times, lead to a more extreme test statistics. In this particular example, the Wilcoxon test leads to a significant p-value at the 5% significance level while the logrank test does not.

Another possible choice of weights is to consider $w(y_{(i)}) = \hat{S}(y_{(i)})$ with $\hat{S}(.)$ an estimate of the common survival function of both groups. This leads to the so-called Peto and Peto test and will also give more weight to the early differences compared to the late differences, but independently of the number of individuals still at risk. In the example above, this leads to a test statistics equal to 8.67 corresponding to a p-value of 0.004.

Other weight functions have been proposed and will allow to put more emphasis on certain part of the data, e.g., early or late differences between the two survival curves. See for example [154] who proposed a general weight function, including the weights seen above as special cases. As we have seen, we may obtain very different p-values depending on the choice of the weights and it is of upmost importance to appropriately choose and specify this choice a priori (i.e., before analysing the data) based on the research question.

This U-test, and in particular the logrank test, can be generalized to the case of a comparison between more than two groups, as well as a to a test for trend, in which case a specific ordering of the survival functions is specified

Time	R_j	d_j	R_{1j}	d_{1j}	e_{1j}	$d_{ij} - e_{1j}$	v_{1j}	$R_j(d_{ij} - e_{ij})$	$R_j^2 v_{1j}$
1	60	1	30	1	0.5	0.5	0.25	30	900
2	59	2	29	2	0.98	1.02	0.49	60	1710
3	57	4	27	4	1.89	2.11	0.94	120	3066.43
4	53	2	23	2	0.87	1.13	0.48	60	1353.46
5	50	1	20	0	0.4	−0.4	0.24	−20	600
6	48	2	20	2	0.83	1.17	0.48	56	1096.17
8	45	1	17	1	0.38	0.62	0.24	28	476
9	44	2	16	2	0.73	1.27	0.45	56	875.16
10	41	3	14	1	1.02	−0.02	0.64	−1	1077.3
11	38	2	13	1	0.68	0.32	0.44	12	632.43
12	35	1	12	1	0.34	0.66	0.23	23	276
13	33	2	10	1	0.61	0.39	0.41	13	445.62
17	28	3	8	0	0.86	−0.86	0.57	−24	444.44
21	25	3	8	1	0.96	0.04	0.6	1	374
22	22	1	7	0	0.32	−0.32	0.22	−7	105
23	20	3	7	1	1.05	−0.05	0.61	−1	244.26
24	17	4	6	1	1.41	−0.41	0.74	−7	214.5
25	13	3	5	0	1.15	−1.15	0.59	−15	100
26	10	2	5	1	1	0	0.44	0	44.44
29	8	3	4	1	1.5	−0.5	0.54	−4	34.29
30	5	4	3	2	2.4	−0.4	0.24	−2	6
Total:		49		25	19.89	5.11	9.83	378	14075.52

TABLE 2.5

Computation of the logrank and Wilcoxon test statistics for the data from the 60 hypothetical patients from Figure 2.6

in the alternative. Another extension of the U-test is to consider a stratified test. Such tests are used if we want to compare two (or more) groups while adjusting for a categorical variable. The idea is to perform the comparison within each strata defined by the K levels of the categorical variable and to combine the results in a single test statistic. In particular, the stratified logrank test is obtained by computing for $k = 1, \ldots, K$, the value of U_k and V_k defined by (2.11) and (2.12) but computed only for the observations in the kth strata. Under the null hypothesis $H_0 : S_{1k}(t) = S_{2k}(t)$ for all $t \leq y_{(r)}$ and $k = 1, \ldots, K$,

$$\frac{\left(\sum_{k=1}^{K} U_k\right)^2}{\sum_{k=1}^{K} V_k^2} \approx \chi_1^2.$$

We can for example use such a stratified test to compare the survival of the patients in two treatment groups while adjusting for the gender or the presence of a given mutation. It is however important to realize that such a test obviously do not provide any information about the impact of the variable used to stratify. Depending on the situation, it may sometimes be more interesting to model the impact of both the variable defining the groups and the variable defining the strata via a regression models as we will see in the next section.

2.5 Modeling survival data

While hypothesis tests will lead to a p-value, it is usually advised not to rely only on a p-value when analyzing data. It is indeed more informative to present such a p-value, together with a plot of the estimated survival curves by group, as well as a quantification of the difference between the two survival curves (together with a confidence interval). Such a quantification of the difference between two (or more) survival curves can be obtained via modeling.

Regression models are multivariate statistical methods that allow to analyse simultaneously several independent covariates. For example, in the context of a clinical trial, such regression models are often used to estimate the treatment effect while adjusting for (potential) heterogeneity and imbalances in baseline characteristics or important prognostic factors. Furthermore, these models are particularly useful in the context of observational studies where it is of upmost importance to adjust for confounding factors.

As often in statistics, one can consider parametric, semi-parametric, and non-parametric models. In the field of survival data, fully non-parametric models are hardly used in practice and will not be considered further in this book. On the other hand, semi-parametric models are widely spread, and tends to supplant parametric models in most applications.

The two most often encountered families of models are the proportional hazards (PH) models and accelerated failure time (AFT) models. However, other class of models have also been proposed such as the proportional odds (PO) models.

2.5.1 Proportional hazards models

A major advantage of the one-to-one relationship between the hazard function and the survival function is that the effect of a covariate on the hazard translate directly into its effect on the survival function. Regression models in survival analysis are therefore usually set up at the level of the hazard function. Relative risks models that assume a multiplicative effect of the covariates on the hazard scale are commonly encountered.

Considering a set of covariates $\mathbf{X}^t = (X_1, \ldots, X_p)$ the proportional hazards model writes down the hazard function of individual $i(i = 1, \ldots, n)$ with covariates values $\mathbf{x}_i^t = (x_{i1}, \ldots, x_{ip})$ as the product of a baseline hazard function common to all individuals, $h_0(t)$, and a multiplying factor depending of the value of $\mathbf{X}$. Since this factor must be positive, it is common to use the exponential of a (linear) combination of these covariates. The proportional hazards (PH) models is then given by

$$h_i(t) = h(t \mid \mathbf{x}_i) = h_0(t) \exp(\beta^t \mathbf{x}_i) \tag{2.14}$$

where $\mathbf{x}_i$ is the $p \times 1$ observed vector of covariates for subject i and β is the associated $p \times 1$ unobserved parameters vector. On the log-hazard scale this model writes down

$$\log h_i(t) = \log(h(t \mid \mathbf{x}_i)) = \log h_0(t) + \beta^t \mathbf{x}_i \tag{2.15}$$

Therefore this model assumes that the covariates have a multiplicative effect on the hazard of an event, and the coefficient β_j associated with the covariate X_j represents the change in the log-hazard when X_j increases of one unit, all the other covariates being constant.

Using the relationship (1.3), the PH model can also be written as

$$S_i(t) = S(t \mid \mathbf{x}_i) = S_0(t)^{\exp(\beta^t \mathbf{x}_i)} \tag{2.16}$$

where $S_0(t) = \exp\left(-\int_0^t h_0(u)du\right) = \exp(-H_0(t))$ is the baseline survival function.

The main assumption of this model is the *proportional hazards assumption*, that is, the fact that the ratio of the hazards for two subjects with covariate values $\mathbf{x}_i$ and $\mathbf{x}_l$ is constant over time:

$$\frac{h(t \mid \mathbf{x}_i)}{h(t) \mid \mathbf{x}_l} = \frac{\exp(\beta^t \mathbf{x}_i)}{\exp(\beta^t \mathbf{x}_l)} \tag{2.17}$$

which does not depend on time. In other words, all the time dependency is captured by the baseline hazard function which is common to all observations. Considering the case where the two individuals i and l differs only by one unit of jth covariate, the right hand-side of (2.17) further simplifies to $\exp(\beta_j)$. Therefore, $\exp(\beta_j)$ represents the ratio of the hazards for a one unit change in X_j at any time t while keeping all the other covariates constant. This quantity is therefore often referred to as the hazards ratio (HR).

Continuous and/or categorical covariates can be included, as well as interactions between covariates and non-linear terms.

From (2.1), one can easily obtain the likelihood function as

$$L(h_0(.), \beta) \propto \prod_{i=1}^n \left[h_0(y_i) \exp\left(\beta^t \mathbf{x}_i\right)\right]^{\delta_i} \exp\left(-H_0(y_i) \exp\left(\beta^t \mathbf{x}_i\right)\right) \tag{2.18}$$

There have been various proposals regarding the choice of the baseline hazard function. A first option is to assume a parametric distribution for the event times, and to consider the corresponding expression for the hazard in (2.14) leading to a fully parametric PH model. On the other hand, this baseline hazard function can be left totally unspecified leading to the so-called "semi-parametric Cox PH model" or simply "Cox model" [89].

Fully parametric PH models

Once a given distribution have been chosen for T, one can plug in the corresponding value for $h_0(t)$ and $H_0(t)$ (see Table 2.1) in the likelihood expression (2.18). Estimates of the model parameters, so the β's and the parameters of the parametric event times distribution, can be obtained by maximizing this likelihood function. This maximization is typically performed with the Newton-Raphson algorithm [21]. Approximation of the asymptotic variance-covariance matrix of the estimators can be obtained from the observed information matrix.

For example, let's assume that T follows a Weibull distribution with parameters λ and ρ, then $h_0(t) = \lambda \rho t^{\rho-1}$ and (2.14) becomes

$$h_i(t) = \lambda \rho t^{\rho-1} \exp(\beta^t \mathbf{x}_i) \tag{2.19}$$

and

$$S_i(t) = \exp(-\lambda \exp(\beta^t \mathbf{x}_i) t^\rho) \tag{2.20}$$

Interestingly, we see from this expression that the event time of the ith subject is characterized by a Weibull distribution with scale parameter $\lambda \exp(\beta^t \mathbf{x}_i)$ and shape parameter ρ. Plugging (2.19) and (2.20) in (2.1), we obtain the likelihood function which can then be maximized with respect to λ, ρ, and the vector β. Once estimates have been obtained, they can be plug in (2.19) and (2.20) to obtain a fully parametric model-based estimation of the hazard and survival function.

A more flexible alternative can be achieved by considering a parametric but very flexible specification of the baseline hazard for example specifying the baseline hazard as a piecewise constant function or using splines [159, 320, 335, 338]. Considering a piecewise constant hazard, the idea is then to specify

$$h_0(t) = \sum_{q=1}^{Q} \psi_q I(\tau_{q-1} < t \leq \tau_q)$$

for some partition of time $0 = \tau_0 < \tau_1 < \ldots < \tau_Q$ with ψ_q, the value of the baseline hazard over the interval $(\tau_{q-1}, \tau_q]$ and $I(.)$ the indicatrice function. To have a more flexible estimation of the baseline hazard, we should increase the number of intervals (or the number of *knots* $\tau_1, \ldots, \tau_Q$). Note that the limiting case where we have enough intervals so that each interval contains a single true event time (assuming no ties), comes back to leaving $h_0(.)$ completely unspecified and estimating it using non-parametric maximum likelihood estimation. An alternative is to model the baseline hazard function using splines. For example, we can expand the log baseline hazard function into B-spline basis functions

$$\log h_0(t) = \kappa_0 + \sum_{q=1}^{Q} \kappa_q B_q(t, \tau)$$

where $\kappa^t = (\kappa_0, \kappa_1, \ldots, \kappa_m)$ are the splines coefficients, and $B_q(t, \tau)$ is the qth basis function of a B-splines basis with knots $\tau_1, \ldots, \tau_Q$, and q the degree of the B-splines. Again, when the number of knots increase, the flexibility of the approximation of the baseline hazard increases. Position of the knots is typically based on the percentiles of the event times (either the true event times or the observed event times), but other approaches have also been proposed. While in both approaches we can gain flexibility by increasing the number of knots, we should however be careful that it also increases the number of parameters to be estimated, and one should keep a balance between bias and variance and avoid over-fitting. A popular rule of thumb is that the total number of parameters to be estimated (including the parameters from the baseline hazard and the regression parameters) should not exceed between 1/10 and 1/20 of the total number of events observed in the sample [153].

Semi-parametric PH model

In the early seventies, Sir David Cox proposed a PH model (2.14) in which the baseline hazard function $h_0(t)$ was left totally unspecified and showed that we can still obtain estimators for the β parameters [89, 90]. When the baseline hazard function $h_0(t)$ is left unspecified, the likelihood function (2.18) can not anymore be directly maximized to find the estimates of β. The idea is then to maximize a *partial likelihood* which does not contain $h_0(t)$ anymore with respect to β. When there are no ties, this partial likelihood can be derived as a profile likelihood and is given by

$$L_{part}(\beta) = \prod_{i=1}^{r} \frac{\exp(\beta^t \mathbf{x}_{(i)})}{\sum_{l \in \mathfrak{R}(y_{(i)})} \exp(\beta^t \mathbf{x}_l)} \qquad (2.21)$$

in which $\mathbf{x}_{(i)}$ is the vector of covariates for the subject with the ith ordered event time and $\mathfrak{R}(y_{(i)})$ is the risk set at the ith ordered event time. Therefore the sum in the denominator is on all the subjects who are still at risk at time $y_{(i)}$ and the contribution of censored observations is therefore only through this denominator. We can also notice that this partial likelihood only depends on the order of the events (via the definition of the risk set in the denominator) and not on the timing of these events. Therefore this partial likelihood is sometimes described as a measure of how well the model can order the subjects with respect to their event time. We refer to [78] for an intuitive derivation of this partial likelihood which is based on the idea that the intervals between successive event times convey no information about the effect of the covariables on the hazard of event, and to [90, 186] for a more formal derivation of this likelihood as a profile likelihood considering $h_0(.)$ as a nuisance parameter. The general idea behind profile likelihood is to express the nuisance parameter of the model as a function of the other parameters so that it does not appear anymore in the likelihood to be maximized. So, in a first step, we estimate $h_0(.)$ non-parametrically considering β as known while in a second step we replace $h_0(t)$ by its non-parametric estimator in the likelihood function and we then obtain a function depending only on β.

Although tied event times are not possible in theory, given the continuous nature of T, they can however occur in practice. Indeed, while event times are continuous in theory, in practice they are often discrete, being measured in days, weeks, or even sometimes months or years depending on the application. The partial likelihood (2.21) can not be used in case of tied event times. Kalbfleish and Prentice [180] have proposed an appropriate expression of the partial likelihood for the case of ties, but this expression is complex to use. Therefore, several approximations have therefore been proposed [46, 89, 108], see [186] or [372] for an overview of these different approximations.

While this (approximated) partial likelihood is not a real full likelihood, it can be treated as such to obtain maximum partial likelihood estimators $\hat{\beta}$. It has been shown that these estimators are consistent and asymptotically normally distributed with mean β and variance given by the inverse of the expected Fisher information matrix [181]. In practice, maximization of this partial likelihood is usually performed via a Newton-Raphson algorithm and the variance-covariance matrix of $\hat{\beta}$ is approximated by the inverse of the information matrix evaluated at $\hat{\beta}$. Based on asymptotic normality, one can also easily construct a $100(1 - \alpha)\%$ CI for a particular β parameter as

$$\hat{\beta}_j \pm z_{\alpha/2} se(\hat{\beta}_j)$$

where $z_{\alpha/2}$ is the $\alpha/2$ percentile of the standard normal distribution and $se(\hat{\beta}_j)$ is the standard error of $\hat{\beta}_j$ obtained as the squared root of the (jj) entry of the approximated variance-covariance matrix.

Similarly to what we have seen for the fully parametric model, the hazard ratios between two individuals whose covariates values differ only by one unit in covariate X_j is given by $exp(\hat{\beta}_j)$ and a $100(1 - \alpha)\%$ CI can be obtained by exponentiating the confidence limits of for β_j.

We can also build a test statistic for the null hypothesis $H_0 : \beta_j = 0$ given by

$$W = \frac{\hat{\beta}_j}{se(\hat{\beta}_j)}$$

which follows a $N(0, 1)$ distribution under H_0. This is equivalent to consider

$$W^2 = \frac{\hat{\beta}_j^2}{var(\hat{\beta}_j)}$$

which follows a chi-square with one degree of freedom under H_0. This test is often referred to as the Wald test. This test however consider only one particular coefficient, adjusted for the presence of the other covariates in the model.

In some situation, one may be interested to test simultaneously for a subset of β coefficients being all equal to zero. Considering a subset of q coefficients, and without loss of generality considering that there are the last q parameters in β, the idea is then to compare model $M1$

$$h(t \mid X) = h_0(t) \exp(\beta_1 X_1 + \cdots + \beta_p X_p + \beta_{p+1} X_{p+1} + \cdots + \beta_{p+q} X_{p+q})$$

to the reduced model $M2$ (model under H_0)

$$h(t \mid X) = h_0(t) \exp(\beta_1 X_1 + \cdots + \beta_p X_p)$$

Since model $M2$ is nested within model $M1$, we can use a likelihoods ratio test whose statistic is given by

$$LRT = -2log(\hat{L}_2) + 2log(\hat{L}_1) = -2log\frac{\hat{L}_2}{\hat{L}_1}$$

where $\hat{L}_1$ is the value of the partial likelihood for model $M1$ computed for the data at hand with the β coefficients set at the value of their maximum likelihood estimator $\hat{\beta}_1, \ldots, \hat{\beta}_{(p+q)}$ and similarly with model $M2$ for $\hat{L}_2$. The idea is that a large difference between these two likelihoods would indicate that indeed the additional q covariates $X_{p+1}, X_{p+2}, \ldots, X_{p+q}$ in model $M1$ indeed improve the fit of the model. Given that $\hat{L}_k$, $k = 1, 2$ is always smaller than one (since it is a product of probabilities), $-2log(\hat{L}_k)$ is always positive and for a given dataset the smaller the value of $-2log(\hat{L}_k)$ the better the fit of the model. So, a large value of LRT would lead to the conclusion that $M1$ better fit the data than $M2$. The null hypothesis that $H_0 : \beta_{p+1} = \beta_{p+2} = \ldots = \beta_{p+q} = 0$ can then be tested by comparing the value of LRT to the appropriate percentile of a chi-square distribution with q degrees of freedom (asymptotic result).

The Akaike information criterion (AIC) is another tool commonly used to compare models and can be computed for a given model as

$$AIC = -2log(\hat{L}) + \alpha p$$

where p is the number of parameters in the model considered and α is a predefined constant with value of 2 being most often used. The second term therefore acts as a "penalization" for (unnecessary) parameters in the model. This criteria can be used to compare non necessarily nested model, with a smaller value corresponding to a better model.

Since the baseline hazard is considered as a nuisance parameter and is not estimated, the Cox PH model can not be used to directly obtain an estimator of the survival curves of subjects with specific covariate values. The baseline hazard has to be estimated and one proposal is to extend the NA estimator to the case of covariates

$$\hat{H}_0(t) = \sum_{j:y_{(j)} \leq t} \hat{h}_{0(j)} = \sum_{j:y_{(j)} \leq t} \frac{d_{(j)}}{\sum_{k \in \Re(y_{(j)})} \exp(\hat{\beta}^t \mathbf{x}_k)}$$

The survival function for subjects with covariates values $\mathbf{x}_i$ is then estimated by

$$
\begin{aligned}
\hat{S}_i(t) = S(t \mid \mathbf{x}_i) &= \exp(-\hat{H}_0(t) \exp(\hat{\beta}^t \mathbf{x}_i)) \\
&= \left(\hat{S}_0(t)\right)^{\exp(\hat{\beta}^t \mathbf{x}_i)}
\end{aligned} \tag{2.22}
$$

with $\hat{S}_0(t) = \exp(-\hat{H}_0(t))$.

Over the last decades, the Cox PH model became probably the most popular regression models for time-to-event outcome and is widely used. In case of proportional hazards, an advantage of this model is that it summarizes the effect of each covariate by a single summary measure, the hazards ratio. For example, in a clinical trial with a time-to-event endpoint, it is very common to express the treatment effect as a hazards ratio. However the PH assumption is not always realistic and in particular in medicine it has been challenged over the last years by the apparition of new types of treatment having different mechanisms of action. In oncology for example, it is expected from immunotherapy to have a delayed treatment effect and comparison with a more standard treatment in a clinical trial will most probably lead to a violation of the proportional hazards assumption. As will be discussed in Chapter 4, therapies having a curative effect and therefore leading to a fraction of cure patients (i.e., patients that will not experience the event of interest), with or without delaying the occurrence of the event for the non-cure patients, may also lead to a non-proportional hazards situation.

The Cox model has been extended to the stratified semi-parametric Cox PH model, which can in some cases be a solution to the problem of non-proportional hazards. The idea is to consider a categorical variable defining "strata" in the population and to consider a different (unspecified) baseline hazard function in each strata. So, the hazard of individual $i(i = 1, \dots n_j)$ in strata $j(j = 1, \dots, J)$, with covariates values x_{ij} is now given by

$$
h_{ij}(t) = h_{0j}(t) \exp(\beta^t \mathbf{x}_{ij}). \tag{2.23}
$$

The strata can for example be defined based on the gender, and such a stratified model then allows a different baseline function for male and female patients, while leaving these two hazard functions unspecified. While this may be convenient in some applications, it is important to note that we then "loose" all the information about the stratification factor in the sense that this model does not provide any information on the effect of the stratification variable. This model makes the assumption of proportional hazards but within strata and not between the different levels of the variable defining the strata. It is also important to note that in expression (2.23) the β's coefficients are assumed to be the same in all strata.

A relatively unknown (or ignored) drawback of the Cox PH model is the sensitivity of the parameters estimates to omission of covariates. Indeed, several authors have reported that omission of important prognostic covariates can lead to (severe) bias in the estimation of the β parameters [47, 231, 348, 350, 365]. The main reason is that our sample actually evolves over time, with individuals with higher risks being taken out of the risk set earlier. The distribution of known but also unknown covariates therefore evolves with the risk set being composed more and more of stronger individuals as time goes by. In fact, the hazard function, as modeled by (2.14) is conditional on (and only on) the covariates included in the model and should not be interpreted at the individual level. Indeed, this hazard is actually *marginal* with respect to the covariates not included in the model, in the sense that $h(t \mid \mathbf{x})$ actually represents a weighted average of the individual hazards of the individuals still in the risk set at time t, with the weighting being dependent on the distribution of the covariates affecting the event times but not included in the model [27]. We will come back to this idea in Chapter 3 where we will see that we can actually model these unobserved covariates via the introduction of random effects.

Model checking for the PH model

Given the popularity of the (Cox) PH model, we sometimes tend to forget that it relies on some assumptions that needs to be checked. In particular, the proportional hazards assumption is often overlooked.

Model checking for the PH assumption is usually based on the inspection of a log-cumulative hazard plot. Indeed, it is easy to see that model (2.14) can be re-written as

$$\log(H(t \mid \mathbf{x}_i)) = \log H_0(t) + \beta^t \mathbf{x}_i$$

or equivalently

$$-\log(-\log S(t \mid \mathbf{x}_i)) = -\log(-\log(S_0(t)) - \beta^t \mathbf{x}_i$$

It follows that, if the PH assumption is indeed valid, then we expect a plot of $\log(\hat{H}(t \mid \mathbf{x}_i))$ and $\log \hat{H}_0(t)$ versus time to exhibit parallel curves. If we further assume that the survival times follow a Weibull distribution, we can see from equation (2.19) and following the same reasoning that a plot of $\log(\hat{H}_i(t \mid \mathbf{x}_i))$ versus log time should give parallel straight lines for different values of $\mathbf{x}_i$.

This approach only requires estimating $H_i(t \mid \mathbf{x}_i)$ or $S_i(t \mid \mathbf{x}_i)$ non-parametrically, for example via the Nelson-Aalen or the Kaplan-Meier estimator, for the groups of patients defined by the different values of the covariate(s) under study. While this approach on the other hand is mainly useful when we have a limited number of (categorical) covariates and sufficient number of observation per level. Note that $H_i(t \mid \mathbf{x}_i)$ or $S_i(t \mid \mathbf{x}_i)$ can also be estimated while adjusting for other variables for which the PH assumption have already been assessed, for example via (2.22). The estimated log-cumulative hazard curves can therefore be drawn and inspected over different levels of one specific covariate, based on an estimator considering only this variable or adjusting for other variables for which we assume they respect the PH assumption.

That these estimated curves will usually be step functions due to the nature of their estimator, and might be rather poorly estimated for the levels of the variable with less observations. To decide whether these curves are indeed parallel will obviously always be subject to some subjectivity. A commonly adopted attitude is to assume that the PH assumption is satisfied unless these curves show a strong deviation to parallel curves. Continuous covariates can also be considered but must first be categorized to be able to apply this methods and this categorization may have an impact on what we observe. It is usually recommended to consider a reasonably low number of categories, keeping sufficient observations in each category, and ideally considering as meaningful categories as possible. While in theory this approach can be used to evaluate the PH assumption for several covariates at the same time, one has to realize that inspecting all possible combinations of the various levels of each of these covariates will quickly lead to a lot of small "bins" and concluding about parallelism of the estimated curves may quickly become really difficult.

Another possibility to evaluate the PH assumption graphically is simply to compare, for each level of the covariate, a non-parametric estimator of the survival curve obtained based on the patients with that level of the covariate with a parametric PH model-based estimate of this survival curve for each variable category. (Strong) discrepancies between the "observed" non-parametric estimated curves and the "expected" model-based curves will also indicate a problem with the PH assumption. This approach is however mainly useful for parametric PH model and when considering only few categorical covariates (with few levels).

Beside such diagnostic plots, checking the PH assumption is also often based on residuals (see below) or by adding a time-dependent variable in the model, see Section 6.2 of Chapter 6. These two options can be used to build a formal goodness of fit test for the hypothesis of proportional hazards.

While model checking based on residuals is well developed and widely used in the context of linear regression models, it is unfortunately more complex in when dealing with time-to-event data due to the presence of censoring. However several proposals have been developed to account for censoring. They aim to check the PH assumption and the linearity of the covariates effect on the log-hazard, but also include diagnostic checks to detect outliers and influential observations in the data. We provide here a short overview, more details can be found for example in [78, 186, 260].

Cox-Snell residuals – The so-called Cox-Snell residuals are probably the most often used and are actually a particular case of the more general residuals originally proposed by Cox and Snell [92]. The Cox-Snell residual for the ith observation is given by

$$r_i^C = \exp(\hat{\beta}^t \mathbf{x}_i) \hat{H}_0(y_i)$$

where $\hat{H}_0(y_i)$ is generally estimated using the Nelson-Aalen estimator given by (2.5) if left unspecified in the model considered. We can write equivalently

$$r_i^C = \hat{H}_i(y_i) = -\log \hat{S}_i(y_i)$$

The general idea behind these residuals is that if the model considered is correct, than $\hat{S}_i(y_i)$ should be close from the true value $S_i(y_i)$. On the other hand, one can show that if $S(t)$ is the survival function of T then the new variable $\tilde{T} = -\log S(t)$ has a unit mean exponential distribution and this whatever the distribution of T (see for example [78] for an outline of the proof). Therefore, if the model fit our data correctly, we can expect the $r_i^C, i = 1, \ldots, n$ to behave as the realizations of a unit mean exponential distribution. This means that contrarily to the residuals used in linear regressions, they will all be positive and have a highly skewed distribution.

One could then think of plotting these residuals versus the observation number or versus the observed survival time or the rank ordered of these observed time, but such plots are usually not really useful. A better idea to assess the overall fit of a model is to plot $\hat{H}(r_i^C)$ versus r_i^C (*cumulative hazard plot*) or $\log(\hat{H}(r_i^C))$ versus $\log(r_i^C)$ (*log-cumulative hazard plot*). Indeed, if U has a unit exponential distribution then $S(u) = \exp(-u)$ and thus $H(u) = -\log S(u) = u$. So if indeed the residuals are a sample from a unit exponential distribution, we expect the cumulative hazard plot to exhibit a straight line through the origin.

To draw these plots, one can estimate the survival distribution function of the r_i^C using the KM estimator and then compute $\hat{H}(r_i^C) = -\log(\hat{S}(r_i^C)$. Unfortunately, since we have to plug in the estimator of β and $H_0(t)$ to compute the residuals, these estimated residuals do not necessarily follow a unit exponential distribution and this approximation may even be quite poor especially in small sample, and this even if the model under consideration is correct. On the other hand, it may also happen that we indeed observe a straight line even if the model considered is incorrect. In particular, the null model (containing no covariates) will lead to such a straight line even if covariates with a substantial impact on the hazard have been omitted. In practice, the model considered must in fact be seriously wrong to observe a deviation from unit slope straight line [78]. This is less a problem in parametric models where the cumulative hazard can be estimated parametrically.

One has to pay attention to the fact that for censored observations, the corresponding value of the Cox-Snell residuals will also be censored. Therefore the residuals are actually expected to be a censored sample from a unit mean exponential distribution. This has led to the development of the modified Cox-Snell residuals to explicitly take censoring into account. These residuals are given by

$$\tilde{r}_i^C = 1 - \delta_i + r_i^C$$

and are derived based on the lack of memory property of the exponential distribution [78]. We can see that they will be equal to r_i^C for observations corresponding to an event and to $1 + r_i^C$ for censored observations. They will also be all positive with a highly skewed distribution.

Martingale residuals - The martingale residuals have actually been derived from martingale theory from which they borrow their name and from the counting process theory underlying the Cox PH model (see for example [13] or [372] for more details on the martingale theory applied to time-to-event data analysis). They can however be computed as a simple transformation of the Cox-Snell residuals

$$r_i^M = \delta_i - r_i^C$$

Therefore they take value between $-\infty$ to 1, with a negative value for censored observations. It can be shown that they sum to zero and that for large samples, they are uncorrelated to each other with expected value zero.

Given that $r_i^C = \hat{H}_i(y_i)$, a nice interpretation of these residuals is that they corresponds for each observation to the difference between the observed number of events for this observation (δ_i) and the expected number of events for this observation in the interval $(0, y_i)$ as estimated from our fitted model ($\hat{H}_i(y_i)$).Therefore, an observation with a large negative value (resp. a positive value close to 1) of the residual indicates an individual who experienced a longer (resp. shorter) event time than what was expected based on his covariates values. Therefore, an index plot of the residuals versus the observation number will allow to identify the observations whose event times is not well fitted by the model considered. Furthermore, one could plot these residuals versus event times or rank order of these event times, or also against the value of a covariate to identify whether there is a range of time, or of the covariate value, for which the model does not fit the data appropriately. More generally, the residuals can be plotted against the value of the risk score $\hat{\beta}^t \mathbf{x}_i$ for each observation.

These martingale residuals can also be used to investigate the functional form of a covariate. Indeed, an important assumption of the PH model is the linear functional form of the covariates. However in some cases, a transformation of a covariate may be necessary to improve the fit, considering for example a non-linear effect of age or of some biological marker. To investigate this for a given covariate, one can plot the value of the martingale residuals from a model including no covariate (or only covariates for which the functional form is not under question) versus the value of this covariate. Indeed, one can show that this plot will display the functional form required for the covariate under scrutiny [375]. In particular, a straight line will indicate that a linear term is indeed appropriate. To ease the interpretation of this plot, which will usually be quite noisy, it has been proposed to add a smooth curve fitted to the plotted values (such as a LOWESS or LOESS smoother, [76]). Unfortunately, unless a linear pattern or an easy transformation, such as a log transform, is appropriate, the plot will usually be too noisy to really identify the functional form needed.

Deviance residuals – The fact that the martingale residuals are not symmetrically distributed around zero even when the fitted model is correct, is often seen as a disadvantage as it will make the plot of these residuals more difficult to interpret. Therefore, Therneau et al. [375] have proposed a modification of these residuals which have the property to be more symmetrically distributed around zero. These deviance residuals are defined for the ith observation as

$$r_i^D = sgn(r_i^M) \left[-2(r_i^M + \delta_i \log(\delta_i - r_i^M)) \right]^{1/2}$$

with $sgn(.)$ the sign function (equal -1 if its argument is negative and $+1$ otherwise), and they therefore have the same sign as r_i^M. They take their names from the fact that they can be shown to be components of the deviance

$$D = -2(\log \hat{L}_c - \log \hat{L}_f) = \sum_i^n (r_i^D)^2$$

with $\log \hat{L}_c$ and $\log \hat{L}_f$ respectively the maximum partial likelihood of the model considered and of a full model. This deviance can be seen as a generalization of the residual sum of squares and a smaller value indicates a better fit of the model. Plots similar to those discussed for martingale residuals can be drawn and used in the same way. Given that these deviance residuals are more symmetrically distributed, these plots are usually easier to interpret. However, these residuals can not be used to investigate the functional form of the covariates and therefore martingale residuals are still often preferred in practice.

Schoenfeld residuals – For all the residuals mentioned above, one residual is computed for each observation and computing these values require the the estimation of the cumulative hazard function (and therefore different values will be obtained if another estimator is used). On the other hand, the Schoenfeld residuals, also called partial residuals, will produce for each observation one value per covariate included in the model. For the jth covariate, the value of the Schoenfeld residuals for the ith observation is given by

$$r_{ji}^P = \delta_i(x_{ji} - \hat{a}_{ji})$$

with x_{ji} the value of the jth variable for the ith observation and

$$\hat{a}_{ji} = \frac{\sum_{l \in \Re(y_i)} x_{jl} \exp(\hat{\beta}^t x_l)}{\sum_{l \in \Re(y_i)} \exp(\hat{\beta}^t x_l)}$$

and thus do not require the estimation of the cumulative hazard.

As we can see, the residuals pertaining to censored observations will have a zero value (since $\delta_i = 0$ in this case), as well as residuals corresponding to the largest observation if it corresponds to an event time (as in this case $\hat{a}_{ji} = x_{ji}$). We can obtain r_{ji}^P as an estimate of the ith component of the first derivative of the log partial likelihood (2.21). These residuals sum to zero, and in large sample, they are uncorrelated to each other and have expected value zero.

A scaled or weighted version has also been proposed and shown to be more effective in detecting departures form the model considered. These scaled Schoenfeld residuals are given by

$$r_i^{P^*} = d\,Var(\hat{\beta})\mathbf{r}_i^P$$

where $\mathbf{r}_i^P = (r_{1i}^P, r_{2i}^P, \ldots, r_{pi}^P)^t$ is the vector of Schoenfeld residuals for the ith observation and the p covariates in the model and d is the total number of observed events.

The scaled Schoenfeld residuals are mainly known as they offer a tool to check the PH assumption. Indeed, Grambsch and Therneau [143] have shown that the expected value of the ith component of the scaled Schoenfeld residuals for the jth covariate can be approximated by

$$E(r_{ji}^{P^*}) \approx \beta_j(y_i) - \hat{\beta}_j$$

where $\beta_j(y_i)$ is a time-varying coefficient for the covariate X_j evaluated at the ith event time. Therefore, an approximate estimate for $\beta(t)$ is obtained by simply adding $\hat{\beta}$ to the value of the scaled Schoenfeld residuals computed at the event time of each observation. It follows that a plot of $r_{ji}^{P^*} + \hat{\beta}_j$ against time will depict the approximate relationship between $\beta_j(t)$ and t. In particular, an horizontal straight line will suggest a constant β coefficient and thus the appropriateness of the PH assumption. As above, it may be useful to add to the plot a smooth curve fitted on the scatterplot, or even fitting a straight line. Although we may be tempted to simply test for a zero slope in such a regression line, one however has to remind that a non-linear dependency in time may also result in no significant departure from an horizontal straight line.

Score residuals - The score residuals are also obtained from the first derivative of the log partial likelihood but following a slightly different reasoning (see for example [78] for more details). They are defined for the jth covariate of the ith observation as

$$r_{ji}^S = r_{ji}^P + \exp(\hat{\beta}^t\mathbf{x}_i) \sum_{y_r \leq y_i} \frac{(\hat{a}_{jr} - x_{ji})\delta_r}{\sum_{l \in \Re(y_r)} \exp(\hat{\beta}^t\mathbf{x}_l)}$$

These scores will also sum to zero but the value associated to a censored observation will not anymore be necessarily zero.

The score residuals are used to identify influential observations. These are usually defined as observations having a strong impact on the inference for the model. One possibility to identify these observations is simply for each of the n observations to fit the model under consideration on all but this observation (so on the $n-1$ observations obtained by removing the one considered) and compare the results obtained from these n models. However, such a procedure may unpractical when n increases largely. Considering a particular covariate X_j, the amount by which the estimate of β_j would change by omitting each observation $\Delta_i \hat{\beta}_j = \hat{\beta}_j - \hat{\beta}_{j(-i)}$ can be approximated by $r_{ji}^S Var(\hat{\beta})$ [57]. An index plot of this quantity versus the value of each covariate can be used to easily pick up observations with a large absolute value as influential observations. Note that plotting a standardized version $\Delta_i \hat{\beta}_j / se(\hat{\beta})$ will highlight observations having a strong impact on the significance of the parameter estimate. The influence of each observations on a set of parameter estimates, rather than a single coefficient, can be obtained by considering $(\mathbf{r}_i^S)^t Var(\hat{\beta}) \mathbf{r}_i^S$ [296].

As a conclusion, it is usually recommended to start by plotting the deviance residuals versus the risk score as this will give an overall picture on how well the model fit the data while considering all covariates in the model. This can then be further investigated with some more specific plots. The PH assumption will, in practice, rarely be perfectly met and minor violations have been shown to only have a marginal effect on the inference for the model parameters. Therefore, a formal test, either based on the residuals or based on an extension of the PH model to the inclusion of time-dependent covariates (see Section 6.2 of Chapter 6), should be interpreted with care. It is therefore usually recommended to check this assumption by a visual inspection of the log cumulative hazard plot and can be further investigated considering the scaled Schoenfeld residuals.

2.5.2   Accelerated failure time models

The accelerated failure time (AFT) model is often considered as an alternative to the (Cox) PH model if the proportional hazards assumption does not hold although this is probably too restrictive [403]. The AFT model is often described as a log-linear model for the event times but is also naturally described in terms of the survival function.

Considering the log-linear representation, the idea is to model the impact of the covariates directly on T but using a *log* link function since T is a positive variable. The AFT model is then defined as

$$\log T = \mu + \alpha^t \mathbf{X} + \sigma \epsilon \tag{2.24}$$

where μ and σ are location and scale parameters, α is the $p \times 1$ vector of covariate parameters and the error terms e are usually assumed to follow a (flexible) parametric distribution, leading them to a parametric AFT model.

The name accelerated failure time model is better understood from the survival representation of this model. Consider two groups of patients, for example one exposed group with survival $S_E(.)$ and one control group with survival $S_C(.)$, the idea of the AFT model is that

$$S_E(t) = S_C(\Phi t)$$

for some *acceleration factor* $\Phi > 0$, so that the survival of the exposed patients at time t is the one of the control patients at time Φt (and is therefore lower or equal since $S(.)$ is a monotone decreasing function). In a more general setting, one can write $\Phi = \exp(\beta^t \mathbf{x}_i)$, with $\mathbf{X}$ including an intercept term, and the AFT model is then

$$S_i(t) = S(t \mid \mathbf{x}_i) = S_0\left(\exp(\beta^t \mathbf{x}_i)t\right) \qquad (2.25)$$

where $S_0(.)$ is a baseline survival function. We can clearly see from this expression that the effect of the covariates is to change the time scale, so to make the time pass more (resp. less) faster for observations with a larger positive (resp. negative) value of $\beta^t \mathbf{x}_i$. From this expression, we can see that the covariates actually acts multiplicatively on t (via an exponential link), meaning that they either "accelerate" or "slow down" the time scale.

We can make the link between expression (2.24) and (2.25) of this model. Indeed, from (2.24), we have that

$$T = \exp(\mu + \alpha^t \mathbf{X})\exp(\sigma\epsilon)$$

The survival function of T is then

$$
\begin{aligned}
S(t \mid X) = P(T > t \mid X) &= P(\exp(\mu + \alpha^t \mathbf{X})\exp(\sigma\epsilon) > t) \\
&= P\left(\exp(\sigma\epsilon) > \frac{t}{\exp(\mu + \alpha^t \mathbf{X})}\right) \\
&= S_0\left(t\exp(-\mu - \alpha^t \mathbf{X})\right)
\end{aligned}
$$

where $S_0(.)$ is the survival function of $\exp(\sigma\epsilon)$.

Expression (2.25) in turns, leads to an equivalent expression at the level of the hazard function:

$$h_i(t) = \exp\left(\beta^t \mathbf{x}_i\right) h_0(\exp(\beta^t \mathbf{x}_i)t). \qquad (2.26)$$

We can easily see from this expression that the AFT model does not rely on the proportional hazards assumption. Indeed, if we consider the hazards ratio for two subjects with covariates values $\mathbf{x}_i$ and $\mathbf{x}_j$, we obtain

$$\frac{h_i(t)}{h_j(t)} = \frac{\exp(\beta^t \mathbf{x}_i)h_0(\exp(\beta^t \mathbf{x}_i)t)}{\exp(\beta^t \mathbf{x}_j)h_0(\exp(\beta^t \mathbf{x}_j)t)}$$

which is generally not constant over time.

AFT models are usually fully parametric, assuming a particular parametric form for the baseline hazard function $h_0(t)$ in (2.26) or equivalently for the baseline survival function $S_0(t)$ in (2.25). Alternatively, we can also assume a parametric distribution for T or ϵ in the log-linear representation. The most frequently used parametric AFT models consider a normal or a logistic distribution for ϵ, leading respectively to log-normal or a log-logistic distribution for T. Another popular choice is to assume a Gumbel distribution for the error term ϵ. In this case the event times then follow a Weibull distribution and one can show that such an AFT model is equivalent to the Weibull PH model. Indeed, if ϵ follows a Gumbel distribution, i.e. $f_\epsilon(e) = \exp(e - \exp(e))$, then the density function of the transformed variable $z_i = exp(\epsilon_i)$ is

$$f_Z(z) \quad = \quad \frac{\exp(\log z - \exp(\log z))}{z} = \exp(-z)$$

which corresponds to an exponential distribution with mean one. From (2.24), the survival function from the log-linear representation of the AFT model is given by

$$
\begin{aligned}
S_i(t) = P(T_i \geq t) \quad &= \quad P(\log T_i \geq \log t) \\
&= \quad P\left(\mu + \alpha^t \mathbf{x}_i + \sigma \epsilon_i \geq \log t\right) \\
&= \quad P\left(\exp(\epsilon_i) \geq \exp\left(\frac{\log t - \mu - \alpha^t \mathbf{x}_i}{\sigma}\right)\right)
\end{aligned}
$$

Since $\exp(\epsilon_i)$ has a unit mean exponential distribution, we have $P\left(\exp(\epsilon_i) \geq z\right) = \exp(-z)$ such that

$$S_i(t) = \exp\left(-\exp\left(\frac{\log t - \mu - \alpha^t \mathbf{x}_i}{\sigma}\right)\right) \qquad (2.27)$$

Comparing this expression with the survival function obtained for the Weibull PH model (2.20), we can see that these two survival functions are equivalent but with a different parametrization:

$$
\begin{aligned}
\lambda \quad &= \quad \exp(-\mu/\sigma) & (2.28) \\
\rho \quad &= \quad \sigma^{-1} & (2.29) \\
\beta_j \quad &= \quad -\alpha_j/\sigma & (2.30)
\end{aligned}
$$

The AFT model (2.24) assuming a Gumbel distribution of the error term, or equivalently the AFT model (2.25) assuming a Weibull distribution of the event times are therefore equivalent to the Weibull PH model. This means that in this particular case, the AFT model also assumes proportional hazards. This equivalence is important to keep in mind as the *survival* R package actually uses the log-linear representation (2.25) and its parametrization to fit a Weibull parametric PH model (see Section 2.6). Given this equivalence, one can conclude that the Weibull distribution of the event times possess both the PH and the AFT property [78].

Another interesting distribution of the event times in the context of a parametric AFT model is the log-logistic distribution. The survival function associated to a variable U following a log-logistic distribution with parameter λ and κ is

$$S_0(u) = \left(1 + e^\lambda u^\kappa\right)^{-1}$$

From (2.25), we have that according to an AFT model, the survival function of individuals with covariates value $\mathbf{x}_i$ (including an intercept) is

$$\begin{aligned} S_i(t) = S(t \mid \mathbf{x}_i) &= \left[1 + e^\lambda (\exp(\beta^t \mathbf{x}_i)t)^\kappa\right]^{-1} \\ &= \left(1 + \exp(\lambda + \beta^t \mathbf{x}_i)t^\kappa\right)^{-1} \end{aligned} \tag{2.31}$$

meaning that the survival function of the event times given the covariates is also log-logistic with parameter $\lambda + \beta^t \mathbf{x}_i$ and κ. One therefore says that the log-logistic distribution has the accelerated failure time property. However, one can show that this distribution does not have the PH property (as was the case for the Weibull distribution). To do so, we have to note that since the baseline hazard function associated with a log-logistic distribution is

$$h_0(u) = \frac{e^\lambda \kappa u^{\kappa-1}}{1 + e^\lambda u^\kappa}$$

the hazard function of individuals with covariates value $\mathbf{x}_i$ according to an AFT model is

$$h_i(u) = h(t \mid \mathbf{x}_i) = \frac{e^{\lambda + \beta^t \mathbf{x}_i} \kappa t^{\kappa-1}}{1 + e^{\lambda + \beta^t \mathbf{x}_i} t^\kappa}$$

From this expression, we can check that the ratio of the hazard functions of two individuals with different covariates values is usually not constant.

It is important to note that more flexible distributions have also been proposed, eventually encompassing the distributions mentioned above as special case, and allowing much more flexible hazard functions. For example the general gamma distribution [88] which can be further extended to the generalized F distribution [181] have been studied, while [195] proposed a flexible AFT model with an error distribution specified via splines (estimated via penalized maximum likelihood to ensure a smoothed error distribution).

Although less often used in practice, one can also consider a semi-parametric AFT model

$$\log T = \alpha^t \mathbf{X} + \epsilon \tag{2.32}$$

in which the distribution of ϵ is left unspecified. This model usually does not include an intercept, which is difficult to estimate from censored data [177, 403] but $E(\epsilon)$ is then not constrained to zero. The main difficulty in estimating such a model is that the score equation $U(\alpha) = 0$ are in general not easy to solve as

U is neither continuous nor componentwise monotone in α. Various estimation methods have been proposed, see for example [48, 71, 177, 178], and some have been implemented in standard software leading to the semi-parametric AFT model being now practically feasible (see for example the `aftgee` R package [70, 72]).

For a long time, the lack of easy implementation of the semi-parametric AFT model has been seen as a disadvantage of the AFT model over the Cox PH model who is still much more popular. However, besides the fact that the AFT model do not assume proportional hazards, it has also been shown to be more robust to omission of covariates [183].

2.5.3 Proportional odds models

Another alternative to the PH model is the proportional odds (PO) model. This models express the odds of an individual surviving beyond some time t as

$$\frac{S(t \mid \mathbf{X})}{1 - S(t \mid \mathbf{X})} = \exp(\eta^t \mathbf{X}) \frac{S_0(t)}{1 - S_0(t)} \qquad (2.33)$$

where $S_0(t)$ is the baseline survival function, which can be left unspecified or specified parametrically. In the first case, Bennett [32] proposes to first estimate $S_0(t)$ non-parametrically and then to obtain maximum likelihood estimators for the η coefficients. If $S_0(t)$ is specified parametrically, then all model parameters can be estimated via maximum likelihood.

In this model, the covariates therefore act multiplicatively, via the exponential function, on the odds of survival beyond time t. This model can easily be re-written

$$logit(S(t \mid \mathbf{X})) = \log\left(\frac{S(t \mid \mathbf{X})}{1 - S(t \mid \mathbf{X})}\right) = \eta_0(t) + \eta^t \mathbf{X}$$

where $\eta_0(t)$ is the logit transform of the baseline survival function, corresponding to the baseline odds of an event beyond time t. Similarily to what is seen in the Cox PH model, all the time dependency is assumed to be captured by the baseline odds. If we fix a timepoint, and consider a binary outcome equal to 1 if the event occurred before this timepoint and zero otherwise, then this model falls down to a logistic regression.

Considering two individuals, $i \neq j$, whose covariate values only depend in one unit of covariate of the kth covariate, we have

$$logit(S(t \mid \mathbf{x}_i)) - logit(S(t \mid \mathbf{x}_j)) = \log\left(\frac{\frac{S(t|\mathbf{x}_i)}{1 - S(t|\mathbf{x}_i)}}{\frac{S(t|\mathbf{x}_j)}{1 - S(t|\mathbf{x}_j)}}\right) = \eta_l$$

showing that η_l represents the log of the ratios of the odds survival beyond time t for an increase in one unit of covariate X_l, keeping all other covariates constant. The η_l coefficient therefore has a direct interpretation as log-odds ratio, and thus $\exp(eta_l)$ can be interpreted as an odds ratio (OR) of survival beyond time t for one unit increase in covariate X_l.

An interesting feature of this model is the *property of convergent hazards*, which is actually quite natural in most practical applications [78]. Indeed, from (2.33), we can easily obtain

$$S(t \mid X) = S_0(t) \left[\exp(-\eta^t X) + (1 - \exp(-\eta^t X)) S_0(t) \right]^{-1}$$

and taking the log on both side and differentiating both sides with respect to time, we obtain after some easy manipulations

$$
\begin{aligned}
h(t \mid X) &= h_0(t) - \frac{(1 - \exp(-\eta^t X)) f_0(t)}{\exp(-\eta^t X) + (1 + \exp(-\eta^t X)) S_0(t)} \\
&= h_0(t) \left(1 - \frac{S_0(t)}{(\exp(\eta^t X) - 1)^{-1} + S_0(t)} \right)
\end{aligned}
$$

remembering that $h_0(t) = \frac{f_0(t)}{S_0(t)}$, and

$$\frac{h(t \mid X)}{h_0(t)} = \left[1 + (\exp(\eta^t X) - 1) S_0(t) \right]^{-1}$$

which takes value $\exp(\eta^t X)$ when $t = 0$ (since $S_0(t = 0) = 1$) and converges to 1 when t tends to infinity (since $S_0(t)$ tends to 0). If we consider for the sake of illustration a single variable X defining to groups ($X = 1$ or $X = 0$) in the population, this property shows that the hazard functions for the patients in each of the two groups will converge with time. Imagine the variable X is a treatment indicator, considering that the hazards of the survivors will converge over time whether the patients have been treated or not may indeed seem very natural in different settings.

It is quite common to consider a fully parametric PO model, in which case estimates of the parameters can be obtained as maximum likelihood estimators after replacing the expression of $S(t \mid X)$ and $h(t \mid X)$ in the likelihood function (2.1).

In the context of a fully parametric PO model, a natural distribution to consider for the survival times is the log-logistic distribution, characterized by

$$S_0(u) = \left(1 + e^\lambda u^\kappa \right)^{-1}$$

with λ and κ two unknown parameters. The baseline odds is then

$$\frac{S_0(t)}{1 - S_0(t)} = e^{-\lambda} t^{-\kappa}$$

and from (2.33) we find that the odds for an individual with covariate value x_i to survive beyond time t is

$$\frac{S(t \mid x_i)}{1 - S(t \mid x_i)} = \exp(-\lambda \eta^t x_i) t^{-\kappa}$$

which gives after re-arranging some terms

$$S(t \mid x_i) = \left(1 + \exp(\lambda - \eta^t x_i) t^\kappa\right)^{-1}$$

showing that the survival times of this individual also follows a log-logistic distribution with parameters $\lambda - \exp(\eta^t x_i)$ and κ. The log-logistic distribution therefore has the proportional odds property.

Furthermore, comparing this expression to (2.31), we see that assuming a log-logistic distribution of the event times leads to an equivalence between the PO and the AFT model, and the estimated coefficients from one model can be obtained from the estimated coefficients of the other model with $\hat{\eta}_j = -\hat{\beta}_j = \hat{\alpha}_j/\hat{\sigma}$. While the PH and the AFT model were equivalent when assuming a Weibull distribution of the event times, the PO and AFT model are equivalent when the event times are assumed to have a log-logistic distribution. The log-logistic distribution therefore has both the PO and the AFT property and is actually the only distribution having both properties [78].

2.6   Software and examples revisited

2.6.1   Available softwares for classical survival analysis

Standard survival analysis methods are implemented in most statistical softwares, such as R [368, 260], SAS [8], Stata [77], SAS JMP, or SPSS.

R has a long history of survival analysis packages, and the main ones can be found on the CRAN Task view on Survival Analysis [7]. The most popular R package for survival data analysis is certainly the survival package, developed by Therneau et al. [372, 374]. It allows to perform most of the survival analysis methods presented in this chapter, including the estimation of survival functions with the Kaplan-Meier and Aalen-Johansen estimators, hypotheses tests and in particular the logrank test, and the fit of several parametric and semi-parametric regression models. Several datasets are also included in the package, and in particular the colon and the retinopathy datasets presented in Section 1.3 of Chapter 1. We illustrate the use of this package in Section 2.6.2 below. The muhaz R package [160] can be used to obtain (smoothed) estimators of the hazard functions via kernel methods . Other packages are available to obtain smoothed estimators of the hazard functions based on splines (e.g., polspline [197] or bshazard [315]). Packages developed primarily for more advanced models, and that will be discussed in the next chapters, can obviously also be used for more standard analyses. For example, the parfm [337] and the frailtypack [329] packages originally developed for frailty models can also serve to fit PH and AFT models.

The principal procedures to perform classical survival analyses in SAS are the proc lifetest and the proc phreg. We will illustrate their use in

Section 2.6.3. These procedures allow to obtain the main results necessary for a standard analysis of survival data including estimation of survival curves, hypotheses tests and standard regression models. Other procedures and macros are available for further analyses.

2.6.2 Colon cancer data

As mentioned in Section 1.3.1 of Chapter 1, the colon dataset contains data on 929 patients recruited in a 3-arms adjuvant clinical trial in colon cancer comparing observation (Obs, $n = 315$) to Levamisole alone (Lev, $n = 310$), and to a combination of Levamisole and 5-Fluorouracil (Lev+5FU, $n = 304$). This dataset is available in the R package survival and is shortly described in Chapter 8 of [372]. The list of variables available as well as the first lines of this dataset and summary statistics of the baseline characteristics have already been presented in Section 1.3.1 of the previous chapter.

To access these data, we first have to load the survival package. We can use the attach() command so that we don't have to specify the name of the dataset to be used in each command.

```
> library(survival)
> attach(colon)
```

For this trial, both time to death and time to recurrence were of interest, although we will concentrate on time to death (overall survival) to illustrate the implementation of the concepts described in this chapter in R. Remember that this dataset contains two rows per patient, one for each type of event considered (death and recurrence), from which we can derive a dataset per type of event

```
colon.OS <- colon[etype==1,]
colon.TR <- colon[etype==2,]
```

The survfit function can be used on a Surv object to estimate the survival curves, either for all patients or by treatment arms. The conf.type option allows to choose the type of confidence intervals (none, plain, log, log-log, or logit) while the conf.int option allows to choose the α level of the confidence interval (default is 95%).

```
> OS.colon.km <- survfit(Surv(time,status)~1, conf.type="log-log"
    ,data=colon.OS)
> OS.colon.km
Call: survfit(formula = Surv(time, status) ~ 1, data = colon.OS,
    conf.type = ''log-log")

       n   events   median  0.95LCL  0.95UCL
     929      468     2018     1446       NA

> OS.colon.km.rx <- survfit(Surv(time,status)~rx, conf.type="log-
    log",data=colon.OS)
> OS.colon.km.rx
Call: survfit(formula = Surv(time, status) ~ rx, data = colon.OS,
    conf.type = ''log-log")
```

```
              n events median 0.95LCL 0.95UCL
rx=Obs      315     177   1236     772    2035
rx=Lev      310     172   1183     742    2018
rx=Lev+5FU  304     119     NA      NA      NA
```

The created object contains information on the number of observations
and events in each treatment group (as defined by the variable `rx` in this
example), the median survival time in each group (computed in the same unit
as the event time data) together with a confidence interval. A total of 468
events (deaths in this example) were observed, 177 (56.2 %) in the control
arm, 172 (55.5 %) in the Lev arm, and 119 (39.1 %) in the Lev+5FU arm.
The median survival time is 1236 days (95% CI: [772 ; 2035]) in the control
arm, 1183 days (95% CI: [742 ; 2018]) in the Lev arm and is not yet reached in
the Lev+5FU arm (as expected since less than half of the patients have died
in this treatment group). The `summary()` function can be used to obtain the
estimated Kaplan-Meier survival curves, together with the pointwise standard
error and a 95% CI at each event time. However, such an output can be very
long, and it is rather advisable to specify at which timepoint we want to see
the estimated survival. For example, if we want to know the 1 and 2 years
survival time in each group, we can obtain it with

```
> summary(OS.colon.km.rx, time=c(365, 730))
Call: survfit(formula = Surv(time, status) ~ rx, data = colon.OS,
        conf.type = ''log-log")

                   rx=Obs
 time n.risk n.event survival std.err lower 95% CI upper 95% CI
  365    227      88    0.721  0.0253        0.668        0.767
  730    178      45    0.576  0.0279        0.519        0.629

                   rx=Lev
 time n.risk n.event survival std.err lower 95% CI upper 95% CI
  365    221      86     0.72  0.0256        0.667        0.767
  730    170      49     0.56  0.0284        0.502        0.613

                   rx=Lev+5FU
 time n.risk n.event survival std.err lower 95% CI upper 95% CI
  365    252      48    0.841  0.0210        0.795        0.878
  730    209      42    0.700  0.0265        0.645        0.749
```

Figure 2.7 plots the Kaplan-Meier estimated survival curves for all patients
(together with a log-log transform 95% confidence intervals) and by treatment
arm (to improve the readability we have removed the confidence-intervals,
specifying `conf.type="none"` in the `survfit` call). This graph is obtained
with the `plot` function

```
par(mfrow = c(1,2))
plot(OS.colon.km, lwd=1,ylab="Survival",xlab="Time (days)")
legend("topright","All patients")
plot(OS.colon.km.rx, lty=c(1,2,3),ylab="Survival",xlab="Time (
    days)")
legend("topright",lty=c(1,2,3), c("Control","Lev","Lev+5FU"))
par(mfrow = c(1,1))
```

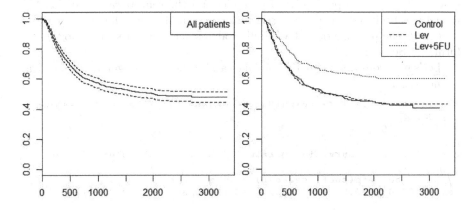

FIGURE 2.7

Colon cancer data: Kaplan-Meier estimates of the survival function for overall survival for all patients with log-log transform confidence intervals (*left*) and by treatment arm without confidence intervals (*right*)

A logrank test can be obtained with the `survdiff` function. For example, we can see that there is no significant difference in the survival of the patient by gender ($p - value = 0.6$)

```
> survdiff(Surv(time,status)~sex)
Call:
survdiff(formula = Surv(time, status) ~ sex)

          N Observed Expected (O-E)^2/E (O-E)^2/V
sex=0 890      444      436     0.136     0.259
sex=1 968      476      484     0.123     0.259

 Chisq= 0.3  on 1 degrees of freedom, p= 0.6
```

On the other hand, the difference in survival by treatment is statistically significant (*p*-value < 0.05). However, as can be seen from the previous results, the difference is mainly driven by the effect of the combination arm (**Lev+5FU**).

```
> survdiff(Surv(time,status)~rx)
Call:
survdiff(formula = Surv(time, status) ~ rx)

                N Observed Expected (O-E)^2/E (O-E)^2/V
rx=Obs        630      345      299      7.01     10.40
rx=Lev        620      333      295      4.93      7.26
rx=Lev+5FU 608        242      326     21.61     33.54

 Chisq= 33.6  on 2 degrees of freedom, p= 5e-08
```

While the logrank allows us to compare the survival between different groups, it does not allow to quantify the effect of each variable on the survival of the patients. As we have seen in Section 2.5, several models are available to reach this goal. The parametric PH model and the semi-parametric Cox PH model can be fitted with the `coxph` function. One however has to be careful that in R, the parametric PH Weibull model is actually fitted in its log-linear form, see Section 2.5.1.

Let's first consider a Cox PH model to assess the effect of gender on survival of the patients

```
> OS.colon.Cox.sex <- coxph(Surv(time, status) ~ sex, data=colon.
    OS)
> OS.colon.Cox.sex
Call:
coxph(formula = Surv(time, status) ~ sex, data = colon.OS)

       coef exp(coef) se(coef)       z     p
sex -0.08361   0.91979  0.09248 -0.904 0.366

Likelihood ratio test=0.82  on 1 df, p=0.3662
n= 929, number of events= 468
```

and a more extended output can obtained with the **summary** function

```
> summary(OS.colon.Cox.sex)
Call:
coxph(formula = Surv(time, status) ~ sex, data = colon.OS)

  n= 929, number of events= 468

       coef exp(coef) se(coef)       z Pr(>|z|)
sex -0.08361   0.91979  0.09248 -0.904    0.366

    exp(coef) exp(-coef) lower .95 upper .95
sex    0.9198      1.087    0.7673     1.103

Concordance= 0.515  (se = 0.012 )
Rsquare= 0.001    (max possible= 0.999 )
Likelihood ratio test= 0.82  on 1 df,    p=0.4
Wald test             = 0.82  on 1 df,    p=0.4
Score (logrank) test = 0.82  on 1 df,    p=0.4
```

We see that the estimated coefficient for gender is -0.084, corresponding to a HR of 0.920 (95% CI: [0.767 ; 1.103]), and is clearly not statistically significant. From such a model, we can therefore not conclude that gender has an impact on the survival of the colon cancer patients included in this trial.

In this study, the variable treatment (`rx`) has three levels (`Obs`, `Lev`, `Lev+5FU`) and is actually defined as a *factor*, thus corresponding to a (nominal) categorical variable, as can be easily check with the function `is.factor()`

```
> is.factor(rx)
[1] TRUE
```

When including such a factor in a model, it will automatically be transformed into *dummy* variables so that each level of the variable (`rx`) is compared to the reference level. So for a categorical variable with 3 levels, 2 dummy variables are created (both with value 0 for the patient in the reference level); the reference level being by default the last one by alphabetical order (so `Obs` in this case). A Cox PH model with the (`rx`) replaced by two dummy variable is then

$$h_i(t) = h_0(t) \exp(\beta_1 x_{1i} + \beta_2 x_{2i})$$

where X_1 is the first dummy variable with value 1 if the patient is in the Lev group (and 0 otherwise), and X_2 takes value 1 if the patient is in the Lev+5FU group (and 0 otherwise), so that patients in the Obs (reference group) have value 0 for both dummy variables. The associated β_1 coefficient therefore represents the effect of Lev over Obs, and the β_2 coefficient the effect of Lev+5FU over Obs, which is exactly the information we are interested in this clinical trial. An "extended output" is obtained, thanks to the summary function, including a confidence interval for each HR, a p-value for two alternative tests of the global model, the Wald test, and the score test. It also provides the value of the concordance C-statistic, which is a measure of the discrimination of the covariates included in the model [153] and its standard error as well as an approximated R^2 based on the general coefficient of determination proposed by [268]. This R^2 statistic is an adaptation from the well-known R^2 in linear regression and can therefore be interpreted as a measure of the improvement in the fit of the model when including the covariates compared with a null model.

```
> OS.colon.Cox.m1 <- coxph(Surv(time, status) ~ rx, data=colon.OS
     )
> summary(OS.colon.Cox.m1)
Call:
coxph(formula = Surv(time, status) ~ rx, data = colon.OS)

  n= 929, number of events= 468

               coef exp(coef) se(coef)       z Pr(>|z|)
rxLev      -0.01512   0.98499  0.10708  -0.141    0.888
rxLev+5FU  -0.51209   0.59924  0.11863  -4.317 1.58e-05 ***
---
Signif. codes:  0 '***' 0.001 '**' 0.01 '*' 0.05 '.' 0.1 ' ' 1

           exp(coef) exp(-coef) lower .95 upper .95
rxLev         0.9850      1.015    0.7985    1.2150
rxLev+5FU     0.5992      1.669    0.4749    0.7561

Concordance= 0.554  (se = 0.013 )
Rsquare= 0.026   (max possible= 0.999 )
Likelihood ratio test= 24.34  on 2 df,   p=5e-06
Wald test            = 22.58  on 2 df,   p=1e-05
Score (logrank) test = 23.07  on 2 df,   p=1e-05
```

These results quantify to which extent the patients in the Lev+5FU have a lower risk of death, with a HR of 0.599 (95% CI: [0.474 ; 0.756]) compared to patients in the control group (Obs). This corresponds to a $1/0.599 = 1.669$ higher risk of deaths for the patients in the control group. As can be seen, this treatment effect for the Lev+5FU group compared to the control group is highly significant. On the other hand, the estimated coefficient for the Lev group compared to the `Obs` group is very close to 0, resulting in a HR very close to one with a 95%CI containing one. This confirms our findings that while there is a significant benefit in terms of overall survival for the patients in the `Lev+5FU` group compared to the control, this is not the case for the patients in the `Lev` group.

The standard error of the estimation of the coefficients are also provided (`se(coef)`), allowing us to compute confidence intervals, as well as the z-value (`z`) for each of these coefficients which are obtained as $\hat{\beta}_j / \sqrt{v\hat{a}r(\hat{\beta}_j)}$. The output also provides the results from a likelihood ratio test comparing this model to a *null model* (i.e. a model including no covariates), based in this case on 2 degrees of freedom (since they are a difference of 2 covariates between the considered model and the null model), and leading to a highly significant *p*-value indicating that the inclusion of these two (dummy) covariates significantly increases the likelihood. Note that the value of the likelihood ratio test statistics can also be easily computed as

```
> 2*(OS.colon.Cox.m1$loglik[2]-OS.colon.Cox.m1$loglik[1])
[1] 24.34347
```

If we are not happy with the default choice of the reference level, we can easily change it by using the `relevel` function. For example, if we are rather interested to have `Lev+5FU` as reference, we can do

```
> new.rx <- relevel(rx,ref="Lev+5FU")
> coxph(Surv(time, status) ~ new.rx)
Call:
coxph(formula = Surv(time, status) ~ new.rx)

               coef exp(coef)  se(coef)      z        p
new.rxObs  0.44101   1.55427   0.08391  5.256  1.47e-07
new.rxLev  0.42011   1.52213   0.08451  4.971  6.67e-07

Likelihood ratio test=35.23  on 2 df, p=2.233e-08
n= 1858, number of events= 920
```

These results are now considering the `Lev+5FU` group as the reference, and show a significantly worse survival (HR above 1) for both the control (`Obs`) and the `Lev` group.

We can add additional covariates in the model to adjust the treatment effect. Adding all available covariates, and removing one by one the least significant ones (`age`, `perfor`, `sex`, `adhere`) to keep only the covariates that have a significant impact on overall survival (*backward selection*), we obtain the following model

```
> OS.colon.Cox.adj <- coxph(Surv(time, status) ~ rx+obstruct+
      differ+extent+surg+node4, data=colon.OS)
> summary(OS.colon.Cox.adj)
Call:
coxph(formula = Surv(time, status) ~ rx + obstruct + differ +
      extent + surg + node4, data = colon.OS)

  n= 906, number of events= 458
```

```
(23 observations deleted due to missingness)

               coef exp(coef)  se(coef)       z Pr(>|z|)
rxLev      0.008829  1.008869  0.109119   0.081 0.935509
rxLev+5FU -0.485652  0.615296  0.119707  -4.057 4.97e-05 ***
obstruct   0.231023  1.259888  0.115837   1.994 0.046112 *
differ     0.217782  1.243316  0.095457   2.281 0.022521 *
extent     0.449996  1.568305  0.116132   3.875 0.000107 ***
surg       0.243566  1.275791  0.102160   2.384 0.017118 *
node4      0.834321  2.303249  0.097377   8.568  < 2e-16 ***
---
Signif. codes:  0 '***' 0.001 '**' 0.01 '*' 0.05 '.' 0.1 ' ' 1

          exp(coef) exp(-coef) lower .95 upper .95
rxLev        1.0089     0.9912    0.8146     1.249
rxLev+5FU    0.6153     1.6252    0.4866     0.778
obstruct     1.2599     0.7937    1.0040     1.581
differ       1.2433     0.8043    1.0312     1.499
extent       1.5683     0.6376    1.2490     1.969
surg         1.2758     0.7838    1.0443     1.559
node4        2.3032     0.4342    1.9031     2.788

Concordance= 0.659  (se = 0.013 )
Rsquare= 0.135   (max possible= 0.999 )
Likelihood ratio test= 131.2  on 7 df,   p=<2e-16
Wald test            = 132.2  on 7 df,   p=<2e-16
Score (logrank) test = 138.1  on 7 df,   p=<2e-16
```

It is important to note that 23 observations were not taken into account in this model because of missing value in at least one the covariates included in the model. The adjusted HR for Lev+5FU versus Obs is now 0.615 (95% CI: [0.487 ; 0.778]), so very slightly closer to one but still largely significant. We see that all other things being equal, patients with obstruction of the colon by the tumor (HR 1.260, 95% CI [1.004 ; 1.581]), differentiation of the tumour (HR 1.243, 95% CI [1.031 ; 1.499]), longer time from surgery (HR 1.276, 95% CI [1.044 ; 1.559]) and more than 4 positive nodes (HR 2.303, 95% CI [1.03 ; 2.788]) have a significantly worst outcome for overall survival. Furthermore, the variable extent of local spread (extent) is also significant. Since this variable (with four levels) is not defined in the dataset as a factor, it is introduced as a continuous variable in the model, with only one β coefficient associated, and therefore assuming that the effect of going from the first level to the second is the same as from the second to the third and from the third to the fourth one. In this case the estimated HR consider that moving from one level (e.g. muscle) to the next one (serosa) is associated with an estimated HR of 1.568 (95% CI [1.249 ; 1.969]), corresponding thus to an increased risk of death. In case we don't want to make this assumption (which is probably the case here), we must enter the variable in the model as a factor, then leading to 3 estimated coefficients for comparison of each level to the reference one.

```
> coxph(Surv(time, status) ~ rx+obstruct+differ+as.factor(extent)
     +surg+node4, data=colon.OS)
Call:
coxph(formula = Surv(time, status) ~ rx + obstruct + differ +
```

```
as.factor(extent) + surg + node4, data = colon.OS)

                        coef  exp(coef)  se(coef)        z        p
rxLev                0.01065    1.01070   0.10932    0.097   0.9224
rxLev+5FU           -0.48707    0.61443   0.11973   -4.068 4.74e-05
obstruct             0.23022    1.25888   0.11598    1.985   0.0471
differ               0.21689    1.24221   0.09547    2.272   0.0231
as.factor(extent)2   0.02770    1.02809   0.48040    0.058   0.9540
as.factor(extent)3   0.56832    1.76530   0.45295    1.255   0.2096
as.factor(extent)4   1.00611    2.73495   0.49289    2.041   0.0412
surg                 0.24578    1.27862   0.10222    2.405   0.0162
node4                0.83629    2.30778   0.09763    8.566   < 2e-16

Likelihood ratio test=132   on 9 df, p=< 2.2e-16
n= 906, number of events= 458
  (23 observations deleted due to missingness)
```

Only the patients with extent of local spread to contiguous structure have a significantly worst outcome than the patients with extent only to submucosoa, with a 2.735 higher risk of death (HR 2.735, 95% CI [1.041 ; 7.186]). Patients with extent of local spread to serosa have a 1.765 higher risk of death, however this HR is accompanied by a wide confidence intervals (95% CI [0.727 ; 4.289]) and therefore do not reach statistical significance. Patients with extent to muscle do not seem to have a worst outcome (HR 1.028, 95% CI [0.401 ; 2.636]). Looking at Table 1.1, we see that less than 2.5% of the patients are in the reference category (submucosa), explaining the large width of the confidence intervals. To avoid this, one could have group the first two categories before adjusting the model or choose another reference category.

All the models fitted above are semi-parametric, i.e. they don't make any assumption about the distribution of the event times and therefore leaves the baseline hazard function unspecified. An alternative is to consider a parametric baseline hazard. A common parametric PH model assumes a Weibull distribution of the event times, with a baseline hazard given then by (2.19). This can be achieved with the **survreg** function. One should however be aware that the estimated coefficients corresponds to the log-linear expression of this model, see Section 2.5.2. So, including only treatment as a factor, we actually fit model

$$\log t = \mu + \alpha_1 X_1 + \alpha_2 X_2 + \sigma \epsilon$$

where X_1 and X_2 are the dummy variables defined above, μ is called the *intercept* intercept and σ is the *scale* parameter. As explained in Section 2.5.2, the random error term e_i is in this case assumed to follow a Gumbel distribution. The estimate provided by the **survreg** function should thus either be interpreted as such or back-transformed to the corresponding Weibull model representation using equations (2.28), (2.29), and (2.30).

```
> OS.colon.Weib.m1 <- survreg(Surv(time, status) ~ rx, dist="
    weibull", data=colon.OS)
> summary(OS.colon.Weib.m1)
Call:
```

```
survreg(formula = Surv(time, status) ~ rx, data = colon.OS, dist
    = ''weibull")
                Value Std. Error     z       p
(Intercept) 7.8820       0.1123 70.17 < 2e-16
rxLev       0.0423       0.1566  0.27    0.79
rxLev+5FU   0.8005       0.1752  4.57 4.9e-06
Log(scale)  0.3805       0.0411  9.25 < 2e-16

Scale= 1.46

Weibull distribution
Loglik(model)= -4114.6   Loglik(intercept only)= -4128.2
    Chisq= 27.28 on 2 degrees of freedom, p= 1.2e-06
Number of Newton-Raphson Iterations: 5
n= 929
```

In this log-linear representation, which actually corresponds to an AFT model, we obtain $\hat{\alpha}_1 = 0.0423$ and $\hat{\alpha}_2 = 0.8005$ meaning that the (log-)time-to-event is (slightly and not statistically significantly) increased for patients in the Lev group compared to those in the Obs group, and is increased to a larger (and statistically significant) extent for patients in the Lev+5FU group compared to those in the Obs group. The summary function allows us to obtain the estimated standard error of the estimators and p-values. The results obtained from this parametric model are in line with those obtained above.

Following equations (2.28), (2.29), and (2.30), one can compute $\lambda = \exp(-\mu/\sigma)$, $\rho = 1/\sigma$, and $\beta_j = -\alpha_j/\sigma$ to obtain the estimated value in the Weibull PH model parametrization. Note that the estimated HR obtained are very close from those obtained with a semi-parametric Cox PH model.

```
> lambda <- exp(-OS.colon.Weib.m1$coef[1]/OS.colon.Weib.m1$scale)
> lambda
(Intercept)
0.004572434
> rho <- 1/OS.colon.Weib.m1$scale
> rho
[1] 0.6835486
> beta <- -OS.colon.Weib.m1$coef[-1]/OS.colon.Weib.m1$scale
> beta
      rxLev    rxLev+5FU
-0.02888938 -0.54720043
> HR <- exp(beta)
> HR
    rxLev rxLev+5FU
0.9715239 0.5785673
```

The package parfm, which will be discussed further in Chapter 3, allows to directly fit a Weibull PH model. As expected, we obtain the same results as after back-transforming the estimated value obtained from the survreg command.

```
> library(parfm)
> OS.colon.Weib.par <- parfm(Surv(time, status) ~ rx, dist="
    weibull", frailty="none",data=colon.OS)
> OS.colon.Weib.par
```

```
Frailty distribution: none
Baseline hazard distribution: Weibull
Loglikelihood: -4114.57

            ESTIMATE SE      p-val
rho          0.684   0.017
lambda       0.005   0.001
rxLev       -0.029   0.105 0.783
rxLev+5FU   -0.547   0.117 <.001 ***
---
Signif. codes: 0 '***' 0.001 '**' 0.01 '*' 0.05 '.' 0.1 ' ' 1
> exp(OS.colon.Weib.par[c(3,4)])
[1] 0.9715241 0.5785659
> ci.parfm(OS.colon.Weib.par, level=0.05)
             low     up
rxLev      0.791  1.193
rxLev+5FU  0.460  0.728
```

By changing the `dist` argument, other parametric PH model can be fitted, assuming either a Weibull, and inverse Weibull, a Frechet, an Exponential, a Gompertz, a Log-logistic, a Log-normal or a Log-Skewed-Normal distribution [265].

Another R package that will be further discussed in Chapter 3 is the `frailtypack` package. This package also allows to directly fit a Weibull PH model but do not use exactly the same parametrization of the Weibull distribution as the `parfm` package. Indeed, while the `parfm` package models the hazard as

$$h(t) = \lambda \rho t^{\rho-1}$$

the `frailtypack` package uses the same parametrization as the `rweibull` function and thus models the hazard as:

$$h(t) = \rho \tilde{\lambda}^{-\rho} t^{\rho-1}$$

with ρ the shape (as above) and $\tilde{\lambda}$ the scale parameter. We can easily go from one parametrization to the other using $\lambda = \tilde{\lambda}^{-\rho}$. After loading the `frailtypack` package, the Weibull PH model can be fitted as follows:

```
> frailtypack
> OS.colon.Weib.fr <- frailtyPenal(Surv(time, status) ~ rx,
    hazard = ('Weibull'), data=colon.OS)
Be patient. The program is computing ...
The program took 0.36 seconds
> OS.colon.Weib.fr
Call:
frailtyPenal(formula = Surv(time, status) ~ rx, data = colon.OS,
    hazard = ("Weibull"))

  Cox proportional hazards model parameter estimates
  using a Parametrical approach for the hazard function

            coef exp(coef) SE coef (H)        z            p
```

```
rxLev      -0.0288939   0.971520    0.109746 -0.26328  7.9233e-01
rxLev+5FU  -0.5473475   0.578482    0.121885 -4.49070  7.0988e-06


     chisq df global p
rx 24.6353   2 4.47e-06


      marginal log-likelihood = -4114.57
      Convergence criteria:
      parameters = 1.69e-06 likelihood = 1.19e-07 gradient = 5.23
        e-07


AIC = Aikaike information Criterion      = 4.43334

The expression of the Aikaike Criterion is:
      'AIC = (1/n)[np - l(.)]'


      Scale for the weibull hazard function is : 2649.02
      Shape for the weibull hazard function is : 0.68

The expression of the Weibull hazard function is:
      'lambda(t) = (shape.(t^(shape-1)))/(scale^shape)'
The expression of the Weibull survival function is:
      'S(t) = exp[- (t/scale)^shape]'


      n= 929
      n events= 468
      number of iterations:   13
```

The results are indeed very close from those obtained with `coxph` and `parfm` as we can find back the value of $\rho = \tilde{\rho}$ and $\lambda = \tilde{\lambda}^{-\tilde{\rho}}$

```
> OS.colon.Weib.fr$shape.weib[1]
[1] 0.6835426
> OS.colon.Weib.fr$scale.weib[1]^(-OS.colon.Weib.fr$shape.weib
   [1])
[1] 0.004572732
```

2.6.3   Rectal cancer data

The rectal cancer dataset contains information on 357 resected stage II-III rectal cancer patients recruited in the Intergroup R98 trial. This trial is shortly introduced in Section 1.3.2 of Chapter 1. As we explained there, this trial had to close before reaching its targeted sample size due to slow recruitment. In this trial, patients were randomized after surgery to either a 5FU/LV regimen (control arm, $n = 178$) or to LV5-FU2 plus irinotecan (experimental arm, $n = 179$). One patient randomized to the experimental arm was actually treated with the control treatment. However, according to the intention-to-treat principle, this patient is included in the arm allocated by randomization for all the analyses presented below.

Patients were recruited by 66 centers and it is important to keep in mind that before initiation, each center had to opt for one of two 5FU-LV regimens and all patients randomized to the control arm had to be treated with the

	5-FU/LV control	5FU/LV + Irinotecan
Strata Mayo Clinic (n)	61	56
Strata LV5-FU2 (n)	117	123
Disease-free survival		
N (patients/events)	178 / 92	179 / 89
5-yrs DFS (s.e.)	57.8%(3.7%)	63.2%(3.7%)
HR (95% CI)	0.80 [0.60 ; 1.09]	
p-value (logrank)	0.154	
Overall survival		
N (patients/events)	178 / 72	179 / 63
5-yrs OS (s.e.)	73.5%(3.4%)	75.0%(3.3%)
HR (95% CI)	0.87 [0.62 ; 1.23]	
p-value (logrank)	0.433	

TABLE 2.6
Rectal cancer data: Main results of the R98 Intergroup trial of postoperative irinotecan in resected stage II-III rectal cancer [99]. Results are stratified according to the institutional choice of control 5-FU/LV regimen.

chosen regimen. This resulted into $n = 61$ treated with the Mayo Clinic regimen and $n = 117$ treated with the LV5-FU2 regimen. The protocol foreseen that for all the analyses, the patients should be stratified according to the choice of the control regimen in the center in which they were recruited. Therefore, $n = 56$ patients in the experimental arm were in the strata Mayo Clinic regimen and the remaining $n = 123$ patients in this treatment arm where in the strata LV5-FU2 regimen, leading to a total of respectively $n = 117$ and $n = 240$ patients in each strata, see Table 2.6.

The primary endpoint for this trial was disease-free survival (DFS) and secondary endpoints included overall survival (OS), time to locoregional relapse and time to distant relapse. The main analysis was performed after a median follow-up of 13 years and is based on a total of 173 DFS events. The results, as published [99], are presented in Table 2.6. In this section, we show how we can obtain these results and perform the analyses presented in the previous section in the SAS software.

Note that to improve the readability of the output, we start by assigning a format and a label to the variable treat.

```
PROC FORMAT;
    VALUE Treat_
        0='5FU/LV'
        1='5FU/LV+Irinotecan';
run;
data R98data; set R98data;
    format treat Treat_.;
    label treat="Treatment arm";
run;
```

In SAS, the procedure `proc lifetest` can be used to compute the Kaplan-Meier estimate of the survival curve. So to obtain the KM estimate of DFS based on our data, we use the command

```
proc lifetest data=R98data plot=(s) timelist=(24 48 72 96 120)  ;
title1 ''DFS" ;
time dfsm*censd(1) ;
strata treat;
run ;
```

The `strata` statement is used here to obtain the results by treatment arm. Using the `timelist` option allows to specify a list of timepoints for which the output will provide the estimated KM value, so here we use it to specify that we only need the value of the KM estimate for DFS to be estimated at 24, 48, 72, 96, and 120 weeks. Note that without specifying this option, SAS will output the KM point estimates at all observed event time, which can result in a very long output. The `cens(1)` specifies the value 1 as the indicator of an event, this can be modify if necessary. The `plot=(s)` statement produces a plot of the DFS estimated curves by strata (so by treatment here); note that this graph is more nicely displayed using the ODS output of SAS.

The output is divided into two main parts: first, the results for each level of the variable specified in the strata statement (so for the control treatment 5FU/LV (stratum 1) and then for the experimental treatment 5FU/LV+Irinotecan (stratum 2)) and second, the results pertaining to the comparison of the (two) strata. For each strata, one can find for each requested timepoint (or for all event times if no specific timepoints have been specified), the observed true event at which the last jump of the KM occurs before this timepoint (`dfsm`), the KM point estimate (`Survival`), so $\hat{S}(t)$, the corresponding estimate of the distribution function (`Failure`), so $\hat{F}(t) = 1 - \hat{S}(t)$, the standard error of the $\hat{S}(t)$, as well as a count of the number of individuals having failed up to that time and the number of individuals still at risk. We then have the estimates for the quartile of the DFS distribution together with 95% CI obtained from the log-log transform; other transformations and other confidence level can of course also be obtained. The mean DFS together with its standard error is also provided, together with a note that we should interpret this information carefully due to censoring.

```
The LIFETEST Procedure

Stratum 1: Treatment arm = 5FU/LV
```

				Product-Limit Survival Estimates		
				Survival Standard	Number	Number
Timelist	dfsm	Survival	Failure	Error	Failed	Left
24.000	23.637	0.6935	0.3065	0.0347	54	122
48.000	47.783	0.5955	0.4045	0.0371	71	103
72.000	68.938	0.5540	0.4460	0.0377	78	92
96.000	95.288	0.4877	0.5123	0.0393	87	51

| 120.000 | 110.705 | 0.4540 | 0.5460 | 0.0412 | 90 | 29 |

Summary Statistics for Time Variable dfsm
                    Quartile Estimates
                Point   95% Confidence Interval
Percent   Estimate   Transform   [Lower   Upper)
   75   .   LOGLOG   145.915   .
   50   92.073   LOGLOG   61.449   .
   25   19.040   LOGLOG   14.078   27.214

              Standard
   Mean   Error

  84.902   4.601

NOTE: The mean survival time and its standard error were
   underestimated because the largest observation was censored
   and the estimation
      was restricted to the largest event time.

The LIFETEST Procedure

Stratum 2: Treatment arm = 5FU/LV+Irinotecan

                        Product-Limit Survival Estimates
                                       Survival
                                       Standard   Number   Number
Timelist   dfsm   Survival   Failure   Error   Failed   Left

  24.000   23.859   0.8001   0.1999   0.0302   35   140
  48.000   47.976   0.6791   0.3209   0.0354   56   116
  72.000   61.547   0.6263   0.3737   0.0367   65   103
  96.000   95.880   0.5556   0.4444   0.0389   75   63
 120.000   115.068   0.5079   0.4921   0.0424   79   29

Summary Statistics for Time Variable dfsm

                    Quartile Estimates
                Point   95% Confidence Interval
Percent   Estimate   Transform   [Lower   Upper)

   75   .   LOGLOG   148.584   .
   50   132.906   LOGLOG   88.126   .
   25   36.421   LOGLOG   23.797   47.062

              Standard
   Mean   Error

  96.127   4.470

NOTE: The mean survival time and its standard error were
      underestimated because the largest observation was
         censored and the estimation was restricted to the
         largest event time.

The second part of the output displays for each strata (so here, for each treatment group) a summary of the number of events and of censored observations. Information with regards to the logrank test, the Wilcoxon and the likelihood ratio tests is also provided, together with corresponding *p*-values.

```
        Summary of the Number of Censored and Uncensored Values


                                                          Percent
Stratum   treat                Total   Failed   Censored  Censored

      1   5FU/LV                 178       92         86     48.31
      2   5FU/LV+Irinotecan      179       81         98     54.75
--------------------------------------------------------------------

  Total                          357      173        184     51.54


Testing Homogeneity of Survival Curves for dfsm over Strata


                       Rank Statistics

treat                          Log-Rank      Wilcoxon

5FU/LV                           9.5934        3065.0
5FU/LV+Irinotecan               -9.5934       -3065.0


        Covariance Matrix for the Log-Rank Statistics

treat                      5FU/LV         5FU/LV+Irinotecan

5FU/LV                    43.0886                  -43.0886
5FU/LV+Irinotecan        -43.0886                   43.0886


        Covariance Matrix for the Wilcoxon Statistics

treat                      5FU/LV         5FU/LV+Irinotecan

5FU/LV                    2974199                  -2974199
5FU/LV+Irinotecan        -2974199                   2974199


        Test of Equality over Strata

                                       Pr >
Test           Chi-Square       DF    Chi-Square

Log-Rank          2.1359         1      0.1439
Wilcoxon          3.1586         1      0.0755
-2Log(LR)         2.4010         1      0.1213
```

Finally, Figure 2.8 displays the estimated DFS curves by treatment arm as produced by SAS. From these results, we can see that at the time of the analysis, a total of 173 patients (51.5%) had an observed event (so either persistent or progressive disease or secondary primary colon cancer or death),

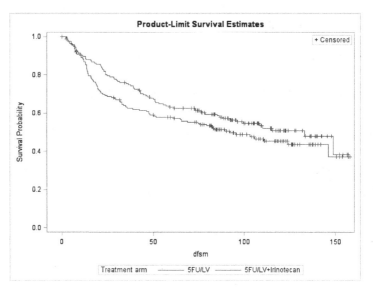

FIGURE 2.8
Rectal cancer data: Kaplan-Meier estimators of the DFS curves by treatment arm for the R98 trial patients as obtained from the `proc lifetest` procedure in SAS

92 in the 5FU/LV arm and 81 in the 5FU/LV+Irinotecan arm. The estimated 2 and 10 years DFS were respectively 69.4% and 45.4% in the $5FU/LV$ arm and 80.0% and 50.8% in the 5FU/LV+Irinotecan arm. Furthermore the median DFS was estimated to be 92.1 months (95% CI: [61.4 ; NYR]) in the $5FU/LV$ arm and 132.9 months (95% CI: [88.1 ; NYR]) in the 5FU/LV+Irinotecan arm. While these results seem to indicate a slight advantage for the experimental arm (5FU/LV+Irinotecan), the effect of treatment on DFS does not reach statistical significance, with a p-value of 0.1439 for the logrank test, and 0.0755 for the Wilcoxon test which put more weight on earlier differences. The choice between the logrank test or the Wilcoxon test should be made before seeing the results, and should ideally be pre-specified in the study protocol or the statistical analysis plan.

Note that for this particular study, it was planned that all analyses should be stratified for the 5FU/LV regimen chosen for the control arm (Mayo Clinic regimen versus LV5-FU2 regimen). This stratification variable, called `strat` in our database can be used to perform such a stratified analysis.

```
proc lifetest data=R98data plot=(s) timelist=(24 48 72 96 120 );
title1 ''DFS" ;
time dfsm*censd(1) ;
strata strat /group=treat;
run ;
```

It will produce KM estimate of DFS for each group (so here each treatment arm as defined by the variable `treat`) within each stratum (defined here by the variable `strat`), as well as a stratified logrank and Wilcoxon test of equality of DFS over group.

```
The LIFETEST Procedure
          Summary of the Number of Censored and Uncensored Values
                                                         Percent
  Stratum strat   treat              Total Failed Censored Censored

        1     1   5FU/LV               61     36      25     40.98
        1     1   5FU/LV+Irinotecan    56     33      23     41.07
Subtotal                              117     69      48     41.03
        2     2   5FU/LV              117     56      61     52.14
        2     2   5FU/LV+Irinotecan   123     48      75     60.98
Subtotal                              240    104     136     56.67
-----------------------------------------------------------------
   Total                              357    173     184     51.54
```

```
The LIFETEST Procedure

Stratified Comparison of Survival Curves for dfsm over Group


              Rank Statistics

treat                   Log-Rank     Wilcoxon

5FU/LV                    9.3579       1760.0
5FU/LV+Irinotecan        -9.3579      -1760.0

      Covariance Matrix for the Log-Rank Statistics
treat                    5FU/LV       5FU/LV+Irinotecan

5FU/LV                   43.0706             -43.0706
5FU/LV+Irinotecan       -43.0706             43.0706


      Covariance Matrix for the Wilcoxon Statistics
treat                    5FU/LV       5FU/LV+Irinotecan

5FU/LV                   968721              -968721
5FU/LV+Irinotecan       -968721              968721


   Stratified Test of Equality over Group
                                   Pr >
Test          Chi-Square    DF    Chi-Square

Log-Rank        2.0332       1      0.1539
Wilcoxon        3.1976       1      0.0737
```

As we can see, the results are in this particular case only slightly impacted by the stratification. Two plots are also produced, representing the estimated DFS survival curve by group (i.e treatment arm) within each stratum. Results obtained are similar to those presented in [99], i.e. a stratified logrank p-value of 0.154. Estimates of the DFS curve per treatment arm within the Mayo Clinic stratum (strata 1) and the LV5-FU2 stratum (strata 2) show that the difference between the two treatment groups is more pronounced in the LV5-FU2 stratum, with globally less good results in the Mayo Clinic stratum (Figure 2.9).

A Cox PH model can be fitted to our data with the `proc phreg` procedure in which a `strata` statement can be added to fit a stratified Cox PH model, see (2.23):

```
proc phreg data=R98data ;
title1 ''Hazard ratio stratified by type of chemotherapy" ;
model dfsm*censd(1)=treat /rl ;
strata strat ;
run ;
```

The `rl` option has been specified to obtained confidence intervals (with rl standing for "risk limits") for our estimated hazards ratio; the level of significance is by default 95% but can of course be changed. A first part of the output (not displayed here) provides some general information on the dataset used, the variables used, the method to handle ties in the partial likelihood (by default Breslow, but it can be changed), the number of events and some model fit statistics. The second part of the output displays the results of the model

```
Hazard ratio stratified by type of chemotherapy

The PHREG Procedure
          Testing Global Null Hypothesis: BETA=0
Test                   Chi-Square    DF    Pr > ChiSq

Likelihood Ratio          2.0306      1       0.1542
Score                     2.0332      1       0.1539
Wald                      2.0290      1       0.1543

                                  Analysis of Maximum Likelihood
                                           Estimates
                    Parameter   Standard                            Hazard
Parameter DF        Estimate      Error   Chi-Square  Pr > ChiSq    Ratio

treat      1        -0.21727    0.15253    2.0290       0.1543      0.805

95% Hazard Ratio
Confidence Limits      Label

  0.597        1.085   Treatment arm
```

The estimated stratified hazard ratio is 0.805 in favor of the experimental treatment arm, but, as expected from the non-significant p-value, the 95% CI [0.597 ; 1.085] does contain the value 1. Removing the `strata` statement fits a non-stratified model, leading to an unstratified hazard ratio of 0.800 with 95% CI [0.594 ; 1.079].

We can also easily add baseline covariates in this Cox PH model. For example, we can adjust the treatment HR for age, gender, localization of cancer, number of involved nodes, preoperative radiotherapy, sphincter conservation,

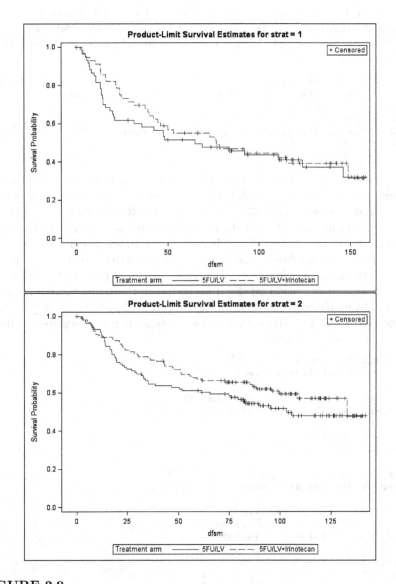

FIGURE 2.9
Rectal cancer data: Kaplan-Meier estimators of the DFS curves by treatment arm for the Mayo Clinic stratum *(top)* and the LV5-FU2 stratum *(bottom)* for the R98 trial patients as obtained from the `proc lifetest` procedure in SAS.

and time of surgery. Removing, one after the other the least significant covariates (*backward selection*), we remain with a model containing the number
of involved nodes and sphincter conservation. To include nominal variables,
the `class` statement must be used, so that the variable is recoded as dummy
variables. We use here the `class` statement to model the 3-categories variable
`ganglenv3` as a factor.

```
proc phreg data=R98data ;
title1 ''Hazard ratio stratified by type of chemotherapy -
   multivariate model" ;
class ganglenv3;
model dfsm*censd(1)=treat ganglenv3 sphincons2 /rl ;
strata strat ;
run ;
```

Note that we can find in the first part of the output the number of observations used, this may be useful in case of the presence of missing data in
the covariates. Indeed, as R, SAS perform by default a complete case analysis,
i.e. discarding all individuals with at least one missing value for the covariates included in the model. The coding of the variables specified in the `class`
statement is also specified in this first part of the output; by default coding is
based on the alphabetical order of the levels. This first part of the output also
provides some information on the convergence of the algorithm, on measures
of model fit with and without covariates as well as the results from three tests
for the global null hypothesis that all coefficients are equal to zero (likelihood
ratio, score, and Wald test).

```
The PHREG Procedure
         Model Information

Data Set                   WORK.R98DATA
Dependent Variable         dfsm
Censoring Variable         censd
Censoring Value(s)         1
Ties Handling              BRESLOW

Number of Observations Read          357
Number of Observations Used          357

        Class Level Information
                       Design
  Class          Value     Variables

  ganglenv3        0        1      0
                   1        0      1
                   2        0      0

        Summary of the Number of Event and Censored Values
                                             Percent
  Stratum      strat     Total    Event   Censored   Censored

         1        1        117       69         48      41.03
         2        2        240      104        136      56.67
-------------------------------------------------------------------
```

```
   Total                   357       173        184      51.54
```

Hazard ratio stratified by type of chemotherapy - multivariate
    model

The PHREG Procedure

```
                        Convergence Status
            Convergence criterion (GCONV=1E-8) satisfied.
```

Model Fit Statistics

Criterion	Without Covariates	With Covariates
-2 LOG L	1652.898	1640.249
AIC	1652.898	1648.249
SBC	1652.898	1660.862

Testing Global Null Hypothesis: BETA=0

Test	Chi-Square	DF	Pr > ChiSq
Likelihood Ratio	12.6495	4	0.0131
Score	13.3725	4	0.0096
Wald	13.1954	4	0.0104

Type 3 Tests

Effect	DF	Wald Chi-Square	Pr > ChiSq
treat	1	2.5929	0.1073
ganglenv3	2	7.5144	0.0233
sphincons2	1	4.4816	0.0343

Hazard ratio stratified by type of chemotherapy - multivariate
    model

The PHREG Procedure

Analysis of Maximum Likelihood Estimates

Parameter		DF	Parameter Estimate	Standard Error	Chi-Square	Pr > ChiSq	Hazard Ratio
treat		1	-0.24636	0.15300	2.5929	0.1073	0.782
ganglenv3	0	1	-0.54657	0.20884	6.8495	0.0089	0.579
ganglenv3	1	1	-0.41700	0.19051	4.7909	0.0286	0.659
sphincons2		1	-0.37853	0.17881	4.4816	0.0343	0.685

95% Hazard Ratio Confidence Limits		Label
0.579	1.055	Treatment arm
0.384	0.872	ganglenv3 0
0.454	0.957	ganglenv3 1
0.482	0.972	

The model fit is not greatly improved by the inclusion of the covariates, with an AIC of respectively 1652.898 and 1647.112 for the model without and with covariates. The null hypothesis of all coefficients being equal to zero is however rejected at the 5% alpha level. As mentioned, we have kept in this model only the covariates for which the Wald test applied on each coefficient separately is significant (except for treatment). The estimated HR for each covariate, together with corresponding 95% CI computed while adjusting for the other variables (multivariate analysis) are provided. All other things being equal, patients with sphincter conservation have a 0.685 times lower risk of event (95%CI [0.482 ; 0.972]); so patients without sphincter conservation have a $1/0.685 = 1.460$ times higher risk of event. As could be expected, the risk of events is lower for patients having no (HR = 0.579, 95% CI [0.384 ; 0.872]) or only one to three (HR = 0.659, 95% CI [0.454 ; 0.957]) nodes involved compared to patients having more than three nodes involved. Adjusting for these factors, the stratified adjusted HR associated with the experimental treatment is now 0.782 (95% CI [0.579 ; 1.055]) in favor of the experimental treatment.

Similar results can be obtained for overall survival (OS) by replacing the dfsm and censd variables in the commands above by the corresponding variables for OS, namely osm and cens.

In this trial, which face recruitment problems, the patients were finally recruited by 66 centers most of which recruited very little number of patients. Furthermore, each center had to choose a priori the type of regimen used in the control arm. Given these circumstances, we will check in Chapter 3 whether this resulted in heterogeneity in outcome between centers.

2.7 Further reading

Survival data analysis has been the subject of several textbooks, amongst which [13, 78, 91, 181, 186, 192, 217, 248, 372]. For a more applied perspective, we can also mention [193] and [260] amongst many other. Modeling of survival data is also sometimes addressed in general books on model building, such as [153, 362, 400], or in textbooks dedicated to clinical trial analysis, see for example [63]. A more advanced public may be interested by the textbooks [13, 125], which concentrates on more methodological aspects, and are based mainly on counting processes and martingales theory. For a broad overview of survival data analysis in a Bayesian context, we refer the reader to [173]. The main references on survival data analysis in the specific context of interval-censored data are [42, 64] and [366]. These books mainly focus on what we have called *classical survival data*. Such data are characterized by a single endpoint of interest (e.g. death from any cause), assuming that this event would be observed for all observations if the follow-up would be long enough and assuming further that all observations are independent or that the population is homogeneous given the observed covariates.

While these methods are applicable in a wide series of practical situations, such classical survival analysis methods do not adequately apply to all situations and several extensions of these methods have been proposed to address specific issues. For example, observations the population may be heterogeneous due to some unobserved factors or observations may be correlated due to the presence of clusters, or observations may be subject to more than one type of event, or may be *non-susceptible* or *cured* for the event of interest. Some of the references mentioned above present one or two chapters to address one of these situations, considering most often the case of correlated survival times or the presence of more than one type of event [78, 181, 186, 248, 260, 372].

3

Frailty Models

3.1 Introduction

The classical methods, seen in the previous chapter, assume that up to the covariates included in the model, the population under study is homogeneous. Individuals with the same value of these covariates are expected to have similar event times. However, in some applications it is more reasonable to consider the population as heterogeneous or as a collection of homogeneous clusters of individuals. Individuals may be exposed to different risk levels, and this even after controlling for known risk factors, or being grouped into clusters so that individuals from the same cluster share some common unobserved exposure. Indeed, for various reasons, one can not measure all risk factors related to the event of interest. This could be for economical or practical reasons (e.g. would require too invasive procedure) or simply due to lack of knowledge about all factors affecting the event. The individuals who are more *frail* due to some unobserved factors will experience the event earlier while the individuals who are *stronger* will remain free of the event for a longer time, leading to more heterogenity than what is taken into account by our model.

The concept of frailty has therefore been developed to handle unobserved heterogeneity in survival data caused by unmeasured covariates. Broadly speaking, the idea is to model this unobserved heterogeneity by adding random effect(s) acting multiplicatively on the hazard function. Frailty models have been developed along two main streams, usually referred to as *univariate* and *multivariate* frailty models.

Univariate frailty models were originally introduced by Vaupel et al. [397] to address the problem of heterogeneity in the population caused by unobserved covariates. Given that individuals are exposed to different risk levels, two sources of heterogeneity can be distinguished: the variability accounted for by observable risk factors and the one caused by unknown or unavailable risk factors. The former are modeled via the introduction of covariates in our model while the latter can be modeled by an unobserved random quantity acting multiplicative on the hazard of each individual. This random effect was then called a frailty, since each individual possesses its own *frailty* (realization of an unobserved random variable) with more frail individuals experiencing the event of interest earlier. While classical survival analysis assumes an homogeneous population, univariate frailty models therefore allow taking into account the unobserved heterogeneity in the study population. The univariate frailty model is usually seen as an extension of the (Cox) PH model in which the hazard function is multiplied by an unobservable random effect. However, one can also see this frailty as a non-observable mixture variable for a population assumed to be a mixture of individuals with (at least partly unknown) different risks [406].

Frailty models have then been used also for "multivariate" or "clustered" survival data. In that context, the study population is divided into clusters and all observations from a same cluster share the same value of the frailty. This frailty term therefore models all the unobserved factors common to all observations of a same cluster (genetic characteristics, socioeconomic environment, exposition factors, ...) and thus model the association between related event times within a cluster. Since all individuals share the same value of the frailty term, this has naturally led to the name *shared* frailty model.

Clustered survival data are actually encountered quite often, although the settings may be quite different. One may have to handle cluster of fixed size (2, 3, 4, ...), as will be the case for example when studying the time to failure of paired organs (fixed cluster size of size 2), or the infection time in the four udder quarter of dairy cows (fixed cluster size of size 4). But in other applications, the cluster size may be varying from one cluster to the other. This is typically the case when considering the patients treated within the same hospital in multi-centers clinical trial or individuals belonging to the same household in a societal study. There might also be nesting in the clustering, with one, two or more nesting levels, considering for example students within classes within school, or households within villages within districts. Also, the observations in a cluster may be ordered (in time or space) or not. Coming back to the examples above, it is difficult to put a meaningful ordering on students in a same classroom or patients treated in a same hospital but such a ordering become obvious when considering repeated events, like recurrent epilepsy crises in young adults or recurrent asthma attack in children. Duchateau and Janssen [107] discuss various examples of clustered survival data, and their characteristics.

It is important to note that the use of the terms *univariate* and *multivariate* frailty models may be confusing. In general, these terms are rather used to specify whether the technique considered include one (univariate) or more than one (multivariate) variables. This is obviously not the case here and one could consider a univariate frailty model including several know risk factors and a multivariate frailty model including only one known risk factors.

Univariate and multivariate frailty models are introduced respectively in Section 3.2 and Section 3.3, followed by a discussion of the most commonly encountered frailty distribution in Section 3.4. It is important to note that besides the shared frailty model, other approaches have been proposed for clustered survival data, such as fixed effects and stratified models, marginal models and copula models. We will also shortly discuss them and discuss their pro's and con's in Section 3.3. Inference for the parametric and semi-parametric frailty models will be presented in Section 3.5. In Section 3.7 we review the available software implementations and we demonstrate how these models can be applied on real data with SAS and R.

Several textbooks specifically on frailty models or discussing these models in length are available, amongst which [107, 167, 372] , and [406]. The frailty models have led to various developments and numerous statistical publications in the last decades (see for example [27] for a recent overview); some important further reading are mentioned in Section 3.8 together with some discussions on extensions of frailty models.

3.2 Univariate frailty models

While classical survival models presented in Chapter 2 assume that the population under study is homogeneous (i.e. given the covariates all individuals have the same risk of events), individual unobserved heterogeneity is often recognized as an important sources of variability in medical and biological applications. If absolutely all risk factors were known, they could (at least in theory) be included in the analysis using for example one of the modeling approach proposed in Section 2.5 of Chapter 1; however this is rarely the case as this information may not be available, either because not collected in the data or even not already identified.

The objective of the univariate frailty model is therefore to model separately the variability accounted for by observable risk factors from the heterogeneity caused by omitted unobserved risk factors. In 1979, Vaupel et al. [397] propose to explicitly model this unobserved heterogeneity (i.e. heterogeneity resulting from unobserved covariates) via the introduction of a multiplicative random effect. A natural way to understand this model, which actually has led to the name of frailty model, is to consider that each individual has its own *frailty*, with the more frail individuals experiencing the event of interest before those who are less frail. Since this frailty is unobserved, the idea is to model it as the realization of a random variable which will impact the hazard of each individual. It has been common to assume that this (time-independent) random effect acts multiplicatively on the hazard. However some alternatives exist, see Section 3.8).

The univariate frailty model is then defined in terms of the conditional hazard of individual $i, i = 1, ..., n$ (given the value of the frailty) as

$$h_i(t \mid U) = h(t \mid U = u_i) = u_i h_0(t) \tag{3.1}$$

In (3.1), u_i is the (unobserved) realization of a random variable from a given density function $f_U(.)$. Since u_i multiplies the hazard function, U has to be non-negative and various frailty distribution has been proposed in the literature and will be discussed later on. A scale factor common to all subjects in the population may be absorbed into the baseline hazard function $h_0(t)$, so that frailty distributions are usually standardized to $E(U) = 1$ (when this mean exists) to avoid identifiability issue [107, 406]. Such a constraint allows to separate the baseline hazard from the overall level of the random frailties.

The variance of this frailty distribution, say $\sigma^2 = V(U)$, is interpretable as a measure of heterogeneity in (unobserved) risks across the population, and will often be referred to as the "heterogeneity parameter". A larger value corresponds to more dispersed value of U and therefore larger heterogeneity in the individual hazards $U h_0(t)$ and smaller value corresponds to values of U more closely concentrated around the mean value 1 and thus less heterogeneity in individual hazards.

A particularity of time-to-event analysis is that we follow our sample over time, and that observations will leave the risk set (either because they experience the event of interest or because they are censored), and that our data therefore dynamically change. The presence of more and less frail individuals in the population will result in our sample in a systematic selection of the more robust individual as the more frail will experience the event (and thus leave the sample) earlier. The remaining individuals at risk will tend to form a selected group with lower risk. The distribution of the covariates among the individuals still at risk will therefore evolves over time, with observations at higher risk leaving the risk set earlier. This phenomenon will distort what is observed in our sample; overall hazard may decline after a while simply due to the fact that the high risk individuals have dropped from our sample earlier on. An estimate of the individual hazard rate without taking into account the unobserved frailty will therefore underestimate the hazard function to an increasingly greater extent as time goes by [406].

Interestingly, this phenomenon leads to another intuitive interpretation of the univariate frailty model. Since our population is fact assumed to be a mixture of more and less frail individuals, one can also see the frailty term in (3.1) as a mixture variable for non-observable levels of risks of the individuals. The univariate frailty model can thus also be seen as a mixture model that explicitly assume that the population is in fact a mixture of individuals with (at least partly unknown) different level of risks. The frailty U modeling the unobserved heterogeneity can therefore also be seen as a mixture variable.

It is important to keep in mind that what we observe is not an individual hazard but the result of a number of individuals with different values of the random variable Z [406]. From (3.1), we can obtain the conditional survival function $S(t \mid U)$ of an individual conditional on the frailty U

$$S_i(t \mid U) = S(t \mid U = u_i) = \exp\left(-\int_0^t h(s \mid u_i)ds\right)$$

$$= \exp\left(-u_i \int_0^t h_0(s)ds\right) = e^{-u_i H_0(t)}$$

where, as before, $H_0(t) = \int_0^t h_0(s)ds$ is the cumulative baseline hazard function. While the univariate frailty model (3.1) is described at the individual level, via the conditional hazard function (conditional on the frailty), this individual model, as well as the corresponding conditional survival, is not observable.

To obtain the global or *population* survival function, the unobserved frailties are integrated out (or "averaged out") such that the population survival function is obtained as the average of the individual survival functions with respect to the frailty distribution.

$$S^p(t) \;=\; E[S(t \mid U)] = E[e^{-U H_0(t)}] \tag{3.2}$$

where the expectation is taken with respect to the frailty distribution.

As pointed originally by Vaupel et al. [397], and further explained in Wienke [406], when assuming the simple frailty model (3.1), the hazard function of the population at time t can be interpreted as the mean of individuals hazards amongst the survivors (i.e. the individuals who have not yet experience the event of interest). We refer the reader to [406] and references therein for an interesting discussion on the consequences of this relationship on the studies of human ageing based on mortality cohort data.

At this stage, it is useful to introduce a mathematical tool known as the *Laplace transform*. The Laplace transform can actually be used to uniquely specified the distribution of a non-negative random variable. For a non-negative variable U with density function $f_U(.)$, the Laplace transform $\mathscr{L}(.)$ is defined by

$$\mathscr{L}(s) = E[\exp(-sU)] = \int_0^\infty e^{-su} f_U(u) du$$

One can show that the qth derivative of this Laplace transform is given by

$$\mathscr{L}^{(q)}(s) = (-1)^q E[U^q \exp(-sU)]$$

From this relation, one can obtain that, if $\mathscr{L}(s)$ exists in a neighborhood of zero, then

$$E[U] \;=\; -\mathscr{L}^{(1)}(0)$$

$$Var[U] \;=\; E[U^2] - (E[U])^2 = \mathscr{L}^{(2)}(0) - \left(-\mathscr{L}^{(1)}(0)\right)^2$$

From (3.2), the population survival function and the corresponding density function for a model with no covariates, can thus be expressed in terms of the Laplace transform of the frailty distribution as

$$S^p(t) \;=\; E[S(t \mid U)] = E[e^{-U H_0(t)}] = \mathscr{L}(H_0(t)) \tag{3.3}$$

$$f^p(t) \;=\; -h_0(t)\mathscr{L}'(H_0(t))$$

where $\mathscr{L}'(.)$ is the first derivative of the Laplace transform. Given that $h(t) =$

$\frac{f(t)}{S(t)}$, we can also write

$$h^p(t) = \frac{-h_0(t)\mathscr{L}'(H_0(t))}{\mathscr{L}(H_0(t))} \tag{3.4}$$

Hougaard [164, 165, 166] was the first one to point out that the frailty density is fully characterized by its Laplace transform and to exploit the fact that the population survival function, and the corresponding population density function, can be expressed in terms of the Laplace transform of the frailty distribution. We will see in Section 3.5 that in the context of parametric frailty models, distribution with an explicit Laplace transform will lead to simpler calculations.

Note that with no parametric assumption on $h_0(t)$ and no covariate included in the model, model (3.1) is in fact not identifiable. However, the model become identifiable if we add covariates under the assumption of a PH structure at the level of the conditional hazard (and considering a finite mean frailty distribution) [115]. The idea is therefore to extend model (3.1) by including covariates, and thus modeling the effect of known observed risk factors, in the conditional hazard of an individual $i, i = 1, ...n$, given the frailty u_i and covariate value $\mathbf{x}_i$ as

$$h_i(t \mid U) = h(t \mid U = u_i, \mathbf{X} = \mathbf{x}_i) = u_i h_0(t) \exp(\beta^t \mathbf{x}_i) \tag{3.5}$$

and one can then see the univariate frailty model as an extension of the Cox PH model. The corresponding conditional survival function is then

$$
\begin{aligned}
S_i(t \mid U) = S(t \mid U = u_i, \mathbf{X} = \mathbf{x}_i) &= \exp\left(-\int_0^t h(s \mid u_i, \mathbf{X} = \mathbf{x}_i)ds\right) \\
&= \exp\left(-u_i \int_0^t h_0(s) \exp(\beta^t \mathbf{x}_i ds\right) \\
&= \exp(-u_i H_0(t) \exp(\beta^t \mathbf{x}_i)
\end{aligned}
$$

By integrating out the frailty with respect to the frailty distribution, we can obtain the corresponding population hazard and survival function for a given vector of covariate values. As previously, these can be expressed in terms of the Laplace transform of the frailty distribution. Indeed, for a given value of $\mathbf{X} = \mathbf{x}$, we have

$$
\begin{aligned}
S^p(t \mid \mathbf{x}) &= \mathscr{L}(H_{\mathbf{x}}^c(t)) \tag{3.6} \\
f^p(t \mid \mathbf{x}) &= -h_{\mathbf{x}}^c(t)\mathscr{L}'(H_{\mathbf{x}}^c(t)) \\
h^p(t \mid \mathbf{x}) &= \frac{-h_{\mathbf{x}}(t)\mathscr{L}'(H_{\mathbf{x}}^c(t))}{\mathscr{L}(H_{\mathbf{x}}^c(t))} \tag{3.7}
\end{aligned}
$$

where $H_{\mathbf{x}}^c(t) = H_0(t)\exp(\beta^t \mathbf{x})$ and $h_{\mathbf{x}}(t) = h_0^c(t)\exp(\beta^t \mathbf{x})$.

The frailty distribution plays an important role in the relationship between the individual survival or hazard and the population survival or hazard function, and in the effect of selection of less frail individuals on the population survival and hazard. Different choices for the frailty distribution have been considered in the literature, including discrete and continuous ones. We give a broad overview of the most commonly used distribution in Section 3.4, for a more detailed discussion on these distribution in the univariate frailty context, we refer the reader to Chapter 3 of the book of Wienke [406].

3.3 Multivariate frailty models

When observations are grouped in clusters, it is often reasonable to assume that the observation in the same cluster share more in common than individuals in different clusters. For example, patients treated in a same hospital share the same environment and are treated more alike than patients from different hospitals, animals from a same litter share genetical material and eventually exposure, ... A particular case of clustered event times are repeated event times, where the event of interest, such as asthma crisis for example, occurs several time within the same individual.

The fact that (unobserved) risk factors are shared by observations in the same cluster create dependence between these observations. The idea is therefore to introduce in the model an unobserved random factor, a frailty, whose value is shared by all individuals from the same cluster. This frailty therefore represents all the unobserved risk factors shared by the observations in the same cluster. This model has been originally by Clayton [75] for bivariate survival models and has been further extended to larger cluster, as well as to the case of clusters of variable sizes.

For subject j, $j = 1, \ldots, n_i$, from cluster i, $i = 1, \ldots, s$, with covariates values $\mathbf{x}_{ij}$ the conditional hazard is given by

$$
\begin{aligned}
h_{ij}(t \mid u_i) &= h_0(t) u_i \exp(\beta^t \mathbf{x}_{ij}) \qquad (3.8) \\
&= u_i h_{ij}^c(t)
\end{aligned}
$$

with $h_{ij}(t)$ the conditional hazard function for subject j from cluster i (conditional on u_i and $\mathbf{x}_{ij}$), u_i the (shared) frailty for cluster i, and $h_{ij}^c(t)$ the hazard for subject j from cluster i after the frailty effect has been factored out. Conditional on the frailty u_i the event times are assumed to be independent (so that the frailty u_i captures all the dependence between observations from the same cluster). We further assume that the u_i are realizations from a density f_U, called the frailty density. Obviously, U is a positive random variable and various choices have been considered in the literature for the frailty distribution. To ensure identifiability of the shared frailty model, one usually restricts the mean of U to equal one when possible. It is also usually assumed that the censoring times are independent of the failures times and of the frailty terms [272].

As in the case of the univariate frailty model, we need to distinguish the conditional hazard and survival function (conditional on belonging to a particular cluster) from the population hazard and survival function. The same relations as those discussed in Section 3.2 still hold and in particular the relationships (3.3) and (3.4) which allow to write the population survival and hazard function in terms of the Laplace transform of the frailty term. Relations (3.6) and (3.7) are also still valid and provide the population survival and hazard function for a given set of covariates values.

The shared frailty model has found several applications, for example in the analysis of multicenter clinical trials [137, 150, 223, 263], the analysis of meta-analyses [334, 389], the validation of prognostic index [221], or in the modeling of spatial survival data [227] amongst other.

Interpretation of the heterogeneity parameter

The variance parameter of the frailty distribution, is often referred to as the "heterogeneity parameter". Indeed, the larger this variance, the more dispersed are the frailty values and therefore the more heterogeneity in the time-to-events of the individuals. Therefore, denoting this parameter θ, large values of θ represents a larger heterogeneity amongst the clusters but also a larger (positive) correlation amongst individuals from the same cluster.

However, the parameter θ is often difficult to interpret as it refers to the variability at the level of the hazard. Therefore it can be interesting to translate this parameter into heterogeneity on a more interpretable quantity. We will see in Section 3.5, that, similarly to what happen in PH model, we can consider a fully parametric or a semi-parametric shared frailty model. If we assume a parametric PH frailty model, we can then easily translate the effect of this heterogeneity parameters on quantities such as the median survival time or the percentage event-free at a given timepoint [106, 221].

Based on the density of U we can obtain the density function for the median survival time over clusters (given $\mathbf{x}$). For example, if we assume a Weibull parametric PH frailty model, then conditional on the frailty value, the event times follow a Weibull distribution $W(\lambda u \exp(\beta^t \mathbf{x}), \rho)$. We can easily obtain that the median survival time for an observation in cluster i given $\mathbf{x}$ is

$$M_{\mathbf{x},i} = [\log 2/(\lambda u_i \exp(\beta^t \mathbf{x}))]^{1/\rho} \tag{3.9}$$

Since $M_{\mathbf{x},i}$ is a monotone transformation of u_i, we can obtain the density function of $M_{\mathbf{x},i}$ for $m \geq 0$ using

$$f_{M_{\mathbf{x},i}}(m) = f_U\left(g^{-1}(m)\right)\left|\frac{d}{dm}g^{-1}(m)\right| \tag{3.10}$$

From (3.9), we have

$$u = \frac{\log 2}{m^\rho \lambda \exp(\beta^t \mathbf{x})} = g^{-1}(m)$$

and thus

$$\frac{d}{dm}g^{-1}(m) = \frac{-\rho \log 2}{\lambda \exp(\beta^t \mathbf{x})} m^{-\rho-1}$$

Given the density function of the gamma distribution, see equation (3.12), we obtain

$$f_{M_{\mathbf{x},i}}(m) = \frac{\rho}{\Gamma\left(\frac{1}{\theta}\right)} \left[\frac{\log 2}{\theta \lambda \exp(\beta^t \mathbf{x})}\right]^{1/\theta} \exp\left(\frac{-\log 2}{\theta m^\rho \exp(\beta^t \mathbf{x})}\right)$$

Such a density function can then be used to visualize the variability of the median time-to-events over the clusters.

Similarly, we can obtain the density function of the percentage of individuals event-free at a given timepoint induced by the frailty distribution. Assuming that the event times follow a Weibull distribution, the percentage of individuals in cluster i with covariates value $\mathbf{x}$ and which are event-free at time t is

$$S_{t,\mathbf{x},i} = \exp(-\lambda t^\rho u_i \exp(\beta^t \mathbf{x}))$$

from which we have

$$u = \frac{-\log s}{\lambda t^\rho \exp(\beta^t \mathbf{x})} = g^{-1}(s)$$

and thus

$$\frac{d}{ds}g^{-1}(s) = \frac{-1/s}{\lambda t^\rho \exp(\beta^t \mathbf{x})}$$

Using (3.10) and (3.12), we obtain the density function for this percentage of event-free individuals over clusters induced by the density of U

$$f_{S_{t,x,i}}(s) = \frac{s^{(\theta \lambda t^\rho \exp(\beta^t \mathbf{x}))^{-1}-1}}{\theta^{1/\theta} \Gamma\left(\frac{1}{\theta}\right) \lambda t^\rho \exp(\beta^t \mathbf{x})} \left[\frac{-\log s}{\lambda t^\rho \exp(\beta^t \mathbf{x})}\right]^{1/\theta-1}$$

We will show in Section 3.7 an example of how we can use such a density function to get an idea of the heterogeneity induced by a given value of the heterogeneity parameter.

Kendall's Tau for association

The Kendall's τ is a rank-based dependence coefficient defined originally for bivariate (complete) observations [184]. However, it has been shown that the Kendall's τ can also be used to describe the association induced by the frailty terms between the event times within the same cluster. While the variance of the distribution of this frailty term can be, as discussed above, used to quantify the degree of dependence within a cluster, the Kendall's τ has the advantage that it can be directly used to compare the degree of dependence implied by two different frailty distributions.

Considering two pairs of bivariate observations (T_1, T_2) and (T_1', T_2'), the Kendall's τ has been originally defined as as the probability that the two pairs are concordant (e.g. if T_1 is smaller than T_1' than T_2 is smaller than T_2') minus the probability that the the two pairs are discordant (e.g. T_1 is smaller than T_1' but T_2 is larger than T_2'). So, we can write

$$\tau = P\left[(T_1 - T_1')(T_2 - T_2') > 0\right] - P\left[(T_1 - T_1')(T_2 - T_2') < 0\right]$$

The Kendall's τ ranges from -1 and 1 and $\tau = 0$ under independence. However, since the Kendall's τ only captures monotonic association, $\tau = 0$ does not necessarily implies independence in general.

In the context of the (shared) frailty model, the dependence between observations of the same cluster is induced by the frailty term. It has been shown that the Kendall's τ can be generalized to that context and can be written in terms of the Laplace transform of the frailty term as (see for example [167], Chapter 7 or [107], Chapter 4)

$$\tau = 4 \int_0^\infty s\mathscr{L}(s)\mathscr{L}^{(2)}(s)ds - 1 \tag{3.11}$$

with $\mathscr{L}^{(2)}(.)$ the second derivative of the Laplace transform of the frailty term $\mathscr{L}(s) = E(\exp(-Us))$.

Based on this expression, the Kendall's τ has become a popular tool to quantify the measure of the dependence of the observations within a same cluster induced by the frailty term, quantifying how concordant or discordant tend to be observations in the same cluster. In particular, it can be used to compare the dependence induced by different choices of the frailty distribution. An advantage of the Kendall's τ is that it is scale invariant, i.e. it is not affected by a monotonic transformation of the random variable considered. So in particular, it will be invariant to a transformation of the time scale. However, one has to keep in mind that the Kendall's τ can only be interpreted as an overall measure of dependence. As mentioned above, the dependence structure change over time due to the selection process (subjects from "frail cluster" will experience the event earlier). The Kendall's τ, on the other hand does not depend on time, and can therefore not be used to quantify such changes in dependence structure over time. For that purpose, local dependence measure, which are functions of time has been proposed. See for example [107, 167] for a detailed discussion on the various way to quantify the effect of the frailty term at different levels.

3.4   Frailty distributions

Both discrete and continuous frailty distribution have been considered in the context of univariate frailty model. Discrete frailty distributions are probably more intuitive when the frailty model is seen as a mixture model. On the other hand, distribution considered in the multivariate case are generally continuous. The set of continuous distributions considered in the univariate and multivariate case are basically the same.

3.4.1 Discrete frailty distribution

The simplest case is the binary frailty model, also called the *two-point frailty model* which considers that the population is composed of two sub-populations with different risks [350, 398]. Imagine for example that individuals with or without a given genetic mutation have different risks for the event of interest, but that for economical (or practical) reasons it is not possible to test the individuals in our sample for this mutation. At the start of the follow-up, each sub-population represent respectively a fraction $\pi_1(0)$ and $\pi_2(0) = 1 - \pi_1(0)$ but these quantities will obviously change over time as a result of the selection process (individuals from the sub-population with the higher risk will experience the event and thus leave the risk set earlier). An interesting special case occurs when the binary frailty is actually dividing the population into a sub-population who is at risk of the event of interest and a sub-population who is actually not at risk of the event of interest. This latter category is then often referred to as *long-term survivors* [119] or *cured individuals* [304]. We will come back to this special case when discussing cure models in Chapter 4.

The binary frailty model can be easily extended to the case where the frailty U actually divide the population in k sub-populations in unknown proportions $\pi_1, ..., \pi_k$, leading then to a *k-point frailty model*. Assuming that the number of sub-populations, and thus of mass-points of the frailty distribution, is known lead to a a parametric model [242]. This will typically be the case for example if we assume that the population is divided according to a known number of possible unobservable genotypes. On the other hand, a non-parametric model in which the number of mass points is an additional parameter to be estimated has also bee proposed [105, 157, 232].

3.4.2 Continuous frailty distribution

Any continuous positive distribution could be considered. Amongst the continuous frailty distributions studied in the literature, the gamma distribution is certainly the most popular. However, this popularity is mainly based on computational and analytical arguments given the simplicity of its Laplace transform. Another very popular continuous distribution is the log-normal frailty, most probably due to its strong link with (generalized) linear mixed models. However, other distributions such as the positive-stable distribution or the inverse Gaussian distribution have also been considered.

While the choice of the frailty distribution is often based on mathematical arguments, the choice of the frailty distribution is not that arbitrary, as different frailty distributions lead to different types of dependence amongst the observations from the same cluster. As already mentioned, the population changes over time since the more frail individuals (or individuals from more frail clusters) will drop earlier, and different frailty distributions will lead to different selection effects. As discussed in Chapter 4 of Duchateau and Janssen [107], the positive-stable distribution implies a very strong dependence initially while at equal global dependence, the gamma distribution leads to stronger dependence at late times. The dependence induced by the inverse Gaussian distribution is somewhat in between the two.

Gamma distribution

The gamma distribution is a two-parameters positive distribution with density function

$$f(u) = \frac{\lambda^\kappa u^{\kappa-1} exp(-\lambda u)}{\Gamma(\kappa)} \qquad \text{with } \kappa, \lambda > 0 \qquad (3.12)$$

where $\Gamma(.)$ represents the gamma function. We can show that

$$E(U) = \frac{k}{\lambda} \qquad \text{with} \qquad Var(U) = \frac{\kappa}{\lambda^2}$$

Note that the parametrization used in R is based on the shape parameter κ and a scale parameter $s = \frac{1}{\lambda}$; the parameter λ is then referred to as the rate. As mentioned earlier, we usually impose $E[U] = 1$ to ensure identifiability of the frailty model and therefore rather consider the one-parameter gamma distribution with $\kappa = \lambda$, whose density function simplifies to

$$f(u) = \frac{u^{\frac{1}{\theta}-1} \exp(-\frac{u}{\theta})}{\theta^{\frac{1}{\theta}} \Gamma(\frac{1}{\theta})} \qquad \text{with } \theta \geq 0$$

with $\theta = 1/\kappa = Var(U)$ the heterogeneity parameter. It is a flexible distribution, with a variety of shapes of the density function depending on the value of its parameter κ. It includes the exponential distribution as special case (when $\kappa = 1$) and tends to a bell-shape form resembling a normal density when κ increases (see Figure 3.1, based on the dgamma function in R).

The corresponding Laplace transform is given by

$$\mathscr{L}(s) = (1 + \theta s)^{-\frac{1}{\theta}}$$

and one can show that

$$\mathscr{L}^{(q)}(s) = (-1)^q (1 + \theta s)^{-q} \left[\prod_{l=0}^{q-1} (1 + \theta s) \right] \mathscr{L}(s).$$

with the product between brackets equal to 1 when $q = 1$. Thanks to the simplicity of its Laplace transform, one can use (3.6) and (3.7) to obtain the

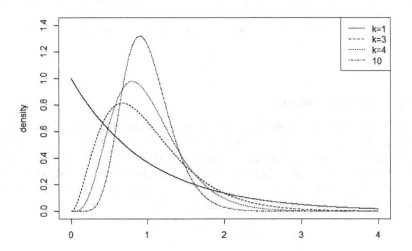

FIGURE 3.1
One-parameter gamma density for different values of the shape parameter κ.

close form expressions for the unconditional (population) survival and hazard function

$$S^p(t \mid \mathbf{x}) \;=\; (1 + \theta H_{\mathbf{x}}^c(t))^{-\frac{1}{\theta}} \tag{3.13}$$

$$h^p(t \mid \mathbf{x}) \;=\; \frac{h_{\mathbf{x}}^c(t)}{1 + \theta H_{\mathbf{x}}^c(t)} = h_{\mathbf{x}}^c(t)(S^p(t \mid \mathbf{x}))^\theta \tag{3.14}$$

where $H_{\mathbf{x}}(t) = H_0(t) \exp(\beta^t \mathbf{x})$ and $h_{\mathbf{x}}(t) = h_0(t) \exp(\beta^t \mathbf{x})$.

Consider now, for the sake of illustration, the case of a single binary covariate X, representing for example the treatment in a randomized clinical trial. Based on (3.8), we can obtain the conditional hazard ratios for this covariate for patients within the same cluster, which is simply

$$HR = \exp(\beta)$$

and is thus obviously constant over time. On the other hand, considering now (3.14), we can obtain the population (or *marginal*) hazard ratio for this covariate, which is now

$$HR^p(t) = \frac{h^p(t \mid x = 1)}{h^p(t \mid x = 0)} = \frac{h_0(t) \exp(\beta) \left(1 + \theta H_0(t) \exp(\beta)\right)^{-1}}{h_0(t) \left(1 + \theta H_0(t)\right)^{-1}}$$

$$= \frac{1 + \theta H_0(t)}{1 + \theta H_0(t) \exp(\beta)} \exp(\beta)$$

So, while the HR is constant at the cluster level, it is not the case anymore at the population level, with a decreasing HR over time when $\beta > 0$ (and thus $\exp(\beta) > 1$).

Given (3.11), the Kendall's τ for a gamma frailty is simply

$$\tau_g = \frac{\theta}{\theta + 2}$$

Log-normal distribution

Another important distribution is the log-normal distribution, which is actually mainly considered in the multivariate frailty context (see Section 3.3). Its popularity has most probably been inherited from the popularity it has achieved in the context of (generalized) linear mixed models. Indeed, as will be discussed below, McGilchrist [253, 254] has developed an estimation method for the following reformulation of the frailty model

$$h_{ij}(t) = h_0(t) \exp(\beta^t x_{ij} + w_i) \tag{3.15}$$

with $w_i = \log u_i$ often called the random effect for cluster i and assuming that the $w_i's$ follows a zero-mean normal distribution with variance σ^2. The mean of W is set to zero to ensure identifiability of the model. This approach, detailed in Section 3.5 has been developed to parallel what is done for classical (linear) mixed models [254, 253, 318, 392].

Based on this, it seems natural for the model (3.8) to consider a log-normal distribution for the frailty U. To ensure identifiability of the model, we constraint $E(U)$ to be equal to 1, leading to the one-parameter log-normal distribution with density

$$f_U(u) = \frac{1}{u\sqrt{2\pi\gamma}} \exp\left(-\frac{(\log u)^2}{2\gamma}\right)$$

with $\gamma > 0$ and one has

$$E(U) = \exp(\gamma/2) \quad \text{and} \quad Var(U) = \exp(2\gamma) - \exp(\gamma)$$

As shown on Figure 3.2 (obtained with the `dlnorm` function in R), the one-parameter log-normal density is an asymmetric density, with increasing asymmetry when γ increases.

As we have mentioned, we constrain $E(W)$ to be equal to zero in model formulation (3.5.2) and $E(U)$ to be equal to 1 in the model formulation (3.8) to ensure identifiability of the model. However, one has to be aware that this is not equivalent; indeed assuming $E(W) = 0$ does not comes back to assuming $E(U) = 1$.

The link with the (linear) mixed model theory can be seen as an advantage. However, a major disadvantage of the log-normal distribution is that it does not have an explicit formulation for the Laplace transform, which makes this distribution less tractable. As a consequence, there is also no explicit formula

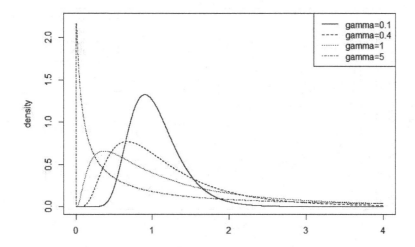

FIGURE 3.2
One-parameter log-normal density for different values of γ.

for the Kendall's τ. However, the value of the Kendall's τ induced by a log-normal frailty can be approximated using for example adaptive quadrature [265].

Positive stable distribution

A common alternative to the gamma frailty distribution is the positive stable frailty model, originally proposed as a frailty distribution by Hougaard [166], and this despite the fact that there is no close form expressions for the probability density and the survival function.

The family of (strict) stable distributions is a family of 2-parameters (a scale $\gamma > 0$ the so-called index $\alpha < 1$) distributions (see Chapter 6 of [121] for a formal definition). By imposing a single parameter $\gamma = \alpha$ to ensure identifiability and considering the single parameter $\nu = 1 - \alpha$, with $\nu \in (0, 1]$ to have a positive distribution, the density function of the one-parameter positive stable distribution is given by

$$f_U(u) = \frac{1}{\pi u} \sum_{k=1}^{\infty} \frac{\Gamma(k(1-\nu)+1)}{k!} (-u^{\nu-1})^k sin((1-\nu)k\pi)$$

This density function have a variety of shapes depending on the value of its parameter ν (see Figure 3.3, based on the R code of [170]).

Although there exists no close form for this density, the Laplace transform has a very simple expression

$$\mathscr{L} = \exp\left(-s^{1-\nu}\right) = \exp\left(-s^{\alpha}\right) \qquad s > 0 \qquad (3.16)$$

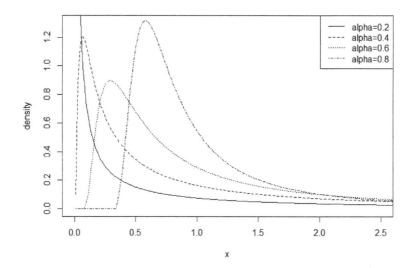

FIGURE 3.3
One-parameter positive stable density for different values of the $\alpha = 1 - \nu$ parameter

Furthermore, one has for $(q \geq 1)$ [402]

$$\mathscr{L}^{(q)}(s) = (-1)^q \left((1-\nu)s^{-\nu}\right)^q \left[\sum_{m=0}^{q-1} \Omega_{q,m} s^{m(1-\nu)}\right] \mathscr{L}(s)$$

where the $\Omega_{q,m}$'s are polynomial of degree m, given recursively by

$$\Omega_{q,0} = 1,$$
$$\Omega_{q,m} = \Omega_{q-1,m} + \Omega_{q-1,m-1}\left[\frac{q-1}{1-\nu} - (q-m)\right] \quad \text{for } m = 1, ..., q-2,$$
$$\Omega_{q,m} = (1-\nu)^{1-q}\frac{\Gamma(q-(1-\nu))}{\Gamma(\nu)} \quad \text{for } m = q-1$$

As for the gamma distribution, the simplicity of the Laplace transform (3.16), lead to a simple close form expressions for the unconditional (population) survival and hazard function

$$S^p(t \mid \mathbf{x}) = \exp\left(-H_{\mathbf{x}}^c(t)^{(1-\nu)}\right) \tag{3.17}$$
$$h^p(t \mid \mathbf{x}) = (1-\nu)h_{\mathbf{x}}^c(t)H_{\mathbf{x}}^c(t)^{-\nu} \tag{3.18}$$

where $H_{\mathbf{x}}(t) = H_0(t)\exp(\beta^t\mathbf{x})$ and $h_{\mathbf{x}}(t) = h_0(t)\exp(\beta^t\mathbf{x})$.

We also have a very simple expression for the Kendall's τ which is simply $\tau_{ln} = \nu$.

An important characteristics of the positive stable distribution is that the mean and variance are both undefined. This means that for this particular distribution, the heterogeneity parameter ν does not correspond to the variance of the frailty. This infinite mean is an important point since it leads to the property that the heteogeneity parameter is independent from the covariate information (Hougaard1988b, Wienke2010).

An other important property of the positive stable frailty model is that the proportional hazards assumption at the level of the condition hazards is preserved at the level of the (unconditional) population hazards, although not with the same proportionality constant [107]. Consider, for the sake of illustration, a single binary covariate X, from (3.18), we can write the population hazards ratio as

$$
\begin{aligned}
HR^p(t) = \frac{h^p(t \mid x = 1)}{h^p(t \mid x = 1)} &= \frac{(1 - \nu)h_0(t) \exp(\beta) \left(H_0(t) \exp(\beta)\right)^{-\nu}}{(1 - \nu)h_0(t) \exp(\beta) H_0^{-\nu}(t)} \\
&= \frac{1 + \theta H_0(t)}{1 + \theta H_0(t) \exp(\beta)} \exp(\beta) \\
&= \exp[(1 - \nu)\beta]
\end{aligned}
$$

which is indeed constant over time.

Inverse Gaussian distribution

Another possible frailty distribution is the Inverse Gaussian, which also benefit from a simple expression of the Laplace transform. Originally it is a 2-parameters family of distributions, but restricting the mean to one to ensure identifiability, the density function can be written

$$
f_U(u) = \frac{1}{\sqrt{(2\pi\theta)}} u^{-3/2} \exp\left(-\frac{(u - 1)^2}{2\theta u}\right) \qquad \theta > 0
$$

with mean 1 and variance θ. The more θ is close to 0, the more it resembles a normal distribution; when θ increases the density function becomes more and more skew (see left panel of Figure 3.4) with the right tail becoming heavier (see right panel of Figure 3.4), thus explaining the larger dispersion.

The Laplace transform is given by

$$
\mathscr{L}(s) = \exp\left(\frac{1}{\theta}(1 - \sqrt{1 + 2\theta s})\right) \tag{3.19}
$$

and for $q \geq 1$, we have [167, 265]

$$
\mathscr{L}^{(q)}(s) = (-1)^q (2\theta s + 1)^{-q/2} \frac{K_{q - \frac{1}{2}}\left((2\theta^{-1}(s + \frac{1}{2\theta}))\right)}{K_{\frac{1}{2}}\left(2\theta^{-1}(s + \frac{1}{2\theta})\right)} \mathscr{L}(s)
$$

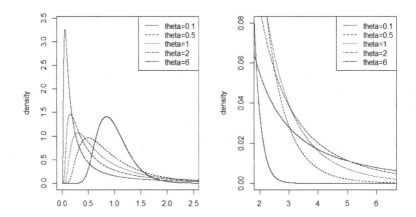

FIGURE 3.4
One-parameter inverse Gaussian density for different values of the θ parameter (*left*), with a zoom on the right tail (*right*).

where $K_\gamma(.)$ is the modified Bessel function of the second kind

$$K_\gamma(\omega) = \frac{1}{2} \int_0^\infty t^{\gamma-1} \exp\left[-\frac{\omega}{2}\left(t + \frac{1}{t}\right)\right] dt \quad \gamma \in R, \omega > 0$$

Given the simple expression of the Laplace transform (3.19) we have for the (unconditional) population survival and hazard function

$$
\begin{aligned}
S^p(t \mid \mathbf{x}) &= e^{\frac{1}{\theta}\left(1 - \sqrt{(1 + 2\theta H_\mathbf{x}^c(t))}\right)} \\
h^p(t \mid \mathbf{x}) &= \frac{h_\mathbf{x}^c(t)}{(1 + 2\theta H_\mathbf{x}^c(t))^{\frac{1}{2}}}
\end{aligned}
$$

where $H_\mathbf{x}(t) = H_0(t)\exp(\beta^t\mathbf{x})$ and $h_\mathbf{x}(t) = h_0(t)\exp(\beta^t\mathbf{x})$.

While the conditional HR is constant, the population hazards ratio is not constant since we can show that considering, for the sake of illustration, a single binary covariate X, we have

$$HR^p(t) = \frac{h^p(t \mid x = 1)}{h^p(t \mid x = 1)} = \frac{(1 + 2\theta H_0(t))^{1/2}}{(1 + 2\theta H_0(t)exp(\beta))^{1/2}} \exp(\beta)$$

Given (3.11), the Kendall'τ for an inverse Gaussian frailty is

$$\tau_{ig} = \frac{1}{2} - \frac{1}{\theta} + 2\frac{\exp(2/\theta)}{\theta^2} \int_{2/\theta}^\infty \frac{exp(-u)}{u} du$$

and one can show that $\tau < 1/2$ [107].

Power variance function distribution

The power variance function distribution has been introduced by independently by Tweedy [390] and Hougaard[166] who derived it as an extension of the positive stable distribution [165]. It contains the gamma, the inverse Gaussian and the positive stable as particular cases. However these distributions are obtained for choices of the parameters at the boundary of the parameter space and asymptotic arguments are needed to actually demonstrate that these distributions indeed belong to the power variance function distribution family. Duchateau and Janssen [107] discuss in detail how to obtain the gamma, inverse Gaussian and positive stable distribution as special cases.

The power variance function distribution is a 3-parameters distribution, and two different expressions, based either on the Aalen parametrization [4] or the Hougaard parametrization are commonly encountered [166]. Following the notations of Wienke [406], we write the density function as

$$
\begin{aligned}
f_U(u) \;=\; & \exp\left(-\lambda(1-\gamma)\left(\frac{u}{\mu}-\frac{1}{\gamma}\right)\right) \\
& \times \; \frac{1}{\pi}\sum_{k=1}^{\infty}(-1)^{k+1}\frac{(\lambda(1-\gamma))^{k(1-\gamma)}\mu^{k\gamma})}{\gamma^k}\frac{\Gamma(k\gamma+1)}{k!}z^{-k\gamma-1}\sin(k\gamma\pi)
\end{aligned}
$$

with $\mu > 0, \lambda > 0$, and $0 < \gamma \le 1$. One can show that $E[Z] = \mu$ and $Var[Z] = \frac{\mu^2}{\lambda}$, when it exists.

Imposing for identifiability purposes $E[Z] = \mu = 1$, and denoting $Var[Z] = 1/\lambda := \theta$ the heteorgenity parameter, it can be shown (although not easy, see [4]) that the Laplace transform is then given by

$$
\mathcal{L}(s) = \exp\left[\frac{1-\gamma}{\gamma\theta}\left(1-\left(1+\frac{\theta s}{1-\gamma}\right)^{\gamma}\right)\right] \tag{3.20}
$$

from which first and second derivatives can be obtained.

We can then derive the (unconditional) population survival and hazard function

$$
\begin{aligned}
S(t \mid \mathbf{x}) \;=\; & \exp\left[\frac{1-\gamma}{\gamma\theta}\left(1-\left(1+\frac{\theta H_{\mathbf{x}}^c(t)}{1-\gamma}\right)^{\gamma}\right)\right] \\
h(t \mid \mathbf{x}) \;=\; & \frac{h_{\mathbf{x}}^c(t)}{\left(1+\frac{\theta}{1-\gamma}H_{\mathbf{x}}^c(t)\right)^{1-\gamma}}
\end{aligned}
$$

Again, the conditional hazard ratio is constant but the population hazards ratio is not constant over time and considering, for the sake of illustration, a single binary covariate X, we have

$$
HR^p(t) = \frac{h^p(t \mid x=1)}{h^p(t \mid x=1)} = \left(\;\right)^{1-\gamma}\exp(\beta)
$$

We can show from the expression of the Laplace transform that the Kendall's τ is given by

$$\tau = (1-\gamma) - \frac{2(1-\gamma)}{\theta}$$
$$- \frac{4(1-\gamma)^2}{\theta^2\gamma} \exp\left(\frac{2(1-\gamma)}{\theta\gamma}\right) \int_1^\infty t^{-(1-\gamma)/\gamma} \exp\left(\frac{-2(1-\gamma)t}{\theta\gamma}\right) dt$$

Compound Poisson distribution

The Compound Poisson distribution was introduced by Aalen [3, 4] as a possible frailty distribution. An interesting feature of this distribution is that it leads to a subgroup of the population with a value zero of the frailty, therefore corresponding to the presence of a *cure fraction* (see Chapter 4), i.e. a fraction of individuals who will never experience the event of interest. Such a distribution will therefore be useful when a part of the individuals are not susceptible to the event of interest, this could be the case for example when studying time to occurrence of a given disease or time to relapse from a curable disease.

This distribution can be constructed as the sum of N independent and identically gamma distributed random variables, with N following a Poisson distribution. One can then see this distribution has being composed of two parts: a positive probability at zero (corresponding to $N = 0$) and a continuous subdensity on the positive real line (corresponding to $N > 0$).

With an appropriate parametrization, one can write this continuous subdensity on the positive real line with exactly same form as the density function of the positive stable distribution but with $\gamma > 1$. One can also show that with an appropriate parametrization, the Laplace transform of the Compound Poisson distribution is the same as the one of the power variance function, except for the range of the parameter γ [107]. As a consequence, the same holds for the expression of the (unconditional) population survival and hazard function.

We can therefore consider a broader class of distributions, defined by (3.20) (when assuming that $E[Z] = 1$) and $\gamma > 0$, and which is divided in two major sub-families according the value of γ, with $\gamma \le 1$ yielding to power variance function distributions and $\gamma > 1$ yielding to the compound Poisson distribution. The limiting case $\gamma = 1$ actually corresponds to a gamma distribution.

However, one has to note that, when $\gamma > 1$ the integral of the hazard function over $[0, \infty)$ is finite, corresponding to an improper survival function. Indeed, one can show that

$$\lim_{t\to\infty} S(t) = \lim_{t\to\infty} \exp\left[\frac{1-\gamma}{\gamma\sigma^2}\left(1 - \left(1 + \frac{\sigma^2\Lambda_0(t)}{1-\gamma}\right)^\gamma\right)\right]$$
$$= \exp\left(\frac{1-\gamma}{\gamma\sigma^2}\right) = P(U = 0)$$

As we will discuss in Chapter 4, this phenomenon is well known in the presence of a fraction of individuals not experiencing the event of interest, and the limiting value $\exp\left(\frac{1-\gamma}{\gamma\sigma^2}\right)$ is often referred to as the cure rate [304].

3.5 Estimation

Although they are used in different contexts, and parameters should be interpreted accordingly, from a modeling point of view, the univariate frailty model is a particular case of the shared multivariate frailty model. Estimation of these two family of models can therefore be considered in a similar way. All the estimation methods discussed here assume that the censoring is independent of the frailty.

The frailty model can be either parametric, in which case, the baseline hazard is specified in a parametric way or semi-parametric if the the baseline hazard is left unspecified. Flexible parametric solution, which for example assume a piecewise constant baseline hazards or use splines to model the hazard have also been proposed and are sometimes referred to as "flexible parametric" approach.

A difficulty in the estimation of the shared frailty model, is that the (conditional) likelihood function depend on the values of the frailty which are unobserved. Estimation is therefore based on the maximization of the marginal likelihood (also sometimes call the full likelihood). This marginal likelihood is obtained after integrating out the frailties from the conditional survival likelihood. The frailties are thus "averaged out" from the conditional likelihood and this marginal likelihood does not contain the frailty anymore.

Within the ith cluster, $i = 1, \ldots, s$, the contribution of each individual follows the same principal as for the likelihood in classical survival analysis (within a cluster, individuals are assumed to be independent). Following (2.1) and based on our model (3.8), the conditional likelihood for the ith cluster is given by

$$L_i(\xi \mid u_i) = \prod_{j=1}^{n_i} \left(h_0(y_{ij})u_i \exp(\beta^t \mathbf{x}_{ij})\right)^{\delta_{ij}} \exp\left(-H_0(y_{ij})u_i \exp(\beta^t \mathbf{x}_{ij})\right) \quad (3.21)$$

where ξ is the vector of parameters containing the regression parameters (β) and the parameters of the baseline hazard when it is specified in a parametric way.

The marginal likelihood for the ith cluster is obtained by integrating out the frailties with respect to their distribution

$$L_{marg,i}(\zeta) = \int_0^\infty \prod_{j=1}^{n_i} \left(h_0(y_{ij})u \exp(\beta^t \mathbf{x}_{ij})\right)^{\delta_{ij}} \exp\left(-H_0(y_{ij}u\beta^t \mathbf{x}_{ij})\right) f_U(u)du$$

$$(3.22)$$

where ζ contains the parameters of interest, i.e. the regression parameters (β), the parameters of the baseline hazard when it is specified in a parametric way, and the parameter(s) from the frailty distribution. The marginal likelihood is then obtained by considering the contribution of all clusters:

$$L_{marg}(\zeta) = \prod_{i=1}^{s} L_{marg,i}(\zeta) \tag{3.23}$$

3.5.1   Parametric frailty models

In parametric frailty models, one assumes a parametric distribution for the event times T. The baseline hazard is therefore assumed to be fully parametrically specified, typically assuming an exponential or a Weibull distribution of the event times, but other choices are possible such as in a classical parametric PH model. In this case, the estimation of such a parametric frailty model can be based on the maximization of the marginal likelihood. The parameters of the baseline hazard are estimated together with the regression coefficients and the parameters of the frailty distribution. The standard errors of the parameter estimates can then be obtained as the diagonal elements of the inverse of the Hessian matrix.

If we consider the case of a gamma frailty and a parametric baseline hazard, the integral in (3.22) can be solved analytically to obtain a close form expression for the marginal likelihood (3.23).

Indeed replacing in (3.22) $f_U(.)$ by the gamma density function,

$$f_U(u) = \frac{u^{1/\theta-1}}{\theta^{1/\theta}\Gamma(1/\theta)} \exp(-u/\theta) \tag{3.24}$$

one can solve this integral to obtain [107]

$$L_{marg,i}(\zeta) = \frac{\Gamma(d_i + 1/\theta) \prod_{j=1}^{n_i} \left(h_0(y_{ij})\exp(\beta^t\mathbf{x}_{ij})\right)^{\delta_{ij}}}{\left(1/\theta + \sum_{j=1}^{n_i} H_0(y_{ij}\exp(\beta^t\mathbf{x}_{ij}))\right)^{1/\theta+d_i} \theta^{1/\theta}\Gamma(1/\theta)} \tag{3.25}$$

and the marginal log-likelihood is then

$$l_{marg}(\zeta) = \sum_{i=1}^{s} \left[d_i log\theta - log\Gamma(1/\theta) + log\Gamma(1/\theta + d_i) \right.$$

$$-(1/\theta + d_i)log\left(1 + \theta\sum_{j=1}^{n_i} H_{ij,c}(y_{ij})\right)$$

$$\left. + \sum_{j=1}^{n_i} \delta_{ij}\left(\beta^t\mathbf{x}_{ij} + logh_0(y_{ij})\right) \right]$$

where $H_{ij,c}(y_{ij}) = H_0(y_{ij})\exp(\beta^t\mathbf{x}_{ij})$.

This marginal log-likelihood can be maximised to obtain the estimators for ζ. The asymptotic variance-covariance matrix of the vector ζ of parameters is the inverse of the Fisher information matrix $I(\zeta) = -E(\mathbf{H}(\zeta))$ and can be estimated as the inverse of the observed information matrix evaluated at $\hat{\zeta}$.

Such an integration is also possible for some other distributions, but lead to a more complex expression. On the other hand, an elegant formulation can be obtained using the Laplace transform of the frailty distribution (3.3). Indeed, the marginal log-likelihood of the observed data can be written [265]

$$
l_{marg}(\zeta) = \sum_{i=1}^{s} \left\{ \left[\sum_{j=1}^{n_i} (\log(h_0(y_{ij})) + \beta^t \mathbf{x}_{ij}) \right] \right.
$$
$$
+ \log \left[(-1)^{d_i} \mathscr{L}^{(d_i)} \left(\sum_{j=1}^{n_i} H_0(y_{ij}) \beta^t \mathbf{x}_{ij} \right) \right]
$$
$$
\left. - \log \left[\mathscr{L} \left(\sum_{j=1}^{n_i} H_0(\tau_{ij}) \beta^t \mathbf{x}_{ij} \right) \right] \right\}
$$

where $d_i = \sum_{j=1}^{n_i} \delta_{ij}$ is the number of events in cluster i and $\mathscr{L}^{(q)}(.)$ is the $q - th$ derivative of the Laplace transform of the frailty distribution.

When the baseline hazard is parametrically specified, estimates of ζ can be obtained obtained by maximizing this marginal log-likelihood; this however requires to compute high order derivatives of the Laplace transform $\mathscr{L}^{(q)}(s)$. Such a maximization will therefore be easy to perform when such high-order derivatives are easy to obtain; as is the case for the gamma, positive stable and inverse Gaussian distribution for which analytical expressions can be found, as shown in Section 3.4.2. Note that the Laplace transform does not exist in a closed form for a log-normal frailty and numerical approximation are required to get the marginal log-likelihood.

3.5.2 Semi-parametric frailty models

In a semi-parametric frailty model, one do not assume any particular distribution for the event times and thus the baseline hazard in model (3.8) is left unspecified. When the baseline hazard is left unspecified, we face the same problem as for the Cox PH model, namely that the marginal likelihood function can not be maximized anymore. We have seen in Chapter 2 that semi-parametric models are typically fitted through partial likelihood maximization. However, we now have to take into account the unobserved random frailty terms. In this situation, we can not apply the partial likelihood approach as such as the integration over the frailties leads to a more complex form of the likelihood (or even to no close form expression for this likelihood).

More elaborated techniques are therefore required to estimate the parameters of interest.

Three main approaches have been proposed, namely the Expectation-Maximization (EM) algorithm [86, 187, 272, 317, 392, 413], originally proposed for the case of a gamma frailty distribution; the penalized partial likelihood approach [253, 254, 318], usually used for the log-normal frailty distribution; and the penalized full likelihood estimation method for the gamma-frailty model [327]. As we will see, these two last approaches are different as the first one is based on a partial likelihood and penalize on the frailty distribution while the second is based on the full likelihood and penalize on the hazard function.

The EM algorithm approach

The EM algorithm has been widely used in various settings in statistics, and in particular when we have to face latent (or unobserved) information [100]. The EM algorithm iterates between an Expectation step (E-Step), in which the expected values of the unobserved information is obtained and a Maximization step (M-Step) maximizing the function of interest after having replaced the unobserved observation with their expected values from the E-Step. The EM algorithm is therefore particularly useful when it is easy to obtain expected values for the unobserved information and to perform the maximization given the expected values of the unobserved information. We will show below that this is indeed the case for the semi-parametric gamma frailty model [107].

In the particular context of the frailty models, the unobserved information corresponds to the frailty terms and the EM algorithm iterates between the computation of the expected values for these frailty terms, conditional on the observed information and the current parameter estimates (E-Step) and the maximization of the likelihood after having replaced the frailty terms by their expected values from the E-Step and considering them to be known. This leads to updated values for the parameter estimates (M-Step) to be used in the next iteration. A nice graphical presentation of the EM algorithm is given in [107].

To implement the EM algorithm, one first has to write down the *complete* likelihood, obtained by assuming that the frailties are actually observed. This complete likelihood is therefore obtained from the joint density of the really observed information $\mathbf{z}$, containing the observed times y_{ij} and the observed censoring indicators δ_{ij}, and of the unobserved frailties $\mathbf{u}$. Denoting ϕ the generic vector of the frailty density parameters, this complete likelihood is given by

$$
\begin{aligned}
L_{comp}(h_0(.), \phi, \beta) &= L_{comp,1}(\mathbf{z} \mid h_0(.), \beta, \mathbf{u}) \times L_{comp,2}(\mathbf{u} \mid \phi) \\
&= L_{comp,1}(h_0(.), \beta) \times L_{comp,2}(\phi) \qquad (3.26)
\end{aligned}
$$

with

$$l_{comp,1}(h_0(.),\beta) = \sum_{i=1}^{s} \sum_{j=1}^{n_i} \left[\delta_{ij} \log \left(h_0(y_{ij}) u_i \exp(\beta^t \mathbf{x}_{ij}) \right) - H_0(y_{ij} u_i \exp(\beta^t \mathbf{x}_{ij})) \right]$$

and

$$l_{comp,2}(\theta) = \sum_{i=1}^{s} \log f_U(u_i)$$

The EM algorithm has mainly been used when considering a gamma frailty model since in this case close form expressions are available for the conditional expectations of the frailties. The maximization step can then be performed using partial likelihood ideas to handle the unspecified baseline hazard. Assuming that the current parameter estimates at iteration k are $\zeta^{(k)} = (h_0^{(k)}(.), \beta^{(k)}, \theta^{(k)})$ the E-step and M-step works as follows:

E-Step: To obtain the expected values for the frailty terms conditional on the observed information and the current parameter estimates, one needs to compute the conditional distribution $f_U(u_i \mid \mathbf{z})$. From the Bayes theorem, we have

$$f_U(u_i \mid \mathbf{z}) = \frac{L_i(h_0(.), \beta \mid u_i) f_U(u_i)}{L_{marg,i}(h_0(.), \beta, \theta)}$$

and after plugging in this expression the conditional likelihood (3.21), the gamma density (3.24), and the expression of the marginal likelihood for a gamma frailty distribution (3.25), we obtain

$$f_U(u_i \mid \mathbf{z}) = \frac{u_i^{d_i + 1/\theta - 1} \exp\left(-u_i(1/\theta + H_{i,c}(y_i)) \right) (1/\theta + H_{i,c}(y_i))^{d_i + 1/\theta}}{\Gamma(d_i + 1/\theta)}$$

where $H_{i,c}(y_i) = \sum_{j=1}^{n_i} H_0(y_{ij}) \exp(\beta^t \mathbf{x}_{ij})$ is the conditional hazard. This can be shown to correspond to a gamma density with parameters $(d_i + 1/\theta)$ and $(1/\theta + H_{i,c}(y_i))$. From the properties of the gamma density, we have

$$E_{(k)}(U_i) = E_{\zeta^{(k)}}(U_i \mid \mathbf{z}) = \frac{(d_i + 1/\theta^{(k)})}{1/\theta^{(k)} + H_{i,c}^{(k)}(y_i)}$$

where $H_{i,c}^{(k)}(y_i)$ is obtained by replacing $H_0(y_{ij})$ and β by $H_0^{(k)}(y_{ij})$ and $\beta^{(k)}$ obtained at the previous step in $H_{i,c}(y_i)$. Also, since the conditional distribution of U_i given $\mathbf{z}$ is gamma, the conditional distribution of $\log(U_i)$ is log-gamma and it is therefore easy to derive the expected value

$$E_{(k)}(\log(U_i)) = \psi\left(d_i + 1/\theta^{(k)}\right) - \log\left(1/\theta^{(k)} + H_{i,c}^{(k)}(y_i)\right)$$

with $\psi(.)$ the digamma function, i.e. the first derivative of the logarithm of the gamma function.

M-Step: One replaces u_i and $\log(u_i)$ by the expected values $E_{(k)}(U_i)$ and $E_{(k)}(\log U_i)$ obtained in the previous E-Step in $L_{comp}(h_0(.), \beta, \theta)$. As can be seen from (3.26) one can maximize separately $l_{comp,1}(\theta)$ to estimate β (with $h_0(.)$ as a nuisance function) and $l_{comp,2}(\theta)$ to estimate θ. To maximize $l_{comp,1}(\theta)$ with respect to β the idea is to profile $l_{comp,1}(h_0(.), \beta)$ to a partial likelihood (by considering the frailties as fixed offset terms). Using the current estimate of β, one can obtain the Nelson-Aalen estimator of the baseline hazard with the frailties considered to be known offset terms, as this value is required in the E-Step. We then move back to the E-Step with the new current parameter estimates $\zeta^{(k+1)} = (h_0^{(k+1)}(.), \theta^{(k+1)}, \beta^{(k+1)})$.

As starting values, θ can be set to 1, and β can be set equal to the values estimated from a Cox PH model. The convergence is usually assessed once the absolute difference between 2 successive values of the marginal log-likelihood below are below a preset value. Estimated variances of the estimators can be obtained from the diagonal elements of the inverse of the observed $(r + p + 1) \times (r + p + 1)$ information matrix of the marginal log-likelihood. Nielsen et al. [272] have shown that the rate of convergence of the EM algorithm can be improved by using a modified profile likelihood.

The EM algorithm can also be used for other choices of the distribution of the frailty, and in particular for normal random effects under the model specification

$$h_{ij}(t) = h_0(t) \exp(\beta^t \mathbf{x}_{ij} + w_i) \tag{3.27}$$

with $w_i \sim N(0, \gamma)$ A difficulty then is that there is usually no close form expression for the marginal likelihood and several versions of the EM algorithm have been proposed, which differ mainly in the way the E-Step is conducted. See for example Cortinas et al. [86] who propose to use the Laplace approximation to compute the conditional expectations in the E-step, and who compare some proposed approach via an intensive simulation study. An alternative approach to estimate the parameters of model (3.27) assuming a normal distribution of the random effects is the penalized partial likelihood approach as discussed below.

The penalized partial likelihood approach

This approach, originally proposed for the log-normal frailty model, is usually described using the formulation of the frailty model

$$h_{ij}(t \mid w_i) = h_0(t) \exp(\beta^t \mathbf{x}_{ij} + w_i)$$

with $w_i \sim N(0, \gamma)$ [253, 254].

This approach is actually based on the same factorization of the complete data likelihood in two parts as (3.26) noting that:

- the first part $L_{comp,1}(h_0(.), \beta)$ corresponds to the conditional likelihood of the data given the frailty;

- the second part $L_{comp,2}(\phi)$ corresponds to the distribution of the random effects which is now seen as a penalty term; the idea being that the values of the random effects that are far away from the mean are associated with a large negative contribution to the full data log-likelihood.

Considering the model expression (3.28), the idea is then to consider the random effects as additional parameters and to replace $L_{comp,1}(h_0(.), \beta)$ by a partial likelihood, similar the one considered from a Cox PH model (see (2.21)). This leads to the penalized partial likelihood

$$l_{ppl}(\gamma, \beta, w) = l_{part}(\beta, w) - l_{pen}(\gamma, w) \tag{3.28}$$

with

$$l_{part}(\beta, w) = \sum_{i=1}^{s}\sum_{j=1}^{n_i} \delta_{ij}\left[(x_{ij}^t\beta + w_i) - \log\left(\sum_{lk \in R(y_{ij})} \exp(x_{lk}^t\beta + w_l)\right)\right]$$

and

$$\begin{aligned} l_{pen}(\gamma, w) &= -\sum_{i=1}^{s}\log f_W(w_i) \\ &= \frac{1}{2}\sum_{i=1}^{s}\left(\frac{w_i^2}{\gamma} + \log(2\pi\gamma)\right) \end{aligned}$$

when we assume that the random effects w_i follows a $N(0, \gamma)$ distribution.

However, one has to take into account the fact that the w_i are in fact unobserved random effect and not fixed effect. So, the maximization then alternates between an inner and an outer loop until convergence, see [107] for a nice graphical representation:

Inner loop: For the current value of γ, a Newton-Raphson algorithm is used to maximize $l_{ppl}(\gamma, \beta, w)$ for β as well as to obtain best linear unbiased predictors (BLUP) of the random effects w.

Outer loop: Following the idea of restricted maximum likelihood (REML) from the (generalized) linear mixed model methodology, the idea is obtain an updated value for γ using the current BLUPs for w.

The inner loop requires the convergence of the Newton-Raphson algorithm and the outer loop is iterated until $|\gamma^{(l)} - \gamma^{(l+1)}|$ is sufficiently small. Asymptotic variances for $\hat{\beta}$ and $\hat{\gamma}$ can be obtained from the V matrix used in the Newton-Raphson procedure [253, 254].

The penalized partial likelihood approach can also be used for other frailty distribution. While the inner loop is generally the same, this is not the case for the outer loop. For the gamma frailty PH model, no REML estimates are available for θ in the outer loop. The maximization of a profile version of the marginal likelihood for θ can be used instead. It has been shown that for a gamma frailty PH model, the PPL approach lead to the same values of the estimators as the EM algorithm [107, 376].

The penalized full likelihood estimation approach

Another possibility is to specify the baseline hazard in a parametric but very flexible way, such as assuming a piecewise constant hazard or using splines to specify the hazard function. This approach has been introduced for gamma frailty model by [327] and further developed in [330, 333] in particular for more complex models including more than one random effect (see Section 3.6)

As already mentioned, one can take advantage of the mathematical convenience induced by the gamma frailty distribution to obtain an analytical expression of the marginal likelihood. However, this marginal likelihood can not be directly maximized due to the presence of the unspecified hazard function. Furthermore, one can not easily transpose the idea of the Cox partial likelihood due to the complexity of this marginal likelihood obtained after integrating out the unobserved frailties. The idea is therefore to replace the baseline hazard by a highly flexible specification and penalizing at the level of the marginal likelihood for the smoothness of the baseline hazard estimation. This approach is therefore different from the approach of the penalized partial likelihood described above and which penalizes on the frailty distribution. Since this approach does not rely on the partial likelihood and actually maximize the "full" marginal likelihood, it is often referred to as the *penalized full likelihood approach* by opposition to the *penalized partial likelihood*. An advantage of this approach is that it allows a "non-parametric" (in reality a "flexible parametric") estimation of the hazard function.

As we have seen in Section 3.5.1, assuming a gamma frailty distribution allows to integrate the random effects out of the conditional likelihood and to analytically obtain the marginal likelihood (3.23). Rondeau et al. [327] actually base their penalized full likelihood estimation approach on a slightly different formulation of the marginal log-likelihood, which has been proposed by [190, 272], and in which the gamma function does not appear anymore making the computations easier

$$l_{marg}(h_0(t), \beta, \theta) = \sum_{i=1}^{s} \left[I_{d_i \neq 0} \sum_{m=1}^{d_i} \left[\log\left(1 + \theta(d_i - m)\right) \right] \right. \tag{3.29}$$

$$-(1/\theta + d_i) log \left[1 + \theta \sum_{j=1}^{n_{ik}} H_0(y_{ij} \exp(\beta^t \mathbf{x}_{ij})) \right] \tag{3.30}$$

$$\left. + \sum_{j=1}^{n_i} \delta_{ij} (\beta^t \mathbf{x}_{ij} + \log h_0(y_{ij})) \right] \tag{3.31}$$

As discussed in Section 3.5.1, if the baseline hazard function is specified parametrically, then the marginal likelihood (3.23), re-expressed here as (3.31), can be maximized to obtain maximum likelihood estimators. The idea here is therefore to specify this baseline hazard in a very flexible way and to jointly estimate the regression parameters β, the frailty parameter θ, and the baseline hazard function $h_0(t)$ assuming the latter to be a smooth function. Classically, this can be achieved by penalizing the likelihood with a term that takes large value for rough functions. Following [179, 275], the *maximum penalized likelihood estimators* (MPnLE) of $h_0(t), \beta$ and θ are then obtained by maximizing

$$l_{pmarg}(h_0(t), \beta, \theta) = l_{marg}(h_0(t), \beta, \theta) - \kappa \int_0^\infty (h_0^{''}(t))^2 dt$$

with $l_{marg}(h_0(t), \beta, \theta)$ the marginal log-likelihood (3.31) defined above, $(h_0^{''}(t))^2$ the squared second derivative of $h_0(t)$ and $\kappa \geq 0$ a positive smoothing parameter. In practice, the integral appearing in the penalization term is computed over the period where at least one subject is still at risk. It is common to see this expression as a trade-off between *faithfulness* to the data, as captured by $l_{marg}(.)$ and *smoothness* of the baseline hazard estimation, as measured by the squared norm of the second derivative of the hazard $(h_0^{''}(t))^2$ [327]. For large values of κ the term $\int_0^\infty (h_0^{''}(t))^2 dt$ will be highly penalizing the likelihood and thus the estimation of the corresponding hazard will be forced to tend to a linear function of time. On the other hand, for small value of κ, the likelihood is less penalized and the main contribution to $l_{pmarg}(.)$ for the estimation of the corresponding hazard comes from $l_{marg}(h_0(t), \beta, \theta)$. The resulting estimate of $h_{0(.)}$ will track the data more closely but will also be more irregular.

While the exact computation of the maximum penalized likelihood estimator of a non-parametric regression functions have been studied in a broader context [354], the exact computation of such a MPnLE of $\hat{h}_0(.)$ is in fact not possible here, and Rondeau et al. [327] therefore propose to approximate it using splines. So, an approximation $\tilde{h}_0(.)$ of the MPnLEs $\hat{h}_0(.)$ is obtained considering a linear combination of polynomial functions (splines), such that

$$\tilde{h}_0(.) = \sum_{l=1}^m \tilde{\eta}_l M_l(.)$$

where the $M_i(.)$ are cubic M-splines [313], i.e. splines of order 4 and m is the number of splines. An approximate estimator of the baseline cumulative hazard can also be obtained with the same coefficients with $\tilde{H}_0(.) = \sum_{i=1}^m \tilde{\eta}_i I_i(.)$, where $I(.)$ are I-splines (or integrated M-splines) defined as $I_i(x) = \int_0^x M_i(s)ds$.

To maximize the penalized marginal likelihood $l_{pmarg}(.)$ with respect to the vector of parameters $\xi = (\eta^t, \beta^t, \theta)$ [327] proposes to use the robust Marquardt algorithm [247] and at each step of the algorithm to restrict all the spline coefficients ζ_l to be positive for numerical convenience.

A point of discussion is of course the choice of the smoothing parameters κ. When applicable, a practical approach consists of heuristically determining the smoothing parameters by considering the survival curves obtained with different values of κ. However, [327] also proposed to determine the smoothing parameter by maximizing a cross-validation score $C\bar{V}(\kappa)$ originally proposed for a Cox PH model [275]. Interestingly, this criterion can in fact be seen as an AIC criterion. Another possible approach, discussed in [327], is to introduce *a priori knowledge* by fixing the number of degrees of freedom to estimate the hazard function. One can then use the relation linking the model degrees of freedom and the smoothing parameter κ given by [51, 146] to evaluate the smoothing parameter. The idea is that it is easier to specify a degrees of freedom to estimate a given curve (e.g., 2 degrees of freedom to estimate a straight line, 3 for a quadratic curve, ...) than specifying a smoothing parameter.

It is important to note that $\tilde{h}_0(.)$ is actually an approximation of the MPnLE $\hat{h}_0(.)$. However increasing the number of knots will make the approximation error as small as we want. The asymptotic normality and consistency of the MPnLE is discussed by [327] who propose two estimators of the asymptotic variance of the estimators of the splines coefficients, of the regression coefficients and of the heterogeneity parameter θ. These can for example be used to obtain pointwise confidence bands for $\tilde{h}_0(t)$. However, these variance estimators do not take into account the variability due to the choice of the smoothing parameter.

Note that this approach easily accommodates a stratified gamma frailty model, i.e. a model allowing a different baseline hazard in different pre-defined strata [327]. The idea is then to use the same basis of spline for all strata and to consider that only the coefficients η_{ki} are different between the strata $k = 1, ..., K$.

3.6   Extensions of the shared frailty model

Several extensions of the frailty model have been proposed. In this section, we shortly present two "main" extensions and references for further extensions are given in Section 3.8. First we consider the case of *nested frailty models*, when observations are grouped into clusters but with two (or more) hierarchical levels of clustering. Such models could be used for example when considering patients grouped in hospitals, and hospitals being grouped in geographical area or countries. We then consider an extension of the shared frailty models which has been proposed to investigate a potential interaction between an known exposition factor (such as the treatment in a clinical trial) and the cluster structure. When we consider data from a multi-center trial, with patients grouped within hospitals (or centers), it may be indeed be interesting to consider not only the heterogeneity between centers but also to study a potential treatment-by-center interaction. Extension of the shared frailty model introducing a random interaction has been proposed and such an *additive frailty model* has been studied by different authors. A similar model can also be used to quantify trial and treatment heterogeneity in individual patient data meta-analysis [334] or in the context of validation of prognostic index [221].

Nested frailty models

The main idea of the shared frailty models is that individuals belonging to the same cluster, e.g. patients treated in the same hospital or members of the same family, share unobserved characteristics that can be modeled via the inclusion of a shared frailty. However, in some situation, they may be two (or more) levels of *hierarchical clustering*, considering for example family members being clustered in households and households being clustered in villages. Another example would be occurrence of recurrent events in patients treated different hospitals in a multi-center clinical trial. Nested frailty models, also called multilevel frailty models, account for this particular structure in the data by including two (or more) nested random effects that acts multiplicatively on the hazard function [107, 328, 333].

Assume we have G clusters, and S_i sub-clusters in cluster i, and denote T_{ijk} the time-to-event for the kth subject ($k = 1, ..., n_{ij}$) from the jth sub-cluster ($j = 1, ..., S_i$) in the ith cluster ($i = 1, ..., G$), and $\mathbf{x}_{ijk}$ the vector of covariates value for this individual. According to the nested frailty model, the conditional hazard for this individual is then given by

$$h_{ijk}(t \mid u_i, z_{ij}) = h_0(t) u_i z_{ij} \exp(\beta^t \mathbf{x}_{ijk}) \tag{3.32}$$
$$= u_i z_{ij} h_{ijk}^c(t) \tag{3.33}$$

In such a model, the frailty z_{ij} captures all the unobserved factors that make the observations of the jth sub-cluster ($j = 1, ..., S_i$) in the ith cluster ($i = 1, ..., G$) more alike (e.g., the factors shared by all the members of a same households such as factors linked to socioeconomics level, life habits, ...) while the frailty u_i represents the unobserved factors common to all sub-clusters belonging to cluster i (such as for example environmental factors common to all households of a village). A larger variance of z_{ij} (resp. u_i) implies a larger heterogeneity across sub-clusters (resp. clusters) and a greater correlation between observations (resp. sub-clusters) within the same sub-cluster (resp. cluster).

Assuming that both the cluster and the sub-cluster random effects are independent and identically distributed (i.i.d.) and follow a one-parameter gamma distribution, the penalized full likelihood estimation approach presented previously can be generalized [328, 333]. However, an additional difficulty arise from the fact although the frailty density at the sub-cluster level can still be integrated out analytically, this is not rue anymore for the integration with respect to the frailty at the cluster level. A possibility is then to compute these integrals (one for each frailty term at the higher cluster level) numerically via Gaussian quadrature. The first and second derivatives of the penalized marginal likelihood, from which the Hessian and therefore the asymptotic variance-covariance matrix is obtained, can also be calculated numerically.

Additive frailty models

It has become quite popular to extend model (3.5.2) by adding a random interaction between the random effect and a covariate:

$$h_{ij}(t \mid w_{0i}, w_{1i}) = h_0(t) \exp(w_{0i} + (\beta + w_{1i})x_{ij}) \tag{3.34}$$

Such a model has been proposed for example to study the heterogeneity in treatment effect over centers in a multi-center clinical trial or the heterogeneity in treatment effect between the different clinical trials included in a meta-analysis. Indeed, in both situations, it may be interesting to have not only an estimate of the global treatment effect over all centers (or trials in a meta-analytic context) but also about the heterogeneity of this treatment effect between centers (or trials). In this case, x_{ij} is the treatment indicator for patient i of cluster j ($i = 1, \ldots, n_i; j = 1, \ldots J$), β is the fixed treatment effect, and $\mathbf{w}^t = (w_0^t, w_1^t)$ the vector of random effect. It is convenient to assume that the random effects follow a bivariate normal distribution with mean 0 and variance-covariance $V(\theta)$. One can interpret w_{0i} as the influence of the ith center (or trial in a meta-analytic context) on the overall underlying baseline risk and w_{1i} as the influence of the ith center (or trial) on the overall treatment effect (β). A larger variance of w_{0i} represents a greater heterogeneity across centers (or trials in a meta-analytic contexts) and a stronger correlation of the event times of the patients treated in the same center. On the other hand, a larger variance of w_{1i} indicates a a larger heterogeneity in the treatment effects over the different centers (or trials in a meta-analytic context), with possibly treatment effect in different directions in the different centers which would obviously be problematic. On the other hand, a zero variance of w_{1i} would indicate that the treatment effect is homogeneous over the different centers (or trials in a meta-analytical context). Of note, these two random effects may be correlated, for example if we expect higher treatment effect in centers already showing better outcomes for the patients.

While the variance θ_0 and θ_1 of these two random effects is of particular interest as they represent respectively the heterogeneity in outcome between the different clusters and the heterogeneity in the (binary) variable X effect between clusters, their value is difficult to interpret. One can therefore translate the impact of the heterogeneity parameters θ_1 and θ_2 on more interpretable quantities following the same idea as in Section 3.5.1. Assuming for example a Weibull baseline hazard ($h_0(t) = \lambda \rho t^{\rho-1}$), we can for the interpretation of θ_1 consider the density function of the median survival time in the group with $x = 0$ (control) given by

$$f_{M_c}(m_c) = \frac{\rho}{m_c \sqrt{2\pi\theta_0}} \exp\left(-\frac{1}{2\theta_0}\left(\ln\left(\frac{\ln 2}{\lambda m_c^\rho}\right)\right)^2\right)$$

Regarding the interpretation of θ_2, we can look at the density function of the hazard ratio over centers given by

$$f_{HR}(h) = \frac{1}{h\sqrt{2\pi\theta_1}} \exp\left(-\frac{1}{2\theta_1}(\ln h - \beta)^2\right)$$

A simultaneous interpretation of both θ_1 and θ_2 is less straightforward. A possibility is to consider the density function of the median survival in the group with $x = 1$ (experimental) for fixed values (for example quantiles) of the center random effect

$$f_{M_e}(m_e) = \frac{\rho}{m_e\sqrt{2\pi\theta_1}} \exp\left(-\frac{1}{2\theta_1}\left(\ln\left(\frac{\ln 2}{\lambda m_e^\rho}\right) - w_0 - \beta\right)^2\right)$$

Model (3.34) can be easily extended to incorporate other covariates, which allow for example to adjust the model for some baseline prognostic factors of the patients [333]. The model can then be written

$$h_{ij}(t \mid w_{0i}, w_{1i}) = h_0(t) \exp\left(w_{0i} + w_{1i}x_{1ij} + \beta^t \mathbf{x}_{ij}\right)$$

where $\mathbf{X}_{ij}$ is a vector of covariates whose first component is the variable x_{1ij} (e.g., treatment) for which we consider an interaction.

The marginal likelihood for model (3.34) and (3.35) can not be obtained in an analytical close form and various estimation procedures have been proposed to overcome this. For example, one can generalize the penalized full likelihood approach described before while approximating the integrals with no analytical solution with a Laplace integration technique; see [87, 150, 196, 223].

3.7 Software and examples revisited

Frailty models can nowadays be fitted in most major standard statistical software such as R , SAS , and Stata. One should however recognized that R is particularly rich in terms of available packages to fit different types of frailty models with various estimation procedures.

In R, the standard package for classical survival analysis survival [374] can actually be used with the usual coxph function to fit a (simple) semi-parametric model with a gamma or log-normal frailty, using the penalized partial likelihood approach. The coxme package [373], which is actually an extension of the survival package for frailty models, allows to fit semi-parametric model with log-normal frailty using the penalized partial likelihood estimation procedure of [318]. While this package is restricted to log-normal frailty, it has the advantage that it allows to consider correlated frailties.

The parfm R package [337] is limited to parametric frailty models but offer some nice features. Various parametric models (exponential, Weibull, Gompertz, log-normal, log-logistic baseline hazard) with various frailty distributions (gamma, inverse Gaussian, positive stable) can be fitted. The objective of this package is to offer a large choice of frailty distribution and parametric baseline hazard. These parametric frailty models are fitted via the maximization of the marginal log-likelihood [265].

The `frailtyEM` R package [24], on the other hand, is as we can understand from his name, based on the EM approach and allows to fit a wide range of parametric (exponential, Weibull, Gaussian, logistic, log-normal or log-logistic) and semi-parametric models with different frailty distribution (gamma, positive stable, and power variance family distribution). This package is specifically dedicated to the analysis of clustered data (and allows in this case left truncation) as well as to the analysis of recurrent events with different data format allowed [25].

An important R package for frailty models is `frailypack` [329], which allows to fit frailty models as well as a wide range of extensions. In the `frailypack` package, parametric (Weibull) and flexible semi-parametric (baseline hazard specified as piecewise constant or via penalized splines) gamma and log-normal frailty model can be fitted. More complex models, such as nested and additive models, as well as correlated random effects models can also be fitted. For several of these models, stratification of the baseline hazard and introduction of time-dependent covariates is possible as well as the handling of left-truncated and interval-censored data. The package also allows to fit (bivariate and trivariate) joint models (see Chapter 6). The estimation is based on the penalized full likelihood estimation approach described in Section 3.5.2. Maximization of the penalized full likelihood is based on the robust Marquardt algorithm [247], which combines a Newton-Raphson algorithm and a steepest descent algorithm [331, 333].

In `SAS`, the standard `proc phreg` procedure for a standard Cox PH model also allows to fit a semi-parametric frailty model with a gamma or a log-normal frailty. Estimation is based on the penalized partial likelihood approach. If we consider parametric frailty model, the main difficulty is actually to integrate out the random effect to obtain the marginal likelihood to be maximized. The `proc nlmixed` can be used to approximate this marginal likelihood by Gaussian quadrature to fit a parametric models with a log-normal frailty.

The `STATA` software also offer possibilities to fit frailty models, for example via the `streg` command which fit a parametric frailty model (but in an AFT formulation) with various choice of hazard (exponential, Weibull, Gompertz, log-normal, log-logistic, and general gamma) and gamma or inverse Gaussian frailty.

A review of main available software to fit a frailty model, with a comparison of some of them is presented in [163], see also [27] for references to more recent R packages.

3.7.1 Diabetic retinopathy data

We come back now to the diabetic retinopathy dataset introduced in Section 1.3.3 of Chapter 1 and available in the R package `survival`. A particularity of this dataset is that it contains information, and in particular time to loss of vision, for both eyes of the patients with one eye treated with the experimental treatment and the other being used as control. This dataset contains 197 patients and is therefore composed of 394 observations (two per patient).

Since these data contains two measurements per patient (one for each eyes), these data are obviously clustered, with all cluster sizes equal to two. Note that we have 80 patients having both eyes censored, 63 patients having an event for the control eye and not for the treated eye, 16 patients with the opposite situations, and 38 patients with an event for both eye. This leads to a total of 155 events.

For the sake of illustration, let's first concentrate only on the treatment effect, with no further adjustment. If we ignore the correlation structure, a Cox PH model can be simply be fitted as

```
> Ret.Cox.trt <- coxph(Surv(futime, status)~trt,data=retinopathy)
> summary(Ret.Cox.trt)
Call:
coxph(formula = Surv(futime, status) ~ trt,data=retinopathy)

  n= 394, number of events= 155

       coef exp(coef) se(coef)      z Pr(>|z|)
trt -0.7766    0.4600   0.1688 -4.602 4.19e-06 ***
---
Signif. codes:  0 '***' 0.001 '**' 0.01 '*' 0.05 ''. 0.1 '' 1

      exp(coef) exp(-coef) lower .95 upper .95
trt        0.46      2.174    0.3304    0.6403

Concordance= 0.59  (se = 0.02 )
Rsquare= 0.055   (max possible= 0.988 )
Likelihood ratio test= 22.37  on 1 df,   p=2e-06
Wald test            = 21.17  on 1 df,   p=4e-06
Score (logrank) test = 22.25  on 1 df,   p=2e-06
```

A parametric model could also be fitted, considering the for example a Weibull baseline hazard. While the `coxph` function would then provide results in a log-linear representation, an alternative is to use the **parfm** package without frailty, as

```
> Ret.Weib.trt <- parfm(Surv(futime, status)~trt, dist="weibull",
     frailty="none",data=retinopathy)
> Ret.Weib.trt

Frailty distribution: none
Baseline hazard distribution: Weibull
Loglikelihood: -836.379

        ESTIMATE SE      p-val
rho       0.810  0.058
lambda    0.032  0.008
trt      -0.790  0.169 <.001 ***
---
Signif. codes:  0 '***' 0.001 '**' 0.01 '*' 0.05 '.' 0.1 ' ' 1
```

```
> ci.parfm(Ret.Weib.trt, level=0.05)["trt",]
   low    up
 0.326  0.632
```

Results are actually very close based either on the semi-parametric or on the Weibull parametric PH model, with a highly significant decrease in the time to loss of vision for the treated eye compared to the control arm.

Any of the two models above, could also be adjusted for other covariates, for example we consider below adjustment for the type of diabetes and the risk score (considered as a numerical variable) in the semi-parametric Cox PH model:

```
> Ret.Cox.trt.adj <- coxph(Surv(futime, status)~trt+type+risk)
> Ret.Cox.trt.adj
Call:
coxph(formula = Surv(futime, status) ~ trt + type + risk, data=
    retinopathy)

               coef  exp(coef)  se(coef)        z         p
trt        -0.78151    0.45772   0.16902   -4.624  3.77e-06
typeadult   0.07017    1.07269   0.16229    0.432   0.66546
risk        0.14702    1.15837   0.05598    2.626   0.00863

Likelihood ratio test=29.51  on 3 df, p=1.746e-06
n= 394, number of events= 155
```

In both models, the treatment effect is about the same with a HR of about 0.458, corresponding to an important reduction in time to blindness for the treated eyes compared to the control eyes. In the adjusted model, the type of diabetes seems to have little impact while the risk score of the eye has a significant impact. Note that the latter has here been considered as a continuous variable, thus assuming the same coefficient for an increase in risk for 6 to 7, as from 7 to 8, and so on. This could be easily relaxed by introducing this variable as a factor in the model, thus replacing `risk` by `as.factor(risk)`.

The results of PH models (containing only the `trt` covariate), leaving the baseline hazard unspecified, assuming a parametric baseline hazard (Weibull or log-normal), or specified in a flexible way (piecewise constant or using splines) are reported in Table 3.1. The estimated treatment effect from all these models are very close, with a slight difference however with the estimated treatment effect obtained from a model assuming a piecewise constant hazard. These results however should be interpreted with care since they assume independence between the observations made on the two eyes of a same patient, a highly improbable assumption in this case. Indeed, it seems quite obvious that the two eyes of a same patients have much more in common than eyes of different patients, and this beyond the measured covariates. Therefore, the measurements made on the same patient are expected to be more correlated than the measurements made on different patients.

We will now see how to analyze these data while taking the clustering in the data into account and how it may, or may not, influence the results obtained and their interpretation.

A first idea could be to add patient as a fixed effect, however this would lead to a huge increase in the numbers of parameters (actually adding 196 parameters in the models) and to problem of convergence. The interpretation would also then be odd, as the patient efixed effect estimated would be specific to the particular patients included in the analysis. A better alternative is to rather consider patient as a stratification factor. This indeed avoid the increase in the number of parameters (at least when leaving the baseline hazard unspecified) and have results somewhat more interpretable. A stratified Cox PH model can be easily fitted in R adding a **strata** term to the **coxph** function from the standard **survival** package.

```
> Ret.Cox.trt.strat <- coxph(Surv(futime, status)~trt+strata(id),
    data=retinopathy)
> Ret.Cox.trt.strat
Call:
coxph(formula = Surv(futime, status) ~ trt + strata(id))

        coef exp(coef) se(coef)       z       p
trt -0.9623    0.3820   0.2016  -4.773 1.82e-06

Likelihood ratio test=25.49  on 1 df, p=4.455e-07
n= 394, number of events= 155
```

However, such an approach may not be optimal. First, one has to be aware that the clusters in which all observations are censored do not contribute to the likelihood, in this case this corresponds to 80 clusters (40.6% of all clusters). We can indeed check that we obtain exactly the same results, when fitting our stratified model on a subset from which observations from clusters without an event have been removed (the vector **Subset.id** contains the id number of the patients in clusters for which at least one event has been reported).

```
> Sub.Cox.trt.strat <- coxph(Surv(futime, status)~trt+strata(id),
    subset=(retinopathy$id %in% Subset.id))
> Sub.Cox.trt.strat
Call:
coxph(formula = Surv(futime, status) ~ trt + strata(id), subset =
    (retinopathy$id %in%
    Subset.id))

        coef exp(coef) se(coef)       z       p
trt -0.9623    0.3820   0.2016  -4.773 1.82e-06

Likelihood ratio test=25.49  on 1 df, p=4.455e-07
n= 234, number of events= 155
```

As we can see, the number of events remain the same (which is expected since we only removed patients with no event) but the number of observations (**cluster**) have now decreased from 394 to 234 (we have 2 observations per patient for 80 patients). Note that with this model, we are not able to adjust further for covariates which have been measured at the cluster level, such as the type of diabetes or the age at diagnosis.

Another possibility is to adjust what is often referred to as a marginal model. Following the generalized estimating equation (GEE) approach, the idea is to fit a Cox PH model under a working assumption of independence (independence working model), but then to correct the estimate of the standard error of the estimated coefficient to take into account, or to correct, for the presence of correlation between the observations from the same cluster. The estimates obtained under this independence working model can be shown to be, under some conditions, consistent even if they ignore correlations (see [107] for a proof the particular setting of bivariate survival data and [359] for the more general setting of multivariate survival data). This can be done using a sandwich-type estimator of the variance [228] and is implemented in the coxph function via the addition of a cluster term in the expression of the model:

```
> Ret.Cox.trt.marg <- coxph(Surv(futime, status)~trt+cluster(id),
    data=retinopathy)
> Ret.Cox.trt.marg
Call:
coxph(formula = Surv(futime, status) ~ trt + cluster(id), data=
    retinopathy)

          coef exp(coef) se(coef) robust se       z       p
trt -0.7766    0.4600    0.1688    0.1475 -5.267 1.39e-07

Likelihood ratio test=22.37  on 1 df, p=2.246e-06
n= 394, number of events= 155
```

As expected, the results in term of estimated coefficients are exactly the same. However, we now have the value of a robust se corresponding to the corrected standard errors. This standard error is slightly lower than the one obtained ignoring clustering. The treatment effect obtained from this marginal model, should be interpreted at the level of the population. It represents the effect of treatment for any two individuals, one from treated with control and one treated with experimental while ignoring the presence of cluster.

While the stratified and the marginal model can be used to account for clustering, they actually do not provide any information about the heterogeneity between the clusters nor on the intra-cluster correlations, which can also be of interest. To do so, we can fit a frailty model with a shared random effect for the two eyes of a same individual. This shared random effects will therefore model all what is common between the two eyes of a same person and which is not captured by the fixed effects included in the model (e.g., genetical material, life habits, ...). A semi-parametric frailty model with a gamma frailty can be fitted with the coxph function specifying a frailty term in the expression of the model.

```
> Ret.SPF.trt.gamma <- coxph(Surv(futime, status)~trt+frailty(id)
    , data=retinopathy)
> Ret.SPF.trt.gamma
Call:
coxph(formula = Surv(futime, status) ~ trt + frailty(id), data=
    retinopathy)
```

```
                 coef se(coef)      se2   Chisq    DF        p
trt            -0.910     0.174   0.171  27.295   1.0  1.7e-07
frailty(id)                             114.448  84.6    0.017


Iterations: 6 outer, 30 Newton-Raphson
      Variance of random effect= 0.854    I-likelihood = -850.9
Degrees of freedom for terms=   1.0 84.6
Likelihood ratio test=201   on 85.6 df, p=3e-11
n= 394, number of events= 155
```

Note that when adding a frailty term in the model, the `coxph` output then produces two different estimates of the standard errors of the coefficients (`se(coef)` and `se2`), the second one being a variation of the sandwich estimator. Based on the work of [376], [260] advises to use the first one. The gamma distribution is the default, but a normal distribution for the random effects can also be used, specifying `frailty(id, distribution="gaussian")`. Results are shown in Table 3.2.

Note that compared to the marginal model above, the interpretation here is conditional on the value of the frailty (so cluster-specific), and the estimated treatment effect is therefore now conditional on a given cluster.

After having loaded the `coxme` package,

```
library(coxme)
```

we can fit a shared random effect in the form (3.5.2) assuming a normal distribution of the random effect

```
> Ret.SPF.trt.normal2 <- coxme(Surv(futime, status)~trt+(1|id))
> Ret.SPF.trt.normal2
Cox mixed-effects model fit by maximum likelihood

  events, n = 155, 394
  Iterations= 10 44
                  NULL Integrated     Fitted
Log-likelihood -867.9858  -851.1569 -769.6065

                  Chisq     df          p   AIC      BIC
Integrated loglik  33.66   2.00 4.9127e-08 29.66    23.57
 Penalized loglik 196.76  73.01 2.6568e-13 50.74  -171.46

Model:  Surv(futime, status) ~ trt + (1 | id)
Fixed coefficients
          coef exp(coef)  se(coef)      z        p
trt -0.8973526 0.4076474 0.1740347  -5.16  2.5e-07

Random effects
 Group Variable  Std Dev    Variance
 id      Intercept 0.8815430 0.7771181
```

The term `(1|id)` in the model formulation indicates that all observations with the same value of `id` are nested in the same cluster. Results are very close from those obtained with `coxph`, see Table 3.2. The output provides the value of the log (partial) likelihood of a null model (without covariates and without random effects), here -867.986, as well as the value of the log (partial) likelihood from which random effects have been integrated out (see (3.28)), here -851.157. These two values can be used to find back the value of the "integrated log-likelihood chi-square test statistics" provided on the next line, indeed if we consider twice the difference we obtain

```
> 2*(Ret.SPF.trt.normal2$loglik[2]-Ret.SPF.trt.normal2$loglik[1])
Integrated
 33.65772
```

and the corresponding p-value (4.912e-08) can be obtained from the `pchisq` function. This is a "global" test for the whole model, including the treatment fixed effect and the patient shared random effect. A test for the random effect only can be obtained by comparing the value of the integrated log (partial) likelihood to the log (partial) likelihood of a model including only treatment as fixed effect:

```
> Test.stat <- 2*(Ret.SPF.trt.normal2$loglik[2]-Ret.Cox.trt$
   loglik[2])
> Test.stat
Integrated
 11.28544
> pchisq(Test.stat,1,lower.tail=F)
   Integrated
0.0007811732
```

Both `coxph` and `coxme` fit semi-parametric models, i.e. leaving the baseline hazards unspecified. In some situations, we may be interested by fitting a parametric model, assuming a parametric distribution for the baseline hazard (see Section 3.5.1), for example if we are interested in predictions, or if we want to easily compare different frailty distributions, or also in the context of simulations. Parametric frailty models can be fitted for a variety of parametric baseline hazards and frailty distributions using the `parfm` package. As usual, the `parfm` package is loaded via the command

```
library(parfm)
```

For example, a shared frailty model assuming a Weibull baseline hazard and a gamma frailty distribution can be obtained from

```
> Ret.Weib.gamma <- parfm(Surv(futime, status)~trt, cluster="id",
   dist="weibull", frailty="gamma",data=retinopathy)
> Ret.Weib.gamma

Frailty distribution: gamma
Baseline hazard distribution: Weibull
Loglikelihood: -827.744

        ESTIMATE  SE      p-val
theta    1.040   0.329
rho      0.948   0.075
lambda   0.028   0.007
trt     -0.960   0.182  <.001 ***
---
```

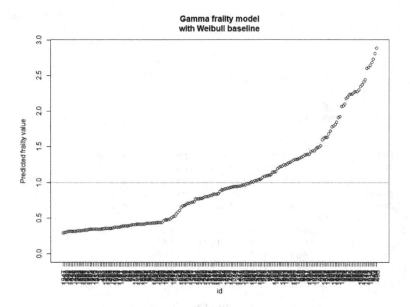

**Gamma frailty model
with Weibull baseline**

FIGURE 3.5
Diabetic retinopathy data: expected values of the frailty from a parametric
(Weibull) PH model with a gamma frailty distribution.

```
Signif. codes: 0 '***' 0.001 '**' 0.01 '*' 0.05 '.' 0.1 ' ' 1

Kendall's Tau: 0.342
```

Note that the output directly provides the estimate of the Kendall's Tau
(0.342) which can be interpreted as an overall measure of dependence. The
parfm package also allows to easily plot the predicted values of the frailties,
see Figure 3.5,

```
u.gamma <- predict(Ret.Weib.gamma)
plot(u.gamma)
```

We can also fit several frailty models assuming different parametric
baseline hazards and different frailty distributions in one call, using the
select.parfm functions and specifying now a vector for the dist and/or
frailty argument. This allows to have a quick look on the fit of these models
and to obtain AIC and BIC value for all these models at once. The following
call fit 16 models, considering either an exponential, Weibull, log-logistic or
log-normal hazard function and a gamma, Inverse Gaussian, Positive Stable
or log-Normal distribution for the frailty.

```
> Ret.frail.parfm <- select.parfm(Surv(futime, status)~trt,
    cluster="id",
+                                         dist=c("exponential","
    weibull","loglogistic","lognormal"),
```

```
+                                                frailty=c("gamma","ingau",
    "possta","lognormal"),
+                                                data=retinopathy)


### - Parametric frailty models - ###
Progress status:
  'ok' = converged
  'nc' = not converged

                    Frailty
Baseline                gamma   invGau  posSta  lognor
exponential.........ok......ok......ok......ok....
Weibull.............ok......ok......ok......ok....
loglogistic.........ok......ok......ok......ok....
lognormal...........ok......ok......ok......ok....
> Ret.frail.parfm
  AIC:            gamma  ingau possta lognor
      exponential  1662   1660   1665   1657
      weibull      1663   1662   1681   1659
      loglogistic  1660   1659   1663   1656
      lognormal    1659   1658   1661   1654


  BIC:            gamma  ingau possta lognor
      exponential  1674   1672   1677   1669
      weibull      1679   1678   1697   1675
      loglogistic  1676   1675   1679   1672
      lognormal    1675   1674   1676   1670
```

As we can see, all these models converged and the value of the AIC and BIC for each model can be easily visualized using

```
plot(Ret.frail.parfm)
```

Looking at the results on Figure 3.6 and keeping in mind that the lower the AIC and BIC the better, a log-normal frailty distribution with a log-normal baseline hazard seems to be a good choice. Results of such a model are given in Table 3.2.

Considering the Gompertz distribution for the baseline hazard in the call above, we would have actually got an error message mentioning that the model has not converged. This may be solved either changing the intial value, with the `iniFpar` argument, or the method of optimization, with the `method` argument, for example, changing the default "BFGS" to the "Nelder-Mead" method. Here, both options lead to a model which now converge.

```
> Ret.Gomp.gam <- parfm(Surv(futime, status)~trt, cluster="id",
    dist="gompertz", frailty="gamma",iniFpar = 1,data=retinopathy)
> Ret.Gomp.gam

Frailty distribution: gamma
Baseline hazard distribution: Gompertz
Loglikelihood: -827.98

        ESTIMATE SE      p-val
theta   1.149    0.352
```

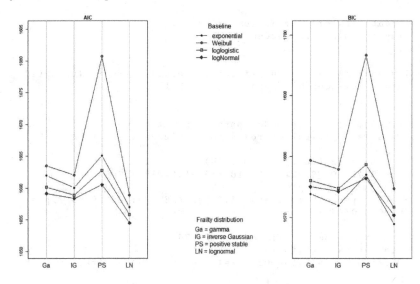

FIGURE 3.6
Diabetic retinopathy data: AIC and BIC values for various parametric shared frailty models with various parametric assumptions for the baseline hazard and for the frailty distribution

```
gamma    0.000   0.006
lambda   0.024   0.004
trt     -0.988   0.186 <.001 ***
---
Signif. codes: 0 '***' 0.001 '**' 0.01 '*' 0.05 '.' 0.1 ' ' 1

Kendall's Tau: 0.365
```

Another, very popular, R package to fit a shared frailty model (and actually also more complex frailty models) is `frailtypack`. Estimation in this package is based on the penalized full likelihood estimation approach described in Section 3.5.2 considering a parametric but very flexible baseline hazard specified via a piecewise constant hazard or splines. This package is loaded with

```
library(frailtypack)
```

and the main function to fit a shared frailty model is `frailtyPenal`, which allows to fit a shared gamma or log-normal frailty model. Note that a parametric baseline hazard can also be considered, with the possibility to fit either a piecewise constant hazard or a Weibull baseline hazard. A parametric shared frailty model with a Weibull baseline hazard and a gamma frailty distribution is obtained via the following code and lead to the same results as those obtained from `parfm` above

```
> Ret.FP.Weib.gamma <- frailtyPenal(Surv(futime, status)~trt +
    cluster(id), hazard = ('Weibull'), data=retinopathy)
```

```
Be patient. The program is computing ...
The program took 0.29 seconds
> Ret.FP.Weib.gamma
Call:
frailtyPenal(formula = Surv(futime, status) ~ trt + cluster(id),
    data = retinopathy, hazard = ("Weibull"))


   Shared Gamma Frailty model parameter estimates
   using a Parametrical approach for the hazard function

        coef exp(coef) SE coef (H)         z          p
trt -0.959742  0.382992    0.182119 -5.26988 1.3652e-07


   Frailty parameter, Theta: 1.04016 (SE (H): 0.329093 ) p =
      0.00078698

      marginal log-likelihood = -827.74
      Convergence criteria:
      parameters = 1.98e-08 likelihood = 1.12e-07 gradient = 5.05
         e-14

   AIC = Aikaike information Criterion      = 2.11103

The expression of the Aikaike Criterion is:
      'AIC = (1/n)[np - l(.)]'

      Scale for the weibull hazard function is : 43.13
      Shape for the weibull hazard function is : 0.95

The expression of the Weibull hazard function is:
      'lambda(t) = (shape.(t^(shape-1)))/(scale^shape)'
The expression of the Weibull survival function is:
      'S(t) = exp[- (t/scale)^shape]'

      n= 394
      n events= 155  n groups= 197
      number of iterations:   12
```

The estimated values for the treatment effect $\hat{\beta}$ and the frailty parameter $\hat{\theta}$ are exactly the same as those obtained with **parfm**. We however have to note that the parametrization used for the Weibull baseline hazard is not the same. Indeed, **parfm** uses the same parametrization as in Chapter 2 (see Table 2.1) while the parametrization used by **frailtypack** is described in the output. We can easily find out that the *shape* corresponds to ρ while the *scale* is actually $1/\lambda$. Applying this transformation, we find that the estimated Weibull parameters are not exactly the same but are very close from those obtained with **parfm**

```
> Ret.FP.Weib.gamma$shape.weib[1]
[1] 0.9475455
> 1/Ret.FP.Weib.gamma$scale.weib[1]
[1] 0.02318564
```

We can also specify a piecewise baseline hazard, either based on percentiles (see below) or based on equidistant intervals (using `"Piecewise-equi"`) and specifying the number of intervals

```
> Ret.FP.cst.gamma <- frailtyPenal(Surv(futime, status)~trt +
    cluster(id), hazard = ('Piecewise-per'),nb.int=10, data=
    retinopathy)
```

Results are summarized in Table 3.2. Using splines for the baseline hazard, we can also choose between splines based on percentiles or equidistant knots. The number of knots needs to be specified and the Rondeau et al. [331, 333] advise to start with a relatively low number of knots (e.g. 7) and to increase it until the graph of the baseline hazard function remains unchanged. An initial value should also be provided for the smoothing parameters of the penalized likelihood; the authors advise to start with a large value (e.g. 10000) and to change it if it does not reach convergence. By setting the `cross.validation` parameters to `TRUE`, a cross-validation procedure is used to choose the value of the smoothing parameter.

```
> Ret.FP.spl.gamma <- frailtyPenal(Surv(futime, status)~trt +
    cluster(id), hazard = ('Splines'), n.knots=7, kappa=10000,
    cross.validation=T, data=retinopathy)

Be patient. The program is computing ...
The program took 0.31 seconds
> Ret.FP.spl.gamma
Call:
frailtyPenal(formula = Surv(futime, status) ~ trt + cluster(id),
    data = retinopathy, cross.validation = T, n.knots = 7, kappa
        = 10000,
    hazard = ("Splines"))


  Shared Gamma Frailty model parameter estimates
  using a Penalized Likelihood on the hazard function

          coef exp(coef) SE coef (H) SE coef (HIH)         z
                    p
trt -0.913031  0.401306    0.153635      0.153635 -5.94287 2.8007
    e-09

    Frailty parameter, Theta: 0.884445 (SE (H): 0.249878 ) p =
        0.00020044

    penalized marginal log-likelihood = -826.7
    Convergence criteria:
    parameters = 2.22e-06 likelihood = 0.000907 gradient = 7.14
        e-05

    LCV = the approximate likelihood cross-validation criterion
          in the semi parametrical case      = 2.12613

    n= 394
    n events= 155  n groups= 197
    number of iterations:  38
```

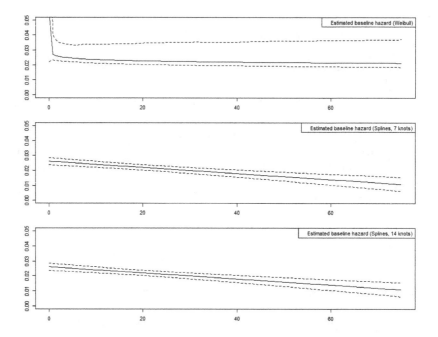

FIGURE 3.7
Diabetic retinopathy data: baseline hazard function estimated by
`frailtypack` either assuming a Weibull baseline hazard (*top*) or using
splines with 7 knots (*middle*) or 14 knots (*bottom*).

```
Exact number of knots used:   7
Best smoothing parameter estimated by
an approximated Cross validation:   2.81511e+11, DoF:   2.00
```

The hazards ratio for the fixed effect parameters are obtained from the
`summary` function:

```
> summary(Ret.FP.spl.gamma)
        hr      95%      C.I.
 trt   0.40 (   0.30 -    0.54 )
```

A plot of the estimated baseline hazard function can be easily obtained
from

```
plot(Ret.FP.Weib.gamma,type.plot="Hazard")
```

See Figure 3.7 where the estimated baseline hazard obtained by assuming a
parametric Weibull hazard or using splines with respectively 7 and 14 knots
are provided. One could also plot the baseline survival function by specifying
`type.plot="Survival"`.

A log-normal frailty distribution can also be specified using the
`RandDist=''` argument (see Table 3.2 for the results.) The `frailtypack`

package also allows (although not for all models) stratification (with up to 6 strata), left-truncation, interval-censoring, as well as more general random effects models (e.g., with nested random effects) and some further extensions of the frailty model.

Results obtained from different models not accounting for clustering were already presented in Table 3.1 and Table 3.2 presents the results from various models taking clustering into account. These models were fitted with R packages mentioned above. The results obtained from the various models are very close for this particular example. As expected, the coefficient for the treatment effect in the marginal model is exactly the same as in a standard Cox model, but its variance has now been corrected to take clustering into account. In the various frailty models, the treatment effect appears even stronger than in standard models, with a hazard ratio of about 0.40, corresponding to 60% lower risk of loss of vision for the treated eyes compared to the control group. This coefficient, and corresponding HR, should however in these models be interpreted as conditional on the cluster. Note that this coefficient is only slightly impacted by the choice of the frailty distribution which is in line with the work of [263] showing that the choice of the frailty distribution has only a slight impact on the estimation of the fixed effects. The estimated frailty parameters are between 0.7854 and 0.884 for gamma frailty models with unspecified or flexible hazards (and slightly outside this range for parametric hazards) and between 0.753 and 1.0211 for log-normal frailty models.

Of note, a possible alternative to analyse such data, with a fixed cluster size of size 2, would be to use copula [12, 107, 138, 269]. This is however out of the scope of this book.

3.7.2 Rectal cancer data

In Section 2.6.3 of Chapter 2, we analyzed the data from the Intergroup R98 rectal cancer trial with classical survival techniques. Remind that this trial included 357 resected stage II–III rectal cancer patients in 66 centers. These patients were randomized after surgery to either a 5FU/LV regimen (control arm, $n = 178$) or to LV5-FU2 plus irinotecan (experimental arm, $n = 179$). Before starting recruiting patients in this trial, each center had to opt for one of two 5FU-LV regimens and all patients randomized to the control arm had to be treated with the chosen regimen. Number of patients in each treatment arm and strata was summarized in Table 2.6.

Our objective here is to illustrate how we can use frailty models to investigate potential heterogeneity over centers. The starting point is that patients treated within the same hospital share more in common than patients from different hospitals and this is not necessarily captured by the available covariates. For example, it is well know that different centers do not attract the same patients, in terms of demographic characteristics, socioeconomic levels, general health status (outside of the condition from which they are treated) ... and this may depend on different characteristics of the hospital such as

Model	Package	Hazard	Cov	$\hat{\beta}$ (s.e)	HR (95% CI)	Hazard
Cox PH	survival	unspecified	trt	-0.777 (0.169)	0.460 [0.330;0.640]	
Parametric PH	parfm	Weibull	trt	-0.790 (0.169)	0.454 [0.326;0.632]	$\hat{\rho} = 0.810$ (s.e. 0.058) $\hat{\lambda} = 0.032$ (s.e. 0.008)
Parametric PH	frailtypack	Weibull	trt	-0.790 (0.169)	0.454 [0.326;0.632]	$1/\hat{\lambda} = 69.87$ $\hat{\rho} = 0.81$
Parametric PH	parfm	Log-normal	trt	-0.783 (0.168)	0.457 [0.329;0.635]	$\hat{\mu} = 3.778$ (s.e. 0.153) $\hat{\sigma} = 1.774$ (s.e. 0.115)
Flexible PH	frailtypack	piecewise cst 10 intervals (perc)	trt	-1.056 (0.169)	0.35 [0.25;0.48]	
Flexible PH	frailtypack	spline - CV 7 knots, $\kappa = 10000$	trt	-0.778 (0.146)	0.46 [0.34;0.61]	

TABLE 3.1

Diabetic retinopathy data: Results for various proportional hazards (PH) models for time to blindness not accounting for clustering in the data (cst: constant, perc: percentile-based, CV: cross-validation).

Model	Hazard	Frailty	$\hat{\beta}$ (s.e)	HR (95% CI)	Hazard	Frailty (s.e)
Stratified Cox PH[1]	unspecified	-	-0.962 (0.202)	0.382 [0.257;0.567]		$\hat{\theta} = 0.854$
Marginal Cox PH[1]	unspecified	-	-0.777 (0.169) robust s.e. 0.1475	0.460 [0.330;0.640] / 0.460 [0.345;0.614]		$\hat{\theta} = 0.753$
Semi-param. frailty[1]	unspecified	gamma	-0.919 (0.174)	0.404 [0.286;0.566]		$\hat{\theta} = 0.777$
Semi-param. frailty[1]	unspecified	log-normal	-0.894 (0.174)	0.409 [0.291;0.572]		$\hat{\theta} = 1.040$ (s.e.0.329)
Semi-param. frailty[2]	unspecified	log-normal	-0.897 (0.174)	0.408 [0.290;0.573]		$\hat{\theta} = 0.772$ (s.e.0.281)
Parametric frailty[3]	Weibull	gamma	-0.960 (0.182)	0.383 [0.268;0.547]	$\hat{\rho} = 0.848$, $\hat{\lambda} = 0.028$	$\hat{\theta} = 0.963$ (s.e.0.309)
Parametric frailty[3]	lognormal	gamma	-0.886 (0.176)	0.412 [0.292;0.582]	$\hat{\mu} = 3.416$, $\hat{\sigma} = 1.544$	$\hat{\theta} = 1.040$ (s.e.0.329)
Parametric frailty[3]	lognormal	lognormal	-0.920 (0.179)	0.398 [0.280;0.566]	$\hat{\mu} = 3.943$, $\hat{\sigma} = 1.653$	$\hat{\theta} = 0.996$ (s.e.0.321)
Parametric frailty[4]	Weibull	gamma	-0.960 (0.182)	0.383 [0.268;0.547]	$\hat{\rho} = 0.95$, $1/\hat{\lambda} = 43.13$	$\hat{\theta} = 0.884$ (s.e.0.250)
Flexible frailty[4]	piecewise cst 10 intervals (perc)	gamma	-0.965 (0.182)	0.381 [0.267;0.544]		$\hat{\theta} = 1.197$ (s.e.0.402)
Flexible frailty[4]	splines - CV 7 knots, $\kappa = 10000$	gamma	-0.913 (0.154)	0.401 [0.297;0.542]		$\hat{\theta} = 1.0211$ (s.e.0.378)
Parametric frailty[4]	Weibull	lognormal	-0.978 (0.186)	0.376 [0.261;0.541]	$\hat{\rho} = 0.98$, $1/\hat{\lambda} = 70.82$	$\hat{\theta} = 0.980$ (s.e.0.302)
Flexible frailty[4]	piecewise cst 10 intervals (perc)	lognormal	-0.929 (0.184)	0.395 [0.275;0.566]		
Flexible frailty[4]	splines - CV 7 knots, $\kappa = 10000$	lognormal	-0.936 (0.168)	0.392 [0.282 ; 0.546]		

TABLE 3.2

Diabetic retinopathy data: Results for various models for time to loss of vision accounting for clustering in the data. All model includes treatment (trt) as the only fixed effect covariate (s.e.: standard error, cst: constant, perc: percentile-based, CV: cross-validation). Models are fitted with [1] survival [2] coxme [3] parfm, [4] frailtypack.

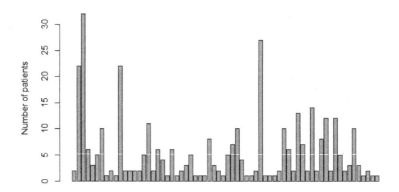

FIGURE 3.8

Rectal cancer data: Number of patients recruited by each center.

localization, size, status (university, public, private, ...). Also, the way patients are globally handled and treated might depend somehow on the procedures put in place in different hospitals, and the management of the patients is therefore more alike for patients treated in the same hospital than for patients treated in different hospitals. Of course, such an heterogeneity should be somehow "controlled" in the context of a clinical trial, for which all patients should be treated according to the same protocol. However, it is not unreasonable to think that some of the heterogeneity remain [222], given that even the more complete protocol can not control or standardize everything.

In this study, the 357 patients were recruited by 66 centers, each recruiting between 1 and 32 patients. The average number of patients recruited by each center was 5.4 and the median was 2.5. A barplot of the number of patients recruited per center is plotted on Figure 3.8.

To investigate the heterogeneity in outcome between centers, a first idea could be to plot the KM estimated curves for DFS and OS by centers. However, with 66 centers having all recruited little (or very little) number of patients, such a graph could not be used to draw any meaningful interpretation. Indeed, the graph would contain way to many curves and each of these 66 KM estimated curve would be estimated based on a very little number of patients. For the same reason, a Cox PH model including center as fixed effect has very little chance to bring interesting information.

Applying a frailty model with a shared frailty for cluster on DFS actually leads to an estimated value of the heterogeneity parameters very close to zero. It seems therefore that based on these data, we are not able to detect any heterogeneity in DFS between centers. We will therefore concentrate for this analysis on OS, for which we will see that there seems to be some heterogeneity between centers.

We start with fitting a semi-parametric frailty model, including only the treatment arm as fixed effect and a shared frailty for the center. Such a model can be fitted in R or in SAS. In SAS, the `proc phreg` procedure can be used to fit a semi-parametric shared frailty model by adding a `random` statement. The variable used to specify the cluster must be declared in the `class` statement. The options of the `random` statement allows to choose between a gamma (`dist=gamma`) or a lognormal distribution (`dist=lognormal`, default). In this later case, we can further choose between a maximum likelihood (`method=ml`) or a restricted maximum likelihood (`method=reml`, default) estimator for the variance of the frailty. We can also use the option to specify initial value for the frailty parameter as well as to control parameters linked to the convergence of the algorithm. It may also be useful to mention the `solution` option which will then displays prediction for the frailty for each cluster (or a selection of clusters to be specified between brackets).

We can therefore fit a frailty model on OS with a gamma shared frailty for center with the following code:

```
proc phreg data=R98data;
   class Centre;
   model osm*event(0)=treat;
   random Centre / dist=gamma;
run;
```

leading to the following output

```
Median Disease Free Survival (months)

The PHREG Procedure

        Model Information

Data Set                    WORK.R98DATA
Dependent Variable          osm
Censoring Variable          event
Censoring Value(s)          0
Ties Handling               BRESLOW
Frailty                     GAMMA


Number of Observations Read      357
Number of Observations Used      357


    Class Level Information for Random Effects

Class      Levels   Values

Centre       66     004 006 009 012 013 015 017 020 021 024 026
                    028 029 032 034 037 042 043 046 047 048 051
                    060 064 072 075 080 084 085 092 096 098 100
                    102 103 106 112 113 114 117 119 120 122 132
                    135 137 138 140 142 143 144 145 148 150 151
                    152 156 157 159 161 163 164 171 172 176 181


Summary of the Number of Event and Censored Values

                              Percent
    Total      Event   Censored   Censored

     357        135       222      62.18
```

```
                         Convergence Status

          Convergence criterion (PCONV=0.0001) satisfied.


Marginal Loglikelihood      -874.82899


                  Testing Global Null Hypothesis

                                    Adjusted
Test                    Chi-Square        DF        Pr > ChiSq

Likelihood Ratio          2.6604        1.92          0.2505
Wald                      1.6961        1.92          0.4100


The PHREG Procedure
Covariance Parameter Estimates

Cov
Parm        Estimate

Centre      0.007350

                          Type 3 Tests

                  Wald                       Adjusted     Adjusted
Effect      Chi-Square    DF    Pr > ChiSq         DF     Pr > ChiSq

treat         0.7234       1      0.3950       0.9981       0.3943
Centre        0.9878       .         .        0.9215       0.2946

                  Analysis of Maximum Likelihood Estimates

                     Parameter     Standard
                        Hazard
Parameter    DF      Estimate        Error    Chi-Square   Pr > ChiSq
    Ratio   Label

treat         1       -0.14700      0.17283     0.7234       0.3950
    0.863   Treatment arm
```

As usual in SAS, the first part of the output provides some general information about the variables used, the number of observations (357 observations)
and of events (135 deaths). The ouput confirms that convergence has been
reached (according to the default parameters here since we did not specify
anything specific) and gives the value of the marginal likelihood computed at
the estimated values of the parameters. Follows two global tests of the model
(not significant in this example) and individual Wald-type test for each of the
fixed effect and the random effect. The usual Wald test, with a one degree of
freedom chi-square distribution under H_0 is provided for the fixed effect. The
Wald test performed for the random effect is the Wald-type test for penalized
models discussed in [372] and based on the Hessian matrix derived from the
partial log likelihood.

We note that the estimated coefficient and HR for treatment is very close
from the one obtained in a model without frailty. The variance of the frailty
is estimated to be 0.0074.

The results obtained in R, with the `emfrail` function from the `frailtyEM` package, and which is based on the EM algorithm leads to about the same results. This function allows to fit a shared frailty models with a gamma, a positive stable or power variance function distribution, and can accommodate left truncated data [25]. The variable defining the cluster should be specified with a `cluster` statement and the frailty distribution (gamma by default) should be specified via the `distribution` statement (note that an initial value for the heterogeneity parameter can also be provided in this statement). An extended output can be obtained with the `summary()` function, which in addition to the model estimates also provide some further information about the model fit and about the frailty distribution such as the Kendall's τ.

```
> R98.Frail.EM <- emfrail(Surv(osm, event)~treat+cluster(Centre),
     distribution = emfrail_dist(dist = "gamma"), data=R98.data)
> summary(R98.Frail.EM)
Call:
emfrail(formula = Surv(osm, event) ~ treat + cluster(Centre),
    data = R98.data)

Regression coefficients:
        coef exp(coef) se(coef) adj. se      z    p
treat -0.147     0.863    0.173   0.176 -0.837  0.4
Estimated distribution: gamma / left truncation: FALSE

Fit summary:
Commenges-Andersen test for heterogeneity: p-val   0.772
no-frailty Log-likelihood: -739.835
Log-likelihood: -739.829
LRT: 1/2 * pchisq(0.0116), p-val  0.457

Frailty summary:
                    estimate lower 95% upper 95%
Var[Z]                 0.007     0.000     0.232
Kendall's tau          0.004     0.000     0.104
Median concordance     0.004     0.000     0.101
E[logZ]               -0.004    -0.121     0.000
Var[logZ]              0.007     0.000     0.261
theta                135.682     4.307       Inf
Confidence intervals based on the likelihood function
```

This output provides the value of two global tests, the Commenges-Andersen test for heterogeneity [79] and the likelihood ratio test, testing whether this model fits better the data than a model without frailty. For this likelihood ratio test, a mixture of chi-square with one and two degrees of freedom must be used, as the model under the null is at the border of the parameter space [74]. Note that both tests are non-significant in this example, and based on these tests, we could rather consider a simpler Cox PH model without frailty. This is in line with the small estimated value of the heterogeneity parameter ($\hat{\theta} = 0.007$) and the corresponding small value of the Kendall's τ ($\hat{\tau} = 0.004$).

Even if the value of the heterogeneity parameter is small, it may be interesting to check its impact on some more relevant medical quantities. Considering the clusters (here the centers) in our study as a sample of a larger population of clusters, we have seen in Section 3.3 that we can translate the impact of a specific value of the heterogenity parameter on the density of some more relevant quantities such as the median survival time or the event-free probability at a given time point over all clusters. For these particular data, as we have seen in Section 2.6.3 of Chapter 2 the median survival is not really meaningful. We will rather concentrate here on the percentage of patients event-free at 48 months. However, to be able to do so, we actually need to assume a parametric baseline hazard. As we have seen in the previous illustration, we can use the `select.parfm()` function from the `parfm` R package to easily try out different parametric distribution as well as different frailty distribution and compare their AIC and BIC. Given the small heterogeneity, the AIC and BIC value are actually the same in this example whatever the choice of the frailty distribution (among gamma, lognormal, inverse Gaussian and positive stable) and we will therefore consider a gamma distribution. In terms of distribution of the events times , we don't see large difference in AIC and BIC. The model with the lowest AIC and BIC is obtained assuming a lognormal distribution of the event time (AIC=1716 and BIC=1731) closely followed by the log-logistic (AIC=1719 and BIC=1735). Given the very little difference between the two, and that the analogous of the formula (3.11) for the density of the survival rate at a given timepoint is much more easy to obtain for the log-logistic distribution we will consider this distribution.

So, we first use `parfm` to fit a parametric shared frailty model assuming a log-logistic distribution of the event times and a gamma frailty density.

```
> parfm(Surv(osm, event) ~ treat, cluster="Centre",dist="
    loglogistic", frailty="gamma",data=R98.data)

Frailty distribution: gamma
Baseline hazard distribution: Loglogistic
Loglikelihood: -855.514

        ESTIMATE SE      p-val
theta   0.032    0.084
alpha  -6.752    0.472
kappa   1.393    0.110
treat  -0.186    0.174 0.284
---
Signif. codes: 0 '***' 0.001 '**' 0.01 '*' 0.05 '.' 0.1 ' ' 1

Kendall's Tau: 0.016
```

With this parametric shared frailty model, both the treatment effect ($\hat{\beta} = -0.186$) and the heterogeneity parameter ($\hat{\theta} = 0.032$) are a bit larger. Assuming a log-logistic distribution of the event times, the survival rate at time t_S given the frailty u_i and covariates values $\mathbf{x}$ is given by (see Table 2.1):

$$S_{t_S,\mathbf{x},i} = \exp\left[-\log(1 + \exp(\alpha)t_S^\kappa)u_i \exp(\beta^{\mathbf{t}}\mathbf{x})\right]$$

and following the same reasoning as in Section 3.3, we can obtain

$$f_{S_{t_S,x,i}}(s) = \frac{(-\log s)^{1/\theta-1} s^{\left(\theta \log(1+\exp(\alpha)t_S^\kappa \exp(\beta^{\mathbf{t}}\mathbf{x}))\right)^{-1}-1}}{\theta^{1/\theta}\Gamma(\frac{1}{\theta})\left[\log(1+\exp(\alpha)t_S^\kappa \exp(\beta^{\mathbf{t}}\mathbf{x}))\right]^{1/\theta}} \qquad (3.35)$$

Using formula (3.35), in which we replaced t_S by 48 months (t_S must be expressed in the same unit as the one used to estimate the hazard function), and the parameter $\theta, \alpha, \hat{\kappa}$, and β by their estimated value $\hat{\theta} = 0.032, \hat{\alpha} = -6.752, \widehat{kappa} = 1.393$, and $\hat{\beta} = -0.186$, we have plotted on Figure 3.9 the density function of the 48-months survival rate for each treatment arm. The top part of the Figure 3.9 displays the survival curves as estimated from a classical KM estimator, with a 4 years survival estimated as 77.0% (95% CI [70.0 ; 82.6]) in the control arm and 80.9% (95% CI [74.23 ; 86.0]) in the experimental arm. Based on the density function in each treatment arm, and using the 5% and 95% percentile, we can conclude that given the heterogeneity we have observed in our data we expect about 90% of the centers to have a 4 years survival between 74.1% and 84.7% in the control arm and between 78.0% and 87.1% in the experimental arm.

Given the little heterogeneity in these data, it is probably not worth pursuing investigating it, for example by trying to explain it with the introduction of fixed effect covariates in the model. Based on these data we can not conclude on the presence of heterogeneity between these centers. It is however not possible to know whether this is really the case (as could explained by the fact that the 66 centers where all in the same country and followed and treat all patients according to the same protocol) or whether we actually don't have enough information (due to the very little number of patients recruited by each center) to put such an heterogeneity in light.

3.8 Further reading

There actually exists a vast literature on frailty models, presenting refinements of the estimation methods proposed here or other methods (see for example the pseudo-likelihood method [140] or the h-likelihood method [150]). Also various applications or other extensions of the models discussed here have been proposed (see below for some references). A big part of these references are actually in a Bayesian framework. We can cite for example [52, 358, 424] amongst many other, and several of the reference given in this section for extension of the frailty model in fact consider a Bayesian approach.

From a modeling point of view, the univariate frailty model is a special case of the shared (multivariate) model, with cluster of size one. However, there are to be used in different contexts. The univariate frailty model has been developed to take into account heterogeneity due to unobserved risk

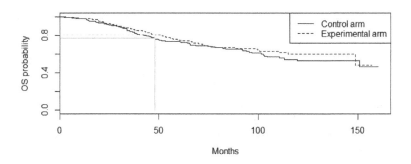

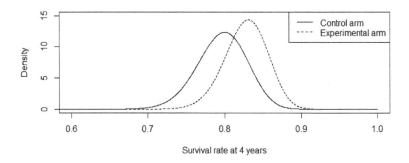

FIGURE 3.9
Rectal cancer data: Density function of the 4 years survival rate over the centers as induced by the estimated frailty value

factors, and the heterogeneity parameter (usually the variance of the frailty distribution) can be interpreted as a measure of overdispersion. However, the use of such an univariate frailty model is debatable as the model requires the inclusion of covariate(s) under the (strong) assumption of proportional conditional hazard to be identifiable. However, given the limited information, it may be difficult to be confident that non-proportionality observed at the level of the population is indeed due to a distortion of the PH effect of the covariates due to unobserved heterogeneity and not due to other reasons [26]. On the other hand, the use of a multivariate frailty model when observations can not be assumed independent due to the presence of clustering in the data is less controversial. The frailty then represents all common unobserved factors shared by individuals in a cluster and therefore creating correlation between these individuals. The more information we have on this correlation, the more confident we can be on the presence of a frailty to explain the non-proportionality at the level of the population [26]. We should however keep in mind that the correlation induced by the introduction of a frailty term can only be positive. Therefore such a model should not be considered if we suspect a negative correlation among observations from the same cluster.

Given that data from meta-analysis or large multi-center trials are often used to identify prognostic factors and build prognostic indices, for example in oncology, the extension of "classical" measures of validity of such prognostic factors, such as the well-known Harrell's C index, to the framework of frailty models have been studied in the literature [221, 252, 395].

Since shared frailty model deals with the correlation between clustered observations, a natural extension of these models is in the context of modeling spatial survival data, see for example [135] who consider a piecewice constant baseline hazard frailty model and [227] who propose using a semiparametric frailty models combining Monte-Carlo simulations and Laplace approximation to handle the intractable integrals in the likelihood function.

While in a shared frailty model, the individuals within a cluster share the same value of the frailty, an interesting extension is to consider, as in the univariate frailty, that each member of the cluster has his own frailty but that the frailty terms within a cluster are correlated. The general idea is that while individuals in a same cluster are more alike than the individuals in the other clusters, their are nevertheless still all different. This idea has led to the development of *correlated frailty models*, mainly in the context of bivariate data [418, 419]. A nice overview is available in [406].

As stated by Wienke [406] in the context of univariate frailty model but also true in the multivariate context, it is clear that the multiplicative frailty model 3.1 represents a rather simplified view of how heterogeneity may act. However, such a simple mathematical models has the merit to provide a way to understand the consequences of heterogeneity. In particular, the assumptions that the frailty is time-independent and acts multiplicatively on the underlying baseline hazard function are arbitrary but have been taken as the basis for most of the subsequent work on unobserved heterogeneity in survival analysis. Neverthless some work has been done on other types of frailty models. For example, one can find work on additive frailty model [326] and proportional odds frailty models [205, 206, 266]. Furthermore, several authors have also considered AFT frailty models, see for example [18, 60, 183, 191, 196]. Developments have also been proposed to extend the frailty model to a time-dependent frailty, although both the estimation methods and the interpretation become more complex. A quite natural context in which time-dependent frailty models have been developed is the one of modeling recurrent events where we can expect the subject-specific time-dependent frailty to change over time [245, 420, 293] given the repetition of the occurrence of the event of interest. An extension to time-dependent frailty could also be interesting when the "cluster effect" is expected to decrease over time. This could be the case for example in a multi-center clinical trials, where the effect of the centers is present as long as the patient is treated (especially for complicated treatment) but would tend to fade away with longer follow-up [264, 410].

The estimation methods described on Section 3.5 deals with right-censored data but can usually also accommodate left-truncation with little adjustments, see for example [327] for the penalized full likelihood approach. Other censoring and truncation scheme are shortly discussed in Chapter 7 of [107]. An example of a shared gamma frailty model applied to current status data, a particular case of interval censored data in which each subject is only observed once (so interval for the time-to-event either includes zero or infinity) is discussed in Chapter 4 of [406]. As already mentioned, the penalized full likelihood approach of [327] for shared gamma frailty models can also be used for stratified shared gamma frailty models. Stratification by a binary variable is also allowed when using this penalized full likelihood approach to fit a nested gamma frailty model or an additive gamma frailty model.

Since repeated events can be seen as a particular case of clustered data, with events occurring in a same individuals being clustered together, the shared frailty model can be used to fit such type of data (see example 2.4 in Chapter 2 of [107] or [27] for a detailed example). A slightly different situation occurs when individuals experiencing recurrent events (e.g., disease recurrences) are also subject to a terminal event (e.g., death), and these events are assumed to be correlated (e.g., several disease recurrences are assumed to increase the risk of death). In that case, the terminal event is considered as informative censoring, and a joint frailty model could be used to jointly model the the hazard function of the recurrent events and the one of the terminal event [200].

As mentioned previously, any positive distribution could in fact be considered for the frailty distribution. The one mentioned in Section 3.4.2 are the most often used, and also the one for which their exist an implementation in easily accessible software (see Section 3.7). Chapter 3 of [406] further discuss the Lévy frailty model (frailty distributions generated by a non-negative Lévy Process) and the log-t frailty model (with the logarithm of a Student distribution as frailty distribution), and other frailty distributions can also be found in the literature.

4

Cure Models

4.1 Introduction

In classical survival analysis, one implicitly assumes that all individuals under study will experience the event of interest if the follow-up is long enough. Indeed, most of the methods developed in classical survival analysis assume that $S(t) = P(T > t)$ is a proper survival function, i.e. that $lim_{t \to \infty} S(t) = 0$ which comes back to assuming that the cumulative hazard function is unbounded, $lim_{t \to \infty} H(t) = \infty$. However, there are many situations in which this assumption is in fact not reasonable, as we can expect a fraction of the population to never experience the event of interest. Many examples exists in different field: in demography one may be interested in time to the second pregnancy for women having already a first child, in sociology in the time to re-arrest after a first stay in prison, or in psychology in the time until a child find the solution of a given problem. There are also numerous examples in medicine, such as the time to relapse after surgery for some specific type of cancer patients, the time to development of HIV in AIDS patients, or the time to mechanical ventilation for hospitalized covid-19 patients. This fraction of individuals, for whom the time-to-event can be considered to be infinite, is often referred to as *cured*, or *immune* or *non-susceptible* individuals in the statistical literature. As already mentioned in the Chapter 1, the event of interest can also be positive to the patients, and in that case the term *cured* appeared particularly inappropriate; for example if we study time to response to a vaccine or a treatment (whatever the way it is defined), it is known that a portion of the subjects under study (we can actually not necessarily speak about "patients" e.g. in a vaccine study) will never show a response. The term *cure* is therefore to be understood as *statistical cure*, i.e. not experiencing the event of interest. Also, when the outcome of interest is overall survival (i.e. time to death) or progression-free survival (i.e. time to progression or death), as is often the case in oncology trials, it is clear that nobody can be "cured" of death. However, for some specific cancer (e.g. early stage melanoma or childhood leukemia), we can nowadays reasonably expect a fraction of long-term survivors to show up amongst patients. One will then be speaking in terms of *long-term survivors* and it is convenient to think of these long-term survivors as *statistically cured* [207, 276, 422].

In the presence of a cure fraction, a mathematical convention is to consider that the time-to-event for a cure individual is in fact $T = \infty$, meaning that the subject will never experience the event of interest. On the other hand, we have $T < \infty$ for a non-cure subject. As we will discuss in this chapter, the presence of a cure fraction has several consequences that led to the developments of particular statistical techniques.

A first one, is that in the presence of a cure fraction, the survival function $S(t) = P(T > t)$ of the population is not proper anymore. Indeed, in the presence of a cure fraction , we have

$$\lim_{t \to \infty} S(t) = 1 - p > 0 \qquad (4.1)$$

and equivalently

$$\lim_{t \to \infty} H(t) = -\log(1 - p) < \infty \qquad (4.2)$$

Therefore the survival function is said to be improper, and the limiting value, which is often denoted $1 - p$ corresponds to the proportion of cure individuals and is therefore often called the *cure rate*. An example of such a survival function is shown in the left panel of Figure 4.1, where we clearly see a proportion of about 40% of observations not experiencing the event. The cumulative hazard is bounded from above, meaning that when t becomes large, the accumulated instantaneous risk of experiencing the event will not become infinite but will rather reach a "plateau", meaning that after some time the remaining subjects will not experience any event anymore.

A second consequence is that quite obviously, in the presence of a cure fraction, this cure rate in itself becomes a parameter of interest. Indeed, if, for example, a new treatment lead to a fraction of cure we would like to be able to quantify it. Going one step further, in a clinical trial comparing two treatments we would be interested by the effect of the new experimental treatment both on the fraction of cure as well as on the time-to-event for the *uncured* patients. Some authors have referred to this as the *long-* and *short-term* effect of the treatment. For some types of cancer, such as pediatric cancers, the primary goal of cancer treatment has actually shifted over the last decades from prolongation of survival towards cure. Indeed, a life-prolonging treatment would only offer a limited benefit in this young population. Also in adults, expressing the advantage of a new treatment not only in terms of delayed death but also in terms of cure is of major importance when such a cure can indeed be achieved. In this new paradigm, the cure rate has become an important measure of long-term survival and unless the disease under study is always fatal, the proportion of cure patients is an important component of the treatment benefit [220, 243].

A third important consequence is that the presence of a cure fraction may lead to non-proportional hazards in the whole population. This will be for instance the case in a clinical trial when studying a treatment having an effect both on the cure fraction and on the time-to-event of the uncured

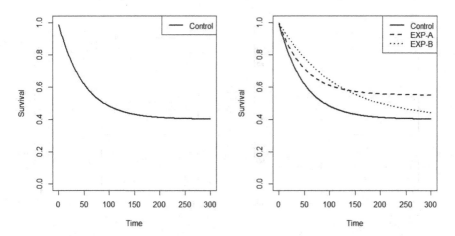

FIGURE 4.1
Survival functions in the presence of cure for a (hypothetical) control group
(*left*) and for a (hypothetical) control group and two (hypothetical) treatment
groups with treatment EXP-A having an effect on the proportion of cure and
treatment EXP-B having an effect on the time-to-event but ultimately not on
the proportion of cure (*right*).

patients. This is illustrated on the right panel of Figure 4.1 representing the
survival function for a control treatment and for two experimental treatment,
one affecting only the probability to be cure (EXP-A) and one affecting only
the time-to-event for the uncured patients (EXP-B). It is obvious from this
plot that the second experimental treatment leads to a non-PH situation.

It is therefore important to take the presence of such a cure fraction into
account when analyzing the data. However, this is not straightfoward. Indeed,
an important difficulty when analyzing survival data with a fraction of cure
observations comes from the presence of right-censoring. In the absence of censoring, one could consider that observations come from two sub-populations
(the "cure" and the "uncured"), and the membership to each of these two sub-
populations would be fully observed. A simple idea would then be to model
our data using a standard mixture model. However, due to right censoring,
the cure status ($I[T < \infty]$) is actually only partially observed. While it is
obvious that individuals experiencing the event of interest are, by definition,
not cure, we can not distinguish the cure status of the right-censored observations. As can be seen from Figure 4.2, the cure status is obviously known for
subjects who got the event during the course of the study (and are therefore
uncured) but is not observed for subjects who are censored during or at the
end of the study. Also, standard survival analysis techniques typically assume
that censored subjects will have the same survival pattern after censoring

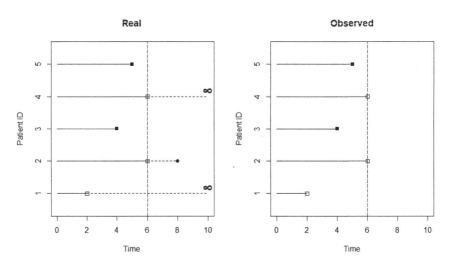

FIGURE 4.2
Example of 5 hypothetical patients. Patients 3 and 5 experience an event
during the course of the study and are therefore uncured. Patient 1 is censored
during the study and patients 2 and 4 are censored at the end of the study.
While patient 2 will actually experience the event (although this will not be
observed due to censoring) this is not the case of patient 4 (*left*). However,
from the observed information (*right*), we are not able to distinguish the cure
status of patient 1, 2, and 3.

that the non-censored subjects, this obviously raise an issue if the censored
observations contains cure ($T = \infty$) and non-cure ($T < \infty$) observations.

Therefore, specific cure models have been developed to study the relationship between the time-to-event T and covariates, while taking into account
the presence of a cure fraction in the population and the presence of censored
observations in the sample. The goal of these models is to study the impact of
these covariates not only on the time to the event of interest but also on preventing the occurrence of this event in a non-negligible part of the population.
While the advances of statistical research on cure models are closely linked
to the progress made in the treatment of cancer, these models have also been
studied in the context of other medical applications, as well as, more broadly,
in other fields. It is interesting to note that these models are often referred to
as *split population models* in economics (highlighting the fact that the population is a mixture of a "cure" and and "uncured" subpopulation) and as
limited-failure population life models in engineering (putting the emphasis on
the fact that $S(t)$ is improper).

The work on cure models have mainly been developed according to two
different axes, leading to two main families of cure models. The first one starts
from the idea that the population is actually a mixture of two sub-populations,

the "cured" and the "uncured" subjects and explicitly models the survival function of the population as resulting from a mixture of these two types of observations. Seminal work is originating from Boag about 70 years ago [175]. He was the first statistician to draw the attention to the presence of cure in the analysis of cancer patient data and proposed at that time a fully parametric model including the cure rate as one of the model parameters and assuming a log-normal model for the failure time of the uncured patients. Few years later, Berkson and Gage [35] proposed a similar model, considering an exponential model for the uncured patients. These models were finally popularized in the late seventies by Farewell [118, 119], who proposed to model the cure rate as a dependent variable in a logistic regression model. This idea have been further developed in the statistical literature and have led to a family of cure models often referred to as *mixture cure models*, which has been widely studied over the last decades. A major advantage of such a model, as we will discuss below, is that it allows to disentangle the effects of the covariates on the probability to be cure and on the event times of uncured patients. While the mixture cure models explicitly model the presence of the two sub-population, the second main family of cure models, called the *promotion time cure models* (or *non-mixture cure models*) is directly link to the observation that the survival function in the global population is improper. The idea, as proposed by by Yakovlev [415] and Tsodikov [383, 384], is to explicitly model the fact that the survival function is improper, or equivalently that the cumulative hazard function is bounded, explaining why this second family of model is also often referred to as *bounded cumulative hazard models*. These two main families of cure models will be discussed respectively in Sections 4.2 and 4.3. Further extensions have been proposed, as well as models that unify these two families of cure models into a single over-arching family of models. However, these are still rarely used in practice and we will refer the reader to [10] for a more complete overview on these unifying models. For an overview of the development of cure models, we refer the reader to [10, 244, 289] and to [220] for an emphasis on the use of cure models in oncology clinical trials.

Since we cannot distinguish the cure observations from the uncured and censored ones, an important issue is when to use a cure model rather than a standard survival model. Obviously, the (medical) context will usually give us some information on whether we can expect a fraction of cure or not. However, we will see in this chapter that this information is not sufficient to safely fit a cure model as we may face identifiability problems. A good hint for the presence of a cure fraction is the presence of a long and stable *plateau* in the right tail of estimated survival curve, with the height of the plateau corresponding to the fraction of cure patients. We will reference some formal results on identifiability of cure models and will link these results to more informal recommendation on when to use a cure model in Section 4.4. A key point is that, we do not only require a "plateau" but we also require follow-up to be long enough to see a "long plateau" containing a "large" number of censored observations. Some real data examples are analyzed in Section

4.5 with an emphasis on the interpretation of the model parameters in the mixture cure model and in the promotion time cure model.

4.2   Mixture cure models

The mixture cure model has originally been proposed by Boag [175], Berkson and Gage [35], and Farwell [119]. This model explicitly takes into the presence of two sub-populations, the cure (or immune or non-susceptible) individuals who will never experience the event of interest and the uncured (or susceptible) individuals who will experience the event of interest. The mixture cure model is then composed of two sub-models, an *incidence model* for the probability to be uncured, and a *latency model* for the event times of the uncured observations.

Following the notations of Amico et al. [10], we denote by B the cure status indicator, with $B = 1$ corresponding to susceptible (i.e. uncured) individuals and $B = 0$ for non-susceptible (cure) individuals. We can then define the probability to be susceptible as $\pi = P(B = 1)$. Assuming that for the cure observations, the event time if infinite $(T = \infty)$, we have that the survival function of this subpopulation is

$$S_c(t) = P(T > t \mid B = 0) = 1 \qquad \text{for all } t$$

corresponding therefore to a degenerate survival function. Then, it is natural to define the mixture cure model by the following unconditional (population) survival function of T:

$$\begin{aligned} S_{pop}(t) = P(T > t) &= (1 - \pi)S_c(t) + \pi S_u(t) \\ &= (1 - \pi) + \pi S_u(t) \end{aligned}$$

where the subscript *pop* indicates that the survival function relates to the whole population and $S_u(t)$ is the (conditional) survival function of the uncured patients defined as

$$S_u(t) = P(T > t \mid B = 1)$$

Note that, this later conditional survival function of the uncured is a proper survival function, i.e. $lim_{t \to \infty} S_u(t) = 0$.

Consider two vectors of covariates $\mathbf{X}$ and $\mathbf{Z}$, we can then build a model for the probability to be susceptible, $\pi(\mathbf{X})$ referred to as the *incidence model* and a model for the time-to-event amongst the susceptible $S_u(t \mid Z)$ referred to as the *latency model*. The mixture cure model, including covariates, is then given by:

$$S_{pop}(t \mid \mathbf{X}, \mathbf{Z}) = (1 - \pi(\mathbf{X})) + \pi(\mathbf{X})S_u(t \mid \mathbf{Z}). \qquad (4.3)$$

As we will see below, $\mathbf{X}$ will usually includes an intercept term while $\mathbf{Z}$ will usually not, depending on the choice of the specific model for each sub-model. Apart for this difference, the two vectors $\mathbf{X}$ and $\mathbf{Z}$ can be the same or different.

While this model has the advantage to take into account the presence of cure individuals, and to explicitly model an improper population survival function, it has also the advantage to convey more information about the covariates effects as would a standard survival model such as the Cox PH model. This model as an appealing mixture model structure and its popularity is certainly linked to the easy interpretation of the model parameters. An interesting feature of this model is that each of the two sub-models is allowed to depend on potentially different covariates, since $\mathbf{X}$ can be identical to $\mathbf{Z}$ (with the exception of the intercept term) or partially or completely different from $\mathbf{Z}$. This model therefore allows to disentangle the effect of covariates on the incidence and on the latency. Typically, in a clinical trial, the treatment indicator will be included in both sub-models to quantify both the short (latency) and long (incidence) term effect of the treatment. On the other hand, the fact that covariates in $\mathbf{X}$ and $\mathbf{Z}$ can be different is in line with the intuition that medical and patient related factors associated with the probability to be susceptible and the time-to-event for the susceptible patients may not be the same.

4.2.1 The incidence and the latency submodels

A choice of model must be made for each sub-model. For the incidence part, modeling the probability of being susceptible, every model for a binary outcome could be considered. However, this part is nearly always modeled through a logistic regression model:

$$\pi(x) = P(B = 1 \mid \mathbf{X} = \mathbf{x}) = \frac{\exp(\gamma^t \mathbf{x})}{1 + \exp(\gamma^t \mathbf{x})} \qquad (4.4)$$

for a given covariate vector $\mathbf{X}$ (including an intercept) and a parameter vector γ to be estimated from the data.

On the other hand, more choices have been proposed in the literature for the incidence part, which model the event times for the susceptible individuals. As is the case for standard survival models, we can distinguish parametric from semi-parametric mixture cure models. In the former, the survival times of susceptible individuals follow a fully-parametric model, while the latter leaves the baseline hazard function of the susceptible individuals unspecified.

The most common choices are either a parametric PH model or a semi-parametric Cox PH model, and the survival function of the susceptible patients can then be written

$$
\begin{aligned}
S_u^{PH}(t \mid \mathbf{Z} = \mathbf{z}, B = 1) &= P(T > t \mid \mathbf{Z} = \mathbf{z}, B = 1) \\
&= (S_{u0}(t))^{\exp(\beta^t \mathbf{z})}
\end{aligned}
$$

with **Z** a vector of covariates (which does not include an intercept) and β the corresponding vector of parameters. The baseline survival function of the susceptible $S_{u0}(t) = S_u(t \mid B = 1) = P(T > t \mid \mathbf{Z} = \mathbf{0}, B = 1)$ is then either specified fully parametrically or left unspecified [201, 117, 283, 285, 367]. This model is sometimes referred to as the *proportional hazard mixture cure model*, this can however be confusing since, as we will see below, this model does actually not possess the proportional hazard structure at the population level.

Among the various parametric models considered, the most popular is probably the Weibull PH model [119] with hazard of the susceptible modeled has

$$h_u(t \mid \mathbf{z}) = \lambda \rho t^{\rho-1} \exp(\beta^t \mathbf{z}). \tag{4.5}$$

with $\lambda > 0$ the shape parameter and $\rho > 0$ the scale parameter ($\rho = 1$ in the case of an exponential model, [136]). This can be translated in terms of the survival of the susceptible as

$$S_u(t \mid \mathbf{z}) = \exp\left(-\lambda t^{\rho} \exp(\beta^t \mathbf{z})\right), \tag{4.6}$$

As discussed in Chapter 2, the Weibull model is fairly flexible and is often considered to provide a good description of survival times in biomedical applications. However, one has to be aware of the assumption of a monotonic baseline hazard function which may be too restrictive in some situations.

The main advantages of a fully parametric cure model is (i) the simplicity of the estimation procedure, relying on the maximization of the likelihood function (see Section 4.2.2) and (ii) the direct estimation of the survival function for a given covariates profile, which is sometimes itself of interest [278]. However, semi-parametric mixture cure models, for which the baseline hazard of the susceptible patients is left unspecified, and in particular considering a Cox PH model for the latency, have gain much more popularity in the statistical literature (see for examples [201, 237, 367, 369] amongst others).

Considering a semi-parametric Cox PH model for the latency, the hazard function of the susceptible patients is given by

$$h_u(t \mid \mathbf{z}) = h_{uo}(t) \exp(\beta^t \mathbf{z}), \tag{4.7}$$

or equivalently in terms of the survival function of these susceptible patients

$$S_u(t \mid \mathbf{z}) = S_{u0}(t)^{\exp(\beta^t \mathbf{z})}, \tag{4.8}$$

where $h_{uo}(t)$ and $S_{u0}(t)$ are respectively the baseline hazard and baseline survival function of the susceptible patients. Remind that these functions are actually conditional on being susceptible, such that for example $S_{u0}(t) = S_u(t \mid B = 1) = P(T > t \mid \mathbf{Z} = \mathbf{0}, B = 1)$.

It is important to realize that while logistic/(semi-)parametric PH mixture cure models assume proportional hazards for the susceptible patients, we don't necessarily observe proportional hazards at the level of the population. This is illustrated in Figure 4.3, representing the population survival functions for two groups of patients (e.g. control and experimental arm of a clinical trial), from a logistic/exponential mixture cure model [220]. Three different situations are considered: (a) the experimental treatment has only a long-term effect by increasing the proportion of cure (incidence) but no effect on delaying the event for the susceptible patients (latency); (b) the experimental treatment only has a short-term effect by delaying the event for the susceptible patients but has no long-term effect on the proportion of cure; (c) the experimental treatment has both a short-term effect on delaying the event for the susceptible and a long-term effect on increasing the proportion of cure. The top panels represent the survival curves of the susceptible patients ($S_u(t \mid z)$) while the bottom panels represent the population (observed) survival curves ($S_{obs}(t \mid z)$). As expected, all susceptible survival curves are proper (goes to 0 when time increases) and follow the proportional hazards assumption (the two curves in setting (a) are superimposed since the treatment has no effect on the time-to-event for the susceptible). On the other hand, looking at the population survival curves, one can see that only the first situation leads to PH, with the two curves attaining their plateau by "running parallel to each other", while to the other situations are violating this PH assumption.

For the latency sub-model, an alternative to the PH model is the AFT model, especially when we can not assume PH in the susceptible patients. In this case, the time-to-event of the susceptible patients T^u are modeled as

$$\log(T^u) = \beta_0 + \beta^t \mathbf{Z} + \sigma \epsilon, \tag{4.9}$$

with β_0 and $\sigma > 0$ the location and scale parameter and ϵ an error term with density function f_ϵ. The corresponding survival function of the susceptible patients

$$S_u^{AFT}(t \mid \mathbf{Z} = \mathbf{z}, B = 1) = S_{u0}(t \exp(-\beta_0 - \beta^t \mathbf{Z}))$$

with $S_{u0}(.)$ the baseline survival function of the susceptibles (so conditional on $B = 1$). As in standard survival analysis, one can consider a parametric distribution for $S_{u0}(.)$ (or equivalently for f_ϵ) leading to a parametric logistic/AFT mixture cure model [286, 351, 416] or left unspecified leading to a semi-parametric logistic/AFT model [224, 238, 429]. Although these models have the advantages of not making any PH assumption, neither at the level of the uncured patients (except when a Weibull distribution is assumed for the event times) nor at the population level, they suffer from the same lack of popularity as the standard AFT model in the medical literature.

4.2.2 Estimation

As mentioned above, the mixture cure models is actually a family of models, encompassing a wide variety of parametric and semi-parametric (and even non-parametric) models with different choice of models for each sub-model.

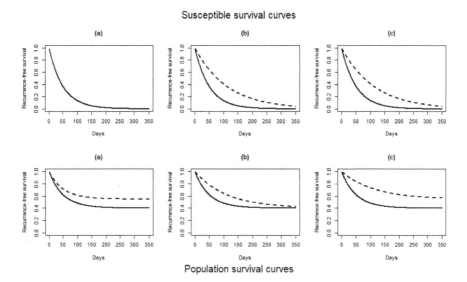

FIGURE 4.3
Survival functions from logistic/exponential PH mixture cure models for a
control (*solid line*) and an experimental treatment (*dotted line*) group. Survival
functions of the susceptible (*top*) and the population survival function (*bottom*)
in three different situations: the experimental treatment (a) only affects the
probability to be susceptible (long-term effect), (b) only affects the survival of
the susceptible patients (short-term effect), and (c) affects both the probability
to be susceptible and the survival of the susceptible (short and long term
effect).

As a consequence, a variety of estimation approaches have been proposed to
cover the various cases. Most of the estimation methods proposed for the
mixture cure models are in a frequentist framework and aim to maximize the
likelihood function (while we will see that most estimation methods proposed
for the second class of cure models are rather based on Bayesian approaches).

Assume we have i.i.d. data $(Y_i, \delta_i, \mathbf{X}_i, \mathbf{Z}_i), i = 1, ..., n$, where n is the number of patients, with $Y_i = \min(T_i, C_i)$ the observed time and $\delta_i = I(T_i \le C_i)$
the censoring indicator. The likelihood function is obtained by considering

- the contribution of uncensored observations; these individuals experienced
  the event and are then not cured. For such an individual i, his contribution
  is

$$f^*(y_i) = \pi(\mathbf{x}_i) f_u(y_i \mid \mathbf{z}_i, B = 1)$$

where $f_u(.)$ is the conditional density function of event time for the uncured
observations.

- the contribution of the censored observations, who are either cure (with probability $1 - \pi(\mathbf{x})$) or uncured (with probability $\pi(\mathbf{x})$. Based on the mixture cure model, the contribution for such an individual i is

$$S^*(y_i) = (1 - \pi(\mathbf{x}_i)) + \pi(\mathbf{x}_i)S_u(y_i \mid \mathbf{z}_i, B_i = 1)$$

The likelihood function is then given by

$$
\begin{aligned}
L^{MCM}(\zeta) &= \prod_{i=1}^{n} f^*(y_i)^{\delta_i} S^*(y_i)^{1-\delta_i} \\
&= \prod_{i=1}^{n} [\pi(\mathbf{x}_i)f_u(y_i \mid \mathbf{z}_i)]^{\delta_i} \\
&\times \prod_{i=1}^{n} [1 - \pi(\mathbf{x}_i) + \pi(\mathbf{x}_i)S_u(Y_i \mid \mathbf{z}_i)]^{1-\delta_i} \quad (4.10)
\end{aligned}
$$

with $f_u(t \mid \mathbf{z}) = -(d/dt)S_u(t \mid \mathbf{z})$ and ζ the vector containing all model parameters (so from the incidence and the latency models). Note that, this likelihood function actually has the same structure as in the classical survival setting (see (2.1) in Chapter 2), but with the density function and the survival function adapted to take into account the presence of a cure fraction according to our mixture cure model.

For a fully parametric model, this likelihood function can be maximized using numerical optimization, such as the Newton-Raphson algorithm. The variance of the estimators can then be obtained from the inverse of the observed Fisher information matrix of second order derivatives of $\log(L^{MCM}(\zeta))$. While classical survival distribution, such as those presented in Chapter 2 can be considered, more flexible models can be considered by extending the fully parametric estimation procedure to wider class of parametric distribution. For example, Yamagushi et al. [416] and Peng et al. [286] have proposed an AFT model for the latency with respectively a generalized gamma distribution for $\log T$ or a generalized F distribution for T.

To avoid the restriction of a parametric conditional survival function, one may prefer to rely on a semi-parametric cure model leaving the distribution of the event times of the uncured patients unspecified. However, estimation of such a semi-parametric model is less straightforward and different proposals have been made.

Let's consider first the case of the logistic/Cox PH mixture cure model. In this case, the baseline survival function $S_{0,u}(t \mid B = 1)$ acts as a nuisance parameter and prevents us from directly maximizing the likelihood (4.10). An additional difficulty is that we can not apply the partial likelihood idea as developed for the Cox PH model. Indeed, since we have non-PH at the level of the population, the ratio of the marginal hazard functions is not constant over time and $h_{0,u}(.)$ can not be isolated. In fact, it is important to realize that the latency, and in particular, $h_{0,u}(.)$ is conditional on the cure status

$B = 1$ and therefore contains information on the incidence of the event. To circumvent this, several approaches have been proposed.

Given that the that cure status is a latent variable (only partially observed), a popular approach is to rely on the EM algorithm [285, 367]. The idea is to first write the complete data likelihood, i.e., the likelihood we would have if the cure status was observed, and then to alternate between an E-step in which the expected value of this cure status is computed given the current value of the parameters and the observed data and a M-Step in which the complete data-likelihood is maximized with respect to the model parameters after having replaced the cure status is its expected value from the E-step. The complete data likelihood distinguish the contribution from the uncensored and thus uncured subjects (for whom $\delta_i B_i = 1$), the censored but uncured subjects (for whom $(1 - \delta_i)B_i = 1$) and the censored and cured subjects (for whom $(1 - \delta_i)(1 - B_i) = 1$) and can thus be written as

$$
\begin{aligned}
L_{comp}^{MCM}(h_0(.), \gamma, \beta) &= \prod_{i=1}^{n} [\pi(\mathbf{x}_i) h_u(y_i \mid \mathbf{z}_i) S_u((y_i \mid \mathbf{z}_i)]^{\delta_i B_i} \\
&\times \prod_{i=1}^{n} [\pi(\mathbf{x}_i) S_u(y_i \mid \mathbf{z}_i)]^{(1-\delta_i)B_i} \times \prod_{i=1}^{n} [1 - p(\mathbf{x}_i)]^{(1-\delta_i)(1-B_i)}
\end{aligned}
$$

where $h(t \mid \mathbf{Z}_i)S_u(t \mid \mathbf{Z}_i)_i$ is the density function of the uncured (cf the general relationship (1.3)). A further reason of the popularity of the EM algorithm in this context, is that the complete likelihood function L_{comp} can be written as the product $L_{comp}^{MCM} = L_{comp,1}(\gamma) \times L_{comp,2}(\beta, S_{u0})$, each of the two elements containing only the parameters of one the two sub-models:

$$
L_{comp,1}(\gamma) = \prod_{i=1}^{n} \pi(\mathbf{x}_i)^{B_i} [1 - p(\mathbf{x}_i)]^{(1-\delta_i)(1-B_i)} \tag{4.11}
$$

$$
L_{comp,2}(\beta, S_{u0}) = \prod_{i=1}^{n} \left[(h_u(y_i \mid \mathbf{z}_i) S_u(y_i \mid \mathbf{z}_i))^{\delta_i B_i} S_u(y_i \mid \mathbf{z}_i)^{(1-\delta_i)B_i} \right] \tag{4.12}
$$

This property obviously simplifies the maximization in the M-step, since one can handle the maximization separately for each set of parameters. Denoting $\zeta = (\gamma, \beta, S_{u0})$, the vector of all model parameters, the EM algorithm iterates between the two following steps:

E-step: At the kth iteration, the expectation of the latent variable B_i given the current values of the parameters $\zeta^{(k-1)}$ and the observed data $\mathcal{O} = (y_i, \delta_i, \mathbf{x}_i, \mathbf{z}_i)$ is given by (see e.g. [10]):

$$
\begin{aligned}
E(B_i \mid \mathcal{O}_i, \zeta^{(k-1)}) &= \delta_i + (1 - \delta_i) \frac{\pi^{(k-1)}(\mathbf{x}_i) S_u^{(k-1)}(y_i \mid \mathbf{z}_i)}{1 - \pi^{(k-1)}(\mathbf{x}_i) + \pi^{(k-1)}(\mathbf{x}_i) S_u^{(k-1)}(y_i \mid \mathbf{z}_i)} \\
&= \omega_i^{(k)}
\end{aligned} \tag{4.13}
$$

where $\pi^{(k-1)}(\mathbf{x}_i)$ is given by (4.4) in which γ have been replaced by the estimated value $\hat{\gamma}^{(k-1)}$ obtained at the previous step and $S_u^{(k-1)}(y_i \mid \mathbf{z}_i)$ is given by (4.8) in which β have been replaced $\hat{\beta}^{(k-1)}$. Since the log of the complete data likelihood is linear in B_i, one can obtain the expected log-complete data likelihood given the current values of the parameters and the observed data by replacing B_i by $\omega_i^{(k)}$ in (4.11). We will also see in Section 4.4 that to ensure the identifiability of the model we need to force the estimated conditional survival function of the uncured to be proper, and thus to go to zero when time goes to infinity. This can be achieved by setting $\omega_i^k = 0$, so considering the observation to be cured, when observation i is censored ($\delta_i = 0$) after the last event time ($Y_i > \tau = Y_{(r)}$).

M-step: We update the estimation of the parameters $\zeta^{(k-1)}$ by maximizing the expected complete data likelihood with respect to the parameters of the model. Given the factorization mentioned above, we can maximize separately $L_{comp,1}(\gamma)$ and $L_{comp,2}(\beta, S_{u0})$. With regard to the incidence, the likelihood to maximize is actually the same as in a classical logistic regression and can be maximized using a Newton-Raphson algorithm. Different methods have been proposed for the latency, so for the maximization of $L_{comp,2}(\beta, S_{u0})$ while leaving the baseline survival function of the uncured unspecified. $L_{comp,2}(\beta, S_{u0})$ indeed corresponds to the likelihood function of a regular Cox PH model with the $\omega_i^{(k)}$ as offset term. An important difference with the standard Cox PH model however is that we need in this M-Step to obtain an estimate of the baseline survival function of the uncured $S_{u0}(.)$ since we need it in the E-Step. The main approaches are based either on a profile likelihood methods (which is now possible since we work only with the part of the complete likelihood related to the latency) [367], on a product-limit type method [367], or on a marginal likelihood approach [285]. While these methods will produce a non-parametric estimate of $S_{u0}(.)$ to be used in the E-Step, this estimator will usually not be smooth. In case, we are interested in a smooth estimate of $S_{u0}(.)$, it has been proposed to consider flexible modeling of $h_{u0}(t)$ using splines [82].

The algorithm then iterates between the E-Step and the M-step until convergence. The resulting estimates have been proven to be consistent and asymptotically normal [117]. Corbiére et al. [84] proposed a non-parametric bootstrap to obtain the standard errors of the estimated parameters. It is interesting to note that once the EM algorithm has reached convergence, the value of the $\omega_i^{(k)}$ can be interpreted as estimator of the probability for an individual with covariate values $(\mathbf{x}_i, \mathbf{z}_i)$ to be uncured (and thus to experience the event) given the observed data for that subject [289].

Besides the EM algorithm, other approaches have been proposed, which includes:

- An approach based on the maximization of the marginal likelihood, as originally proposed for classical survival data [180] and extended to the case of the logistic/Cox PH mixture cure model. The idea is to integrate the likelihood function (4.10) over $y_{(j)}, j = 1, \ldots, r$ the ordered distinct uncensored observations and to then maximize this marginal likelihood with respect to the parameters. However, it is often not possible to compute this marginal likelihood in practice and it should be approximated for example via Monte Carlo approximations [201].

- An approach based on the maximization of a penalized likelihood, in the same spirit as what we discuss in Chapter 3 for the frailty model. The idea is to approximate the conditional baseline hazard by a combination of cubic normalized B-splines and to penalize the likelihood to control via a positive smoothing parameters κ the smoothness of the approximated hazard [82]

$$\log L\left((h_0(.), \gamma, \beta)\right) - \kappa \int_0^\infty \left(h_0''(t)\right)^2 dt$$

where $h_0''(t)$ is the second derivative of $h_0(t)$ with respect to time. One can then maximize this penalized likelihood and compute the variance of the parameter estimates based on the inverse of the matrix of the second derivatives of the penalized likelihood.

- An approach based on the maximization of a non-parametric likelihood function obtained by replacing the baseline conditional hazard in the likelihood by a non-parametric estimator [237].

Regarding the semi-parametric logistic/AFT models in which the latency is given by

$$\log(t) = \mu + \alpha^t \mathbf{Z} + e$$

with the density function of the error term left unspecified, the EM algorithm has been used in a similar way as above, except for the maximization of the component of the complete likelihood containing the parameters of the semi-parametric AFT in the M-step. The proposed methods are directly inspired from the methods proposed for the classical semi-parametric AFT model, based on M-estimator [224], rank estimation method [429], or a profile likelihood approach [238]. However, [289] mentions that the first two approaches may suffer from slow or even lack of convergence and recommend the third one which is computationally more efficient and provides a smooth estimate of the baseline hazard function.

4.2.3 Interpretation

As already mentioned, a major advantage of the mixture cure models is that is allows to disentangle the effect of the covariates on the incidence (i.e. the probability to experience the event) and on the latency (i.e. the time-to-event for those who will experience it). Furthermore, the parameters in each of these two sub-models can be interpreted classically.

For example, if we consider as it is often the case, a logistic regression for the incidence part, parameters from this model will be interpreted as usual. In particular, the exponential of the coefficient corresponding to p^{th} covariate, so

$\exp(\gamma_p)$, corresponds to the odds ratio of experience the event for a one unit increase in X_p. We can also use expression (4.4) to obtain easily a model-based estimation of the cure probability for a given set of covariates values. On the other hand, parameters from the latency models are interpreted as usual in survival analysis, with the exception however that they should be interpreted conditionally on being susceptible. So for example, if we consider a Cox PH model in the latency, the exponential of the coefficient corresponding the pth covariate, so $\exp(\beta_p)$ corresponds to the hazards ratio (and thus the increase in the hazard of the event) for a one unit increase in Z_p among the susceptible individuals.

4.3 Promotion time cure models

The promotion time cure model has been originally proposed by Yakovlev et al. [415, 415] and further formalized by Tsodikov [414, 415]. While the mixture cure models explicitly models the presence of two sub-populations, the cure and the uncured observations, the promotion time cure model is rather focusing on the fact that, due to the presence of a fraction of cure, the population survival function is improper. The idea is therefore to *bound* the cumulative hazard such that $\lim_{t\to\infty} H_{pop}(t) = \theta$, with $\theta > 0$ to force the population survival function to not go to zero when time goes to infinity. This comes back to considering that the cure observations have an infinite event time. It can be achieved by writing this cumulative hazard function as

$$H_{pop}(t) = \theta F(t)$$

where F(t) is a proper distribution function, such that $F(0) = 0$ and $\lim_{t\to\infty} F(t) = 1$.

In the original formulation of the promotion time cure model, covariates are introduced only through θ and the model then takes the form

$$S(t \mid \mathbf{X} = \mathbf{x}) = \exp\{-\theta(\mathbf{x})F(t)\} \tag{4.14}$$

where $\mathbf{X}$ is the vector of covariates, which includes and intercept, and $\theta(.)$ is a positive known link function. In this case

$$\lim_{t\to\infty} S(t \mid \mathbf{X} = \mathbf{x}) = \exp\{-\theta(\mathbf{x})\}$$

and $\exp\{-\theta(\mathbf{x})\}$ represents therefore the cure rate. Since $\theta(\mathbf{x})$ must be positive, Tsodikov [383, 384] proposed to specify

$$\theta(\mathbf{x}) = exp(\beta^t \mathbf{x})$$

The distribution function $F(t)$ can be specified parametrically, e.g. considering an exponential, a Weibull or a gamma distribution [65] or left totally unspecified [383, 384, 385].

Given that the cumulative hazard is bounded, this model is also called the *bounded cumulative hazard model*. By opposition to the mixture cure model of Section 4.2, it is also sometimes called the *non-mixture cure model*. One also speaks about *PH cure models* since this model assumes proportional hazards at the population level. Indeed, from (4.14), we have that the model can be expressed in terms of the hazard function as

$$h(t \mid \mathbf{X} = \mathbf{x}) = \theta(\mathbf{x})f(t) \tag{4.15}$$

where $f(t)$ is the density function corresponding to $F(t)$. So, if we consider two individuals with different covariates values, we have

$$\frac{h(t \mid \mathbf{x}_i)}{h(t \mid \mathbf{x}_j)} = \frac{\theta(\mathbf{x}_i)}{\theta(\mathbf{x}_j)}$$

which is indeed constant over time. This proportionality assumption may of course limit the application of this model in practice. As we will see below, see Section 4.3.3, this can be relaxed by including covariates also in the distribution function $F(t)$.

On the other hand the usual denomination of promotion time cure model is not originating from its mathematical properties but is justified by its seminal biological interpretation [414]. Indeed, this model has a strong biological interpretation linked the modeling of tumor progression (see Section 4.3.2).

4.3.1 Estimation

Estimation of the promotion time cure model has been studied mainly in a Bayesian framework. Indeed, one can show that for this model the posterior distribution of the regression parameters is often proper while using improper non-informative priors, which is a nice property in a Bayesian setting. On the other hand, this is not the case for the mixture cure models [425]. Bayesian estimations methods, which usually rely on Markov Chain Monte Carlo (MCMC) methods to approximate the posterior distribution of the parameters of interest, have been proposed for the fully parametric models (assuming a Weibull distribution for $F(.)$) [65], or a semi parametric model (assuming $F(.)$ to be a piecewise constant function) [172, 185] considering both non-informative and informative priors. In the later case, attention should be paid to the zero-tail constraint (see Section 4.4) which can be implemented via an appropriate choice of the prior on the constant value of $F(.)$, see [172] for more details.

Nevertheless some frequentist estimation methods have also been proposed, and are then based on the likelihood function given by

$$
\begin{aligned}
L^{PTM}(\zeta) &= \prod_{i=1}^{n} [\theta(\mathbf{x}_i)f(y_i)\exp(-\theta(\mathbf{x}_i)F(y_i))]^{\delta_i} \times \{\exp(-\theta(\mathbf{x}_i)F(y_i))\}^{1-\delta_i} \\
&= \prod_{i=1}^{n} \{\theta(\mathbf{x}_i)f(y_i)\}^{\delta_i} \times \{\exp(-\theta(\mathbf{x}_i)F(y_i))\} \tag{4.16}
\end{aligned}
$$

where $\theta(\mathbf{X})$ is usually assumed to be $\exp(\beta_0 + \beta^t(X))$ and ζ is the vector containing all model parameters. This likelihood is obtained as usual in survival analysis by considering the contribution of the uncensored observations and of the censored observations .

When $F(.)$ is parametrically specified, maximum likelihood estimates can be obtained for the parameters in $\theta(\mathbf{X})$ and $F(.)$ by maximizing this likelihood function. Maximum likelihood methods have also been proposed when $F(.)$ is left unspecified, based either on the maximization of the full likelihood via a profiling approach [428] or a backfitting approach [241], or more simply based on the maximization of a profile likelihood [302, 384]. The full or complete likelihood, i.e. the likelihood we would get if we could distinguish the cured from the uncured observation, is obtained as for the mixture cure model from the contributions of the uncensored and thus uncured subjects (for whom $\delta_i B_i = 1$), the censored but uncured subjects (for whom $(1 - \delta_i)B_i = 1$ and the censored and cured subjects (for whom $(1 - \delta_i)(1 - B_i) = 1$, and can thus be written as

$$
\begin{aligned}
L_{comp}^{PTM}(F(.), \beta) & = \prod_{i=1}^{n} [\theta(\mathbf{x}_i)f(y_i)\exp(-\theta(\mathbf{x}_i)F(y_i))]^{\delta_i B_i} \\
& \times \prod_{i=1}^{n} [\exp(-\theta(\mathbf{x}_i)F(y_i))]^{(1-\delta_i)B_i} \\
& \times \prod_{i=1}^{n} [\exp(-\theta(\mathbf{x}_i))]^{(1-\delta_i)(1-B_i)}
\end{aligned}
\tag{4.17}
$$

The idea is to then generally to first obtain a non-parametric maximum likelihood estimator (NPMLE) of $F(.)$, by replacing it by a step function (taking a new value at observed event times) in (4.17). We can then maximize the resulting expression for all models parameters as well as for the jump sizes of the NPMLE of $F(.)$ [428]. The number of dimensions for the maximization therefore increases with the number of uncensored observations and can be very large. Instead of using a Newton-Raphson algorithm, Tsodikov [384] proposes a maximization algorithm which reduce the instability problems encountered when the number of parameters is very large. [241] propose a alternative approach based on backfitting to solve the score equations for the step sizes ΔF_j (at event time $Y_{(j)}, j = 1, .., r$) and the model parameters. Finally, [302] propose to first get a profile likelihood, by replacing $F(.)$ by an explicit expression of its NPMLE for (β_0, β^t) fixed. The idea is then to obtain the estimates of the (β_0, β^t) parameters by maximizing the resulting expression (which does not depend on $F(.)$ anymore) with respect these parameters, and then to plug these values into the explicit expression of the NPMLE of $F(.)$ to obtain an estimate for $F(.)$. Asymptotic and efficiency results for the model parameters in $\theta(.)$ and for the non-parametric estimator of $F(.)$ have been obtained, and a weighted bootstrap procedure have been proposed to obtain a consistent approximation of the asymptotic laws of the estimators [302].

Whatever the approach above, the maximization for the jump sizes ΔF_j (at event time $Y_{(j)}, j = 1, .., r$) is performed under the constraint that

$$F_r = \sum_{j=1}^{r} \Delta F_j = 1$$

which corresponds to the zero-tail constraint (see Section 4.4) and is needed for the identifiability of the model.

It is important to note that the semi-parametric promotion time cure model with an exponential link function can be seen as a generalization of the Cox PH model [302]. Indeed, assuming that $\theta(x) = \exp(\beta_0 + \beta^t x)$, then Equation (4.14) becomes

$$
\begin{aligned}
S(t|\mathbf{X} = \mathbf{x}) &= \exp\left[-\exp(\beta_0 + \beta^t \mathbf{x})F(t)\right] \\
&= \exp\left[-\exp(\beta^t \mathbf{x})\exp(\beta_0)F(t)\right] \\
&= \exp\left[-\exp(\beta^t \mathbf{x})H(t)\right],
\end{aligned}
$$

i.e., a PH model in which $H(t) = \exp(\beta_0)F(t)$ is a *bounded* cumulative hazard function, taking values in $[0, \exp(\beta_0)]$. As we have seen in Chapter 2, in theory the cumulative hazard function of the Cox PH model is not bounded. However, in practice, the estimator of the cumulative hazard function based on the available observations is bounded. So, we have the following links between the estimates from both models:

$$
\begin{aligned}
\hat{\beta}_{PT} &= \hat{\beta}_{PH} \\
\exp(\hat{\beta}_{0,PT}) &= \hat{H}_{PH}(Y_{(n)}) \\
\exp(\hat{\beta}_{0,PT})\hat{F}_{PT}(t) &= \hat{H}_{PH}(t)
\end{aligned}
$$

where the index PT and PH refers to estimates obtained from a promotion time cure model and a Cox PH model respectively, and $Y_{(n)}$ is the largest observed event time. This result is however true uniquely when we assume an exponential link function $\theta(x) = \exp(\beta_0 + \beta^t \mathbf{x})$ and leaves the distribution function $F(.)$ unspecified. A major consequence is that as long as the PH assumption is met at the population level, the Cox PH model do indeed provides reliable results even in the presence of a non-negligible cure fraction. We should however be aware that the parameters should be interpreted in the context of a promotion time cure model, thus taking into account the presence of a cure fraction.

4.3.2   Interpretation

The seminal application of the promotion time cure model is the modeling of cancer relapse [415]. The idea is to assume that after an initial cancer treatment, individual i has N_i carcinogenic cells left active with $N_i \sim$

$Poisson(\theta(\mathbf{X}))$ such that $N_i = 0$ corresponds to cure patients. One further assumes that the time for the carcinogenic cell k from individual i to produce a detectable tumor mass is W_{ik} with the W_{ik} mutually independent, independent of N_i, and with a common cdf $F(t)$. Then, the time until the relapse of cancer (observed time) is $T_i = min(W_1, \ldots W_{N_i})$.

So, we see that the covariates $\mathbf{X}$, through $\theta(\mathbf{X})$ have an impact on the number of cells which can metastasize, and therefore directly influence both the cure probability and also the conditional survival of the uncured patients. Indeed, larger values of $\theta(\mathbf{X})$ corresponds to a larger mean number of carcinogenic cells which can metastasize and are therefore associated with a lower cure probability and a lower event time for the uncured patients (since a larger number of carcinogenic cells induce a smaller activation time). So, $\mathbf{X}$ affects both the probability to be cure (i.e. that $N = 0$) and the time-to-event of the uncured observations. In the common case, where $\theta(\mathbf{x}) = \exp(\beta_0 + \beta^t\mathbf{X})$, a one unit increase in X_p is associated with an $\exp(\beta_p)$ times higher mean number of cells which can metastasize, and therefore a decreased (resp. increased) probability to be cure and a shorter (resp. longer) event time when $\exp(\beta)$ is larger (resp. smaller) than one.

The promotion time model has also been used in settings where the biological interpretation does not (directly) hold. In that case the interpretation of the impact of $\mathbf{X}$ on the probability to be cure is straightforward but a direct interpretation of the impact of $\mathbf{X}$ on the conditional survival of the uncured observations is less straightforward. It can however be recovered, and its is actually possible to re-express the promotion time cure model as a mixture cure model, in which the interpretation of the covariate effects is more straightforward.

Although the promotion time cure model is not equivalent to a mixture cure model, we can express the population survival function with a mixture expression

$$S_{pop}^{PTM} = (1 - \pi(\mathbf{X})) + \pi(\mathbf{X})S_u^{PTM}(t \mid \mathbf{X}) \qquad (4.18)$$

However, a major difference is that we have the same vector of covariates $\mathbf{X}$ in the incidence and in the latency. Since

$$\lim_{t \to \infty} S_{pop}^{PTM} = \exp(-\theta(\mathbf{X})) = 1 - \pi(\mathbf{X}) \qquad (4.19)$$

this quantity corresponds to the cure rate providing an easy interpretation of the impact of $\theta(\mathbf{X})$ on the probability to be cure. We can also show that the survival function for the uncured subject is given by [65]

$$S_u^{PTM}(t \mid \mathbf{X}) = \frac{\exp[-\theta(X)F(t)] - \exp(-\theta(X))}{1 - \exp(-\theta(X))} \qquad (4.20)$$

We see that the covariates $\mathbf{X}$ appears at different places in the conditional survival function of the uncured and the interpretation of the effect of $\mathbf{X}$ on this conditional survival is not straightforward. Obviously, $\theta(\mathbf{X})$ capture both type of effects, the *short term effect* on time-to-event for the uncured and the *long term effects* on the probability to be cure. With such a model, the two effects can not be disentangle.

Figures 4.4 and 4.5 represent, for an hypothetical example, the relation between $\theta(\mathbf{X})$ and the cure probability, the conditional survival of uncured observations and the population survival function. These plots have been obtained from equations (4.19), (4.20), and (4.18) considering a Weibull distribution function $F(.)$ with $\lambda = 0.01$ and $\rho = 0.90$. As we can see, a covariate whose effect is to increase the value of $\theta(\mathbf{X})$ will have a decreasing effect on the probability to be cure and will also lead to shorter survival times for the uncured. Coming back to the biological motivation of the model, this results from the fact that such a covariate whose effect is to increase the value of $\theta(\mathbf{X})$ will increase the mean number of cells that can metastasize. At the level of the population, a higher value of $\theta(\mathbf{X})$ is associated with a survival curve being lower, corresponding to worst prognosis patients.

4.3.3 Extended promotion time cure model

An important extension of the promotion time cure model is to introduce covariates both in θ and in $F(.)$. Considering two vectors of covariates X and Z, the model then writes

$$S(t \mid \mathbf{X} = \mathbf{x}, \mathbf{Z} = \mathbf{z}) = \exp\{-\theta(\mathbf{x})F(t \mid \mathbf{z})\} \tag{4.21}$$

and $\theta(\mathbf{x}) = \exp(\beta_0 + \beta^t \mathbf{x})$ is usually assumed.

Tsodikov [386] and Bremhorst et al. [44, 45] consider

$$F(t \mid \mathbf{z}) = 1 - S_0(t)^{\exp(\gamma^t \mathbf{z})} \tag{4.22}$$

where $S_0(.)$ is a proper baseline survival function, so with $\lim_{t \to \infty} S_0(t) = 0$, which is left totally unspecified. Note that this expression corresponds to a Cox PH model, and as in this model we consider no intercept in $\mathbf{Z}$ (as such an intercept would not be identifiable). Other choices are also possible, for example Tsodikov [386] also studied the case where

$$F(t \mid z) = \frac{\exp(\gamma^t \mathbf{z})F_0(t)}{[1 - \exp(\gamma^t \mathbf{z})F_0(t)]}$$

which corresponds to a proportional odds model.

Coming back to the biological interpretation, since the covariate vector $\mathbf{Z}$ intervene only in the distribution function $F(.)$ it actually affects the time needed for a metastatic cell to produce a detectable tumor mass but the number of such cells. On the other hand, as can be seen from (4.20), the covariate vector $\mathbf{X}$ still affects both the number of cells that can metastasize and the time it takes for such cells to produce a detectable tumor mass. While

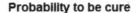

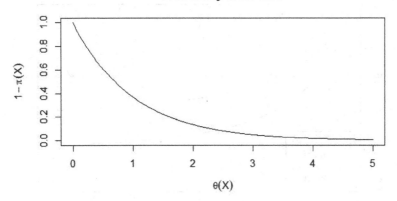

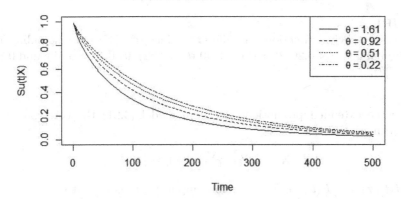

FIGURE 4.4
Representation of the effect of the value of $\theta(\mathbf{X})$ on the cure probability *top* and on the conditional survival function of the uncured *bottom*. The conditional survival function is representing for different values of $\theta(\mathbf{X})$, corresponding to cure probabilities of 0.20 ($\theta(\mathbf{X}) = 1.61$), 0.40 ($\theta(\mathbf{X}) = 0.92$), 0.60 ($\theta(\mathbf{X}) = 0.51$) and 0.80 ($\theta(\mathbf{X}) = 0.22$).

we now have two separate sets of covariates, the covariates effects on the survival of the uncured patients remain difficult to interpret, since the effect of $\mathbf{X}$ via $\theta(\mathbf{X})$ and $\mathbf{Z}$ via $F(t \mid \mathbf{Z})$ can not be disentangled as in the mixture cure models.

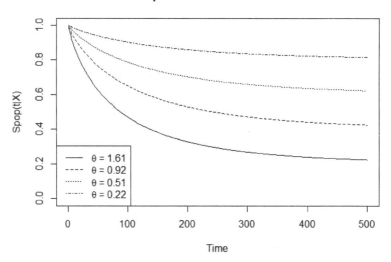

FIGURE 4.5
Population survival function for different values of $\theta(\mathbf{X})$, corresponding to cure probabilities of 0.20 ($\theta = 1.61$), 0.40 ($\theta = 0.92$), 0.60 ($\theta = 0.51$), and 0.80 ($\theta = 0.22$).

For the extended promotion time cure model (4.21) the corresponding hazard function is

$$h(t \mid \mathbf{X} = \mathbf{x}, \mathbf{Z} = \mathbf{z}) = \theta(\mathbf{x})f(t \mid \mathbf{z})$$

with $f(t \mid \mathbf{z}) = \frac{d}{dt}F(t \mid \mathbf{z})$. It is therefore important to note that this extended model does not have a proportional hazards structure anymore, since we have now for two individuals with different values of their covariates

$$\frac{h(t \mid \mathbf{x}_i, \mathbf{z}_i)}{h(t \mid \mathbf{x}_j, \mathbf{z}_j)} = \frac{\theta(\mathbf{x}_i)f(t \mid \mathbf{z}_i)}{\theta(\mathbf{x}_j)f(t \mid \mathbf{z}_j)}$$

Regarding frequentist estimation procedures, the profile likelihood idea mentioned in Section 4.3.1 can also be used although the second step consisting in the maximization of the profile likelihood with respect to the parameters β_0, β, and γ, is more complex [386]. This model has also been studied in a Bayesian framework, considering a P-splines approach to estimate the unspecified baseline hazard function corresponding to $S_0(.)$ in (4.22) and a MCMC algorithm to study the joint posterior density of the parameters [45]. Identifiability issue are discussed in [44, 45], who report that some restrictions on the covariates may be required. In the semi-parametric case (leaving $S_0(.)$

unspecified), estimation procedure needs to ensure that the estimated $F(.)$ is indeed a proper distribution function, which is usually done by imposing the constraint that $\hat{F}(.)$ or $\hat{F}_0(.)$ is indeed equal to one after the last observed event time, which correspond to imposing the zero-tail constraint mentioned in the next section.

4.4   When to use a cure model

Before considering using a cure model, one should ensure that there is some contextual evidence for the existence of a cure fraction. However, this is clearly not enough, as we also need to "see" the presence of this cure fraction in our data. As pointed by Taylor [369], a good hint for the presence of cure in our data can be inferred from the shape of the Kaplan-Meier estimate of the survival function. Indeed, if we see that the survival curve levels-up, with a long plateau containing a "large" number of (right-censored) data points, we can be confident that (almost) all observations in the plateau are in fact cure individuals. Formal identifiability conditions have also be studied (see for example [10]) and some attempts have also been made to test for the presence of cure.

A general and informal rule that holds for all cure models therefore requires the follow-up of the study to be sufficiently long: the estimated survival function should exhibit a long plateau containing many right-censored observations. More formally, the maximum possible event time should be smaller than the maximum possible censoring time. If we denote $\tau_F = \inf\{t : F(t) = 1\}$ and $\tau_G = \inf\{t : G(t) = 1\}$ with G the censoring distribution function, one should have [10] (omitting the covariates for the sake of simplicity)

$$\tau_{F_u} < \tau_G \qquad (4.23)$$

where $F_u = 1 - S_u$ is the conditional distribution function of the uncured. This assumption is actually crucial in most papers on semi-parametric (and non-parametric) mixture cure models. Amico et al. [10] discuss more formally the question of identifiability in mixture cure models and distinguish two definitions of identifiability. The strongest definition states that the model is identifiable if there is a unique set of parameters for which the expected log-likelihood is maximal. In this framework, the censoring distribution plays an important role and one can show that condition 4.23 indeed turns out to be crucial [280, 412].

In a parametric cure model, the parametric assumption made on $S_{u0}(.)$ in a mixture cure model or on $F(.)$ in a promotion time cure model, will ensure in the estimation process that this function will be estimated as a proper survival or distribution function. However, this is not so straightforward in the semi- or non-parametric setting. In a semi-parametric mixture cure model, the baseline survival function in the latency component $S_u(.)$ is left unspecified and estimated non-parametrically. Some additional information is therefore required for the model to distinguish cure from uncured observations amongst the censored ones. A major issue is that even if this model assume that $\lim_{t\to\infty} S_u(t) = 0$, we will often observe in practice that $\hat{S}_u(t) > 0$ when $t > Y_{(r)}$ (the largest observed event time) leading thus to identifiability problem. To solve this, [367] and [369] propose to consider $Y_{(r)}$ as the cure threshold and thus to constraint the survival function of the uncured (or the baseline survival function) to reach 0 at the largest observed event time. This constraint is often referred to as the *zero-tail constraint* and is used in most of the papers (see for example [224, 285, 367]). For example, in the EM algorithm described in Section 4.2.2, this can be achieved by setting in the E-step $\omega_i = 0$ (see (4.13)), so considering the observation to be cured, when observation i is censored ($\delta_i = 0$) after the last event time ($Y_i > \tau = Y_{(r)}$).

The idea behind this zero-tail constraint is actually natural in the contexts in which a cure model is justified, i.e., when such a cure fraction is known to exist and when follow-up is sufficiently long after the largest event time to indeed observe it in our data. However, it may seem less natural to force the conditional survival function to drop suddenly to zero after the last event time, so it has also been proposed to rather estimate parametrically the tail of the conditional baseline survival function once $t > \tau = Y_{(r)}$, according either to an exponential or a Weibull. Such a *tail completion method* allows to force the survival function to decrease smoothly to zero after the largest observed event time, and can in some circumstances reduces bias that would be induced in case event may still occurs after the longest observed time [283].

Considering the promotion time model including covariates only in $\theta(.)$, strong identifiability (i.e. existence of a unique parameter vector β and a unique distribution function $F(.)$ that maximizes the expected log likelihood) has been proved for the general case where $\theta(\mathbf{X}) = \varphi(\beta_0 + \beta^t \mathbf{X})$ for a strictly increasing function $\varphi(.)$, so including the common case of $\varphi(.) = \exp(.)$, and when $F(.)$ is left unspecified [302, 428]. Of note, Bremhorst and Lambert [45] proved a (weaker) identifiability result for the extended models in the case where $\theta(\mathbf{X}) = \exp(\beta_0 + \beta^t \mathbf{X})$ and $F(t \mid Z)$ is given by (4.22). Similar to the case of the mixture cure model, in the semi-parametric promotion time model, since $F(.)$ is left unspecified and estimated non-parametrically, additional information is required to get this identifiability. An equivalent to the zero-tail constraint is imposed in the estimation procedure, by forcing the estimated distribution function $F(.)$ to be one after some threshold τ, often called the *cure threshold* [428]. This comes back to assuming that all individuals with a censoring time larger than τ are cure. In the profile likelihood approach, the estimation procedure actually force the jumps of the NPMLE of $F(.)$ to sum up to one at the last observed event time (see Section 4.3.1); in this case τ is actually the largest observed event time and one assumes that no event can occur after. This is clearly equivalent to the zero-tail constraint of the mixture cure model and, as for this model, one should then use a promotion time model when this assumption is realistic based on the observed data and when a fraction of cure is known to exist.

Forcing $S_{u0}(t)$ in the mixture cure model to be 0 (or to decrease smoothly to 0) after the largest observed event time or forcing $F(t)$ in promotion time model to be 1 after the largest observed event time can be seen as a pragmatic solution to the identifiability problem of these models. As this solution is easy to implement in the estimation algorithms considered it has been widely used in many semi-parametric estimation methods for cure models. Obviously, assuming that no event can occur after the last observed event time is not always realistic. As we have already mentioned, the easiest way to heuristically check that it makes sense to assume that all censored observations after the largest observed event time are cure, is to check whether the Kaplan-Meier estimate of the population survival function indeed show a "long plateau" containing a "large" number of censored observations. This will indicate that we have a follow-up long enough and that we can be confident of the presence of a cure fraction. On the other hand, even if we know that there exists such a cure fraction (e.g., from the medical context) but if we don't have a follow-up long enough to confidently assume that all observations censored after the largest event time are cure, then fitting a cure model relying the zero-tail constraint will lead to biased results.

Given the importance of this assumption, several attempts have been made in the literature to formally test whether we are in the condition to confidently apply a cure model. First, Maller and Zhou [244] proposed a formal test for the presence of a sufficiently long follow-up by testing the identifiability condition

$$\begin{cases} H_0 : \tau_{F_u} \geq \tau_G \\ H_1 : \tau_{F_u} < \tau_G \end{cases}$$

They proposed a test statistic based on the number of censored observations in the tail of the estimated survival curve, however critical values were only provided, based on simulations, for very restrictive settings and this test is therefore not used in practice. Tentatives have also been made to develop test procedures for the presence of a cure fraction. Zhao et al. [433] propose a score test in the context of the logistic/Cox PH mixture cure model for the hypothesis assuming that the incidence does not depend on covariates and a parametric baseline hazard in the latency. They show that the distribution of their score statistics under the null is a mixture of two chi-square (with 0 and 1 degree of freedom) with equal probability. This test has been further extended to the case where the incidence depends on a continuous covariate [169] considering a sup-score test statistics whose distribution under the null hypothesis must be approximated via resampling. Despite these efforts, there is up to now no clear criteria nor widely available hypothesis test for the evidence of a cure fraction, and the current recommendation is to rely on a visual inspection of the tail of the KM estimated survival curve.

Only few proposals have been made with regards to diagnostic checks for the fit of cure models, and most of them have been developed for the mixture cure model. A modification of the Schoenfeld residuals have been proposed to assess the overall fit of a parametric mixture cure model with respect to the covariates included in the model [407]. Other "classical" residuals-based methods have also been extended to the case of either a parametric or semi-parametric mixture cure model. Peng and Taylor [287] investigate martingale and Cox-Snell residuals both for the overall models and for the latency part only, with the aim to check the functional form of the covariates, the presence of outliers, and the fit of the model.

It is important to keep in mind that the promotion time cure model in its original formulation (4.14), so with covariates introduced only via $\theta(\mathbf{X})$ has the proportional hazards property at the population level. So, even if we are in the presence of a cure fraction, if we do not have proportional hazards, the promotion time cure model should not be used. On the other hand, the extended promotion time cure model (with covariates introduced through $\theta(\mathbf{X})$ and $(F(t \mid \mathbf{Z}))$ and the mixture cure model do not assume proportional hazards at the level of the population.

An important characteristic of the promotion time cure model is its strong biological motivation related to the modeling of tumor progression. However, this model has also been used in different context. A drawback is however that we can not disentangle the effect of the covariates on the short (time-to-event for the uncured) and long (probability to be cure) term. On the other hand, the fact that the promotion time cure model with an exponential link and an unspecified $F(.)$ distribution and the Cox PH model are in "in practice" equivalent, and that we can thus simply fit a Cox PH model with any standard software, is obviously an advantage of the promotion time cure model. It is in fact a bit odds that this has not been really exploited in the literature, except maybe by the opponents of the cure models who argue that cure models are not needed since a Cox model can "do the job". We should however keep in mind that (1) this equivalence is only true for one specific cure model and that (2) even if we can indeed use in that case a Cox PH model to obtain the parameter estimates those should still be interpreted in line with the presence of a cure fraction.

A strong advantage of the mixture cure model, is that it allows to differentiate the effects of the covariates on the probability to be cure and on the survival times for the uncured observations. It is even possible to consider different covariates in the incidence and the latency. This reflects the natural intuition that it may not be, for example, the same patient and disease characteristics which impact the short and long term outcome. Note that while the extended version of the promotion time cure model allows to introduce a different vector of covariates in $F(.)$, the interpretation of the models parameters is not as simple as in the mixture cure model and the survival of the uncured will be impacted both by the variables in $\theta(.)$ and in $F(.)$, see (4.20).

Although they are usually not equivalent, there exists some mathematical links between the two modeling approaches. For example, if we assume a Bernoulli distribution for the number of cells that can metastasize and follow the same reasoning as [415], we obtain a promotion time cure model which is actually a mixture cure model [290]. There are other particular situations when the two models are equivalent. This is obviously the case when no covariate at all are considered and both $S_u(t)$ in the mixture cure models and $F(.)$ in the promotion time cure model are left unspecified. The two models are also equivalent when the cure rate, so $\pi(.)$ and $\theta(.)$, do not depend on covariates and the baseline function in $\S_u(. \mid \mathbf{X})$ and $F(. \mid \mathbf{X})$ are left unspecified [290]. On the other hand, as soon as $\pi(.)$ and $\theta(.)$ will depend on covariates will not be equivalent anymore. Nevertheless, the (extended) promotion time cure model can be rewritten as a promotion time cure model using the relation (4.20) for the survival of the uncured and $\exp(-\theta(\mathbf{X})$ for the probability to be cure, having

$$
\begin{aligned}
S_{pop}^{PTM}(t \mid \mathbf{X}, \mathbf{Z}) \;=\; & \exp(-\theta(\mathbf{X})) \\
+ \; & [1 - \exp(-\theta(\mathbf{X}))]\, \frac{\exp[-\theta(\mathbf{X})F(t \mid \mathbf{Z}) - \exp(-\theta(\mathbf{X}))}{1 - \exp(-\theta(\mathbf{X}))}
\end{aligned}
$$

However, we see that the major difference between the two models is the role played by the covariates in the "latency" part of the model.

Legrand and Bertrand [220] conducted a simulation study to investigate the consequences of model mis-specification, either by considering a Cox PH model when there is not cure or considering a mixture cure models when data where generated from a promotion time cure model and vice-versa. The simulation were performed considering a single binary covariate, representing for example the treatment in a clinical trial context. Data were generated from a Cox model (so no cure), with either a short or a long-follow up period, from a promotion time model (with a follow-up long enough to see the plateau) and from a mixture models with a treatment effect only in the incidence, both in the incidence and in the latency, and only in the latency (in each case with a follow-up long enough to see the plateau). These six simulations scenario are represented in Figure 4.6 (taken from [220]).

Each simulated dataset was then analyzed using a semi-parametric Cox PH model, a semi-parametric promotion time model and a semi-parametric mixture cure models (including the treatment covariate both in the incidence and in the latency). As they represent different population parameters, the estimated coefficient can not be directly compared between the models, however comparisons can be made based on the estimated cure fraction and for the estimated conditional survival function of the uncured. The conclusion is that the consequences of model specification can vary largely based on the true underlying model and on the focus of estimation (cure probability, conditional survival function, treatment effect size and significance). As could be expected from the zero-tail constraint, the ability of the cure models to acknowledge the absence of cure if largely impacted by the length of follow up and the amount of censoring. If follow-up is too short, and we therefore don't have a plateau in the tail of the KM estimators of the survival function, fitting a cure model will overestimate the cure fraction and underestimate the

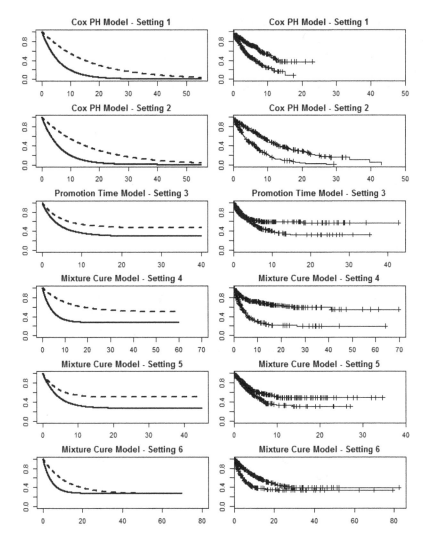

FIGURE 4.6
Survival functions in the simulation settings. *Left:* Theoretical survival functions for each simulation setting. *Right:* Estimated survival functions for a random dataset for each setting. The solid line represents the control group $(X = 0)$ while the dotted line represents the treatment group $(X = 1)$.

conditional survival of the uncured. This can be explained by the fact that all individuals with a censored time longer than the largest observed event time will wrongly be considered as cure (while it still include uncured individuals). So, too many individuals are considered as cure (leading to an over-estimation of the cure probability) and all the individuals with a long event time (longest than the last observed one) are actually considered as cure and therefore not taken into account in the estimation of the uncured survival probability leading to an underestimation of this conditional survival of the uncured. In the presence of cure, the conclusions are mainly driven by the appropriateness of the proportional hazard assumption. When PH holds, all three models seem to recover the treatment effect, but of course only the mixture cure models allow to disentangle short from long term effects. On the other hand, when PH did not hold, the promotion time model seems to recover some part of the treatment effect but the estimated cure rate and conditional survival of the uncured are biased.

4.5 Software and examples revisited

Fitting the simpler forms of cure models does not required any specific software. For example, a non parametric estimator of the cure rate (without covariates) can be obtained from the Kaplan-Meier estimator of the survival function [244] and can thus be obtained from most standard statistical software. Also, fully parametric cure model based on a standard distribution for the survival distribution of the uncured are easily fitted via maximum likelihood estimation, which can usually be coded quite straightforwardly in R or SAS.

However, specific R packages have also been developed to fit cure models, and in particular for the semi-parametric models, see [220, 289] for an overview. The gfcure package (in fact not a real R package, see [284]) allows to fit parametric mixture cure models considering a logistic regression model for the incidence and an AFT model in the latency based on Peng et al. [286]. Obviously, choosing a Weibull distribution of the survival time of the uncured patients will be equivalent to fit a parametric logistic/PH mixture cure model. The most popular R package for (semi-)parametric mixture cure models, allowing both a Cox PH hazard or an AFT model for the latency, is the smcure package [55, 56]. The smcure package allows to fit semi-parametric mixture cure models with various choices for the incidence model (including the logistic model but also other generalized linear models with various link functions) and the choice between a Cox PH or an AFT model for the latency. Estimation is based on the EM algorithm and the variance of the estimated parameters are obtained via bootstrap.

Given the "practical" equivalence between the semi-parametric promotion time cure model (with an exponential link) and the Cox PH model discussed in Section 4.3.1 any standard statistical software fitting a Cox PH model can be used to fit such a promotion time cure model. The semi-parametric promotion time cure models, as well as other models, can also be fitted with the nltm [129]. This package actually can be used to fit different type of models as a special case of a more general non-linear transformation model based on the work of Tsodikov [387]. In particular, it can be used to fit a semi-parametric Cox PH model, the promotion time model as well as its extension to include covariates in the distribution function $F(.)$. The `miCoPTCM` R package [38], originally developed to fit a promotion time model while taking into account measurement error in the covariates can also be used in the case without (or not taking into account) such measurement errors via the backfitting procedure of Ma and Yin [241]. To do so, one should set all the elements of the variance-covariance matrix of the error measurements to zero.

In `SAS`, we can mention the freely available `PSPMCM` macro [83] based on the work of Corbiére [84] which can be used to fit a parametric mixture cure models with an AFT model for the latency or a (semi-)parametric mixture cure model with a PH model for the latency. The choice of the parametric distribution for the survival of the uncured observations includes the exponential, Weibull, log-normal, and log-logistic distributions. For the parametric models, estimation is performed by maximizing the likelihood with a Newton Raphson algorithm (as implemented in `proc nlmixed`). The semi-parametric mixture cure models is fitted using the EM algorithm and standard error of the estimated parameters are obtained from the observed Fisher information matrix computed at the last iteration or via non-parametric bootstrap.

Finally, it is important to note that `STATA` modules have also been proposed, for example `CUREREG` which fits parametric mixture cure models and promotion time cure models [360], and `STPM2`, `STRSMIX` and `STRSNMIX` which are designed specifically for relative survival cure models (see Section 4.6).

4.5.1   Children ALL data

We come back here to the data from the EORTC CLG 58951 trial, presented shortly in Section 1.3.4 of Chapter 1. The design of this randomized phase III clinical trial in children and adolescents with previously untreated acute lymphoblastic leukemia (ALL) was relatively complex as it embeds three main randomizations, each with is own objectives. We concentrate here on the first randomization, aiming thus to compare dexamethasone and prednisolone as induction treatment in childhood ALL and on the patients who started induction treatment ($n = 1941$) [104].

The estimated Kaplan-Meier survival curves by treatment for Overall Survival (OS) and Event Free Survival (EFS) and are displayed in Figure 4.7. These curves have been obtained in `SAS` using the `proc lifetest` procedure specifying the option `atrisk` to see the number of patients still at risk at different timepoints.

```
proc lifetest method=km width=0.5  data=edat58951 plots=survival(
    atrisk=0 to 4000 by 500);
time survt*ssurv(1);
strata trt1n;
run;
```

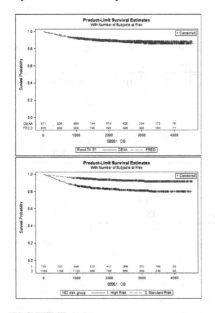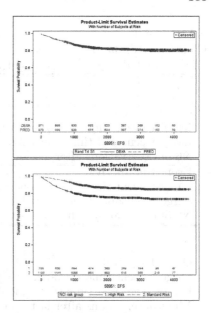

FIGURE 4.7

Children ALL data: Kaplan-Meier estimated overall survival (OS) (*left*) and event-free survival (EFS) (*right*) curves by treatment group (*top*) and by NCI group (*bottom*).

```
proc lifetest method=km width=0.5   data=edat58951 plots=survival(
     atrisk=0 to 4000 by 500);
time efs*sefs(1);
strata trt1n;
run;
```

As we can see, and as is also well known from the medical context, there is obviously a cure fraction for both endpoints, with the OS and EFS survival curves by treatment group leveling of a bit below 90% for OS and at about 80% for EFS and , with in both cases a long plateau observed in each treatment group. We also note that there are numerous censored observations in this plateau for each endpoint. Table 4.1 displays for each endpoint by treatment group and by NCI risk group, the longest observed event time, the longest censored time and the number of censored observation after the last observed event time.

Besides the very good outcomes of these patients, this trial did however not show any benefit of dexamethasone over prednisolone neither for EFS nor for OS with curves for the two treatment group nearly superimposed. This is confirmed by the HR estimated from a Cox PH model obtained from the **proc phreg** procedure:

```
proc phreg data=edat58951;
  model survt*ssurv(1) = trt1n / risklimits;
```

TABLE 4.1

Children ALL data: Observations "in the plateau" of the estimated OS and EFS estimated survival curves by treatment group and by NCI risk group.

	Prednisolone (n=970)	Dexamethasone (n=971)
Overall survival:		
Largest event time (days/months)	3314/108.8	3215/105.6
Largest censored time (days/months)	4530/148.8	4537/149.0
Nb of observations after last event time	225	250
Event-free survival:		
Largest event time (days/months)	3267 / 107.3	3006/98.7
Largest censored time (days/months)	4500 / 147.8	4500/147.8
Nb of observations after last event time	208	266
	NCI Std risk (n=1183)	NCI High risk (n=758)
Overall survival:		
Largest event time (days/months)	3079/101.1	3314/108.8
Largest censored time (days/months)	4537/149.0	4488/147.4
Nb of observations after last event time	377	143
Event-free survival:		
Largest event time (days/months)	3101/101.8	3267/107.3
Largest censored time (days/months)	4500/147.8	4451/146.2
Nb of observations after last event time	280	182

```
run;
proc phreg data=edat58951;
  model efs*sefs(1) = trt1n / risklimits;
run;
```

The estimated treatment effect is -0.037 for EFS, corresponding to a HR of 0.964 (95% CI [0.781 ; 1.190], p-value $= 0.731$) and 0.116 for OS, corresponding to a HR of 1.123 (95% CI [0.859 ; 1.466], p-value $= 0.396$). These results should be interpreted in light of the fraction of cure and, as expected similar results are obtained from a semi-parametric promotion time cure model with an exponential link. Table 4.2 summarizes the results obtained from various cure models and we will see below the commands used in SAS and R to obtain these results. As we can see from these results there is very limited effect of the treatment on EFS or OS, and this is true both for the probability to be cure and for the time-to-event among uncured patients. We will therefore not discuss these results further.

To illustrate on how we can use R and SAS to obtain such results, we will rather consider the variable nci representing the NCI risk group and which is known to be a prognostic factor for these patients. We will further focus on OS, results for EFS can be obtained and interpreted in a similar way.

There are 1183 patients in the NCI Standard Risk group (NSR group) and 758 patients in the NCI High Risk group (NHR group), and respectively 82(6.9%) and 134(17.7%) experienced an event (death). The estimated Kaplan-Meier survival curves by NCI risk group are plotted on Figure 4.7. It is clear from these curves that we can assume a fraction of cure patients in each prognosis group, although this cure fraction is clearly different in the two risk groups. As can be seen below, the estimated survival at 5 and 10 years is respectively 93.7%(95%CI[92.2; 95.0]) and 91.8%(95%CI[89.8; 93.5]) in the NSR group and "only" 83.5%(95%CI[80.6 − 86.0]) and 80.0%(95%CI[76.4; 83.1]) in the NHR group.

```
> OS.ALL.km.nci <- survfit(Surv(survt.m,ssurvn)~nci, conf.type="
  log-log",data=ALL58951)
> summary(OS.ALL.km.nci, times = c(60,120) )
Call: survfit(formula = Surv(survt.m, ssurvn) ~ nci, data =
  ALL58951,
  conf.type = "log-log")

                nci=High Risk
 time n.risk n.event survival std.err lower 95% CI upper 95% CI
   60    464     122    0.835  0.0137        0.806        0.860
  120     91      12    0.800  0.0169        0.764        0.831

                nci=Standard Risk
 time n.risk n.event survival std.err lower 95% CI upper 95% CI
   60    829      71    0.937 0.00722        0.922        0.950
  120    189      11    0.918 0.00923        0.898        0.935
```

We can fit a standard Cox PH model including the NCI risk group as covariate either in R (with the coxph function) function or in SAS (with the coxph procedure), see Section 2.6.1 in Chapter 2.

```
> COX.OS.nci <- coxph(Surv(survt.m,ssurvn)~nci,data=ALL58951)
> summary(COX.OS.nci)
Call:
coxph(formula = Surv(survt.m, ssurvn) ~ nci, data = ALL58951)

  n= 1941, number of events= 216

                      coef exp(coef) se(coef)      z Pr(>|z|)
nciStandard Risk -1.0185    0.3611   0.1403 -7.261 3.84e-13 ***
---
Signif. codes:  0 '***' 0.001 '**' 0.01 '*' 0.05 '.'  0.1 ' '  1

                 exp(coef) exp(-coef) lower .95 upper .95
nciStandard Risk    0.3611      2.769    0.2743    0.4754

Concordance= 0.629  (se = 0.017 )
Rsquare= 0.028    (max possible= 0.808 )
Likelihood ratio test= 54.86  on 1 df,    p=1e-13
Wald test            = 52.72  on 1 df,    p=4e-13
Score (logrank) test = 57.43  on 1 df,    p=4e-14
```

The estimated coefficient is −1.02 corresponding to an estimated HR of 0.36 (95% CI [0.27 ; 0.48]) in favor of the NSR group. The risk of event is therefore 1/0.36 = 2.78 times higher for patients in the NHR group compared to the patients in the NSR group, and this effect is strongly significant (*p*-value

< 0.0001). However, this effect should be in fact be interpreted in light of the presence of a cure fraction in our data.To account for the cure fraction, we fit several cure models to investigate the prognostic value of the NCI risk group while taking the presence if a cure fraction into account (see Table 4.3).

Since the PH assumption seems reasonable we start by fitting a promotion time cure model. Such a model can be fitted using the `nltm smcure` R package or the `miCoPTCM smcure` R package.

The `nltm` package can be used to fit a promotion time cure model as well as different type of models [387]. It is based on a general non-linear transformation model and other possible models that can be fitted include several standard models such as the Cox PH model (`nlt.model = "PH"`) and the proportional odds model (`nlt.model = "PO"`), several types of cure models including the proportional hazards cure model or promotion time model (`nlt.model = "PH"`) and its extension to include covariates in the distribution function $F(.)$ (`nlt.model = "PHPHC"`) as well as a proportional odds cure model (`nlt.model = "PHPOC"`, but also a gamma frailty model (`nlt.model = "GFM"`)). In our case, we specify that we want to fit a "proportional hazard cure model" (PHC)

```
> library(nltm)
> PTCM.NLTM.OS.nci <- nltm(Surv(survt.m,ssurvn)~nci, nlt.model="
    PHC",data=ALL58951)
> summary(PTCM.NLTM.OS.nci)
Call:
nltm(formula1 = Surv(survt.m, ssurvn) ~ nci, data = ALL58951,
        nlt.model = "PHC")

Non Linear Transformation Model: PHC, fit by maximum likelihood

                    coef exp(coef) se(coef)       z        p
nciStandard Risk  -1.02     0.361   0.1403   -7.26 3.7e-13
cure              -1.47     0.230   0.0917  -16.00 0.0e+00

                 exp(coef) exp(-coef) lower .95 upper .95
nciStandard Risk     0.361       2.77     0.274     0.475
cure                 0.230       4.34     0.193     0.276

Likelihood ratio test=785 on 2 df, p=0

n=1941
```

Not surprisingly, these results are similar to what we have found with the Cox PH model, with, as above, an estimated coefficient of -1.02 corresponding to an estimated HR of 0.36 in favor of the NSR patients. This effect take into account both short- and long-term effect. Since $\hat{\beta}$ is negative, patients in the NSR (corresponding to $X = 1$) have a lower value of $\theta(X)$ than patients in the NHR group (corresponding to $X = 1$). These patients will therefore have a lower probability of being uncured (and thus of experiencing death) and a longer event times for those who will experience the event.

Note that the line **cure** corresponds to the estimated coefficient for the intercept of the promotion time cure model and from equation (4.14), we can obtain the estimated cure rate in each risk group as (pay attention that NHR group is the reference):

$$\text{NHR group} \quad : \quad \exp(-\exp(-1.47)) = 0.79$$
$$\text{NSR group} \quad : \quad \exp(-\exp(-1.47 - 1.02)) = 0.92$$

corresponding therefore to an estimated cure rate of 92% for the NSR patients and "only" 79% for the NHR patients. this model-based estimation is very close from what we have observed on Figure 4.7.

The miCoPTCM package has originally been developed to fit a promotion time cure model while taking into account error measurement in the covariate [36, 37]. However, by specifying a null variance-covariance matrix for the assumed (normal) error distribution, this comes back to fitting a promotion time cure model without error in the covariates. Since our model include an intercept and one binary covariate, we have to specify a 2×2 null variance-covariance matrix.

```
> library(miCoPTCM)
> vc <- matrix(nrow=2,ncol=2,0)
> PTCM.miCoPTCM.nci <- PTCMestimBF(formula=Surv(survt.m,ssurvn)~
    nci, varCov=vc, init=runif(2),data=ALL58951)
> summary(PTCM.miCoPTCM.nci)
Call:
PTCMestimBF.formula(formula = Surv(survt.m, ssurvn) ~ nci, data =
    ALL58951,
    varCov = vc, init = runif(2))

                    Estimate    StdErr   z.value   p.value
Intercept          -1.462215  0.091578 -15.9669 < 2.2e-16 ***
nciStandard Risk   -1.021872  0.140052  -7.2964 2.956e-13 ***
---
Signif. codes:  0 '***' 0.001 '**' 0.01 '*' 0.05 '.' 0.1 ' ' 1
```

Despite the fact that the miCoPTCM package is based on a different estimation method, the results we obtain are very similar. Note however that the currently available version of the miCoPTCM package leads to an error message when only one covariate is included into the model but this should be corrected in the next release.

A mixture cure model (MCM) can be fitted with the smcure function from the smcure R package, as long as we include at least one covariate in each sub-model [55]. The required arguments are a formula object specifying the survival model (as usual), the cureform argument specifying the variables to be included in the incidence part of the model (pay attention to not forget the "~" operator to avoid an error message), a model argument, which specifies whether the latency model should be a Cox PH model (model=''ph'') or an AFT model (model=''aft''), and finally a data argument indicating the dataset to be used.

Note that the standard error of the estimated coefficients is obtained by bootstrap with a default of 100 bootstrap samplings. We can modify this number with the optional argument nboot or ask to not compute these estimated standard error by specifying Var=FALSE. This obviously allows the computational time to dramatically decrease, and can be useful for example in a simulation setting where one would be interested just in the estimated values. The model is fitted using the EM algorithm (see Section 4.2), and one can specify a maximum number of iteration via the emmax argument (50 by default) as well as the convergence criterion using the eps argument ($1e - 7$ by default). It may be interesting to check whether these parameters do not need to be increased, e.g. by checking that the estimates do not really change when we increase these default values.

After loading the smcure package, we can therefore fit a MCM with a Cox PH model for the latency and a logistic regression model for the incidence, each including the NCI risk group as covariate, and considering 300 resamplings for the bootstrap while leaving the other arguments at their default value

```
> library(smcure)
> MCM.PH.nci <- smcure(Surv(survt.m,ssurvn)~nci,cureform=~nci,
    model="ph",nboot=300,data=ALL58951)
Program is running..be patient... done.
Call:
smcure(formula = Surv(survt.m, ssurvn) ~ nci, cureform = ~nci,
    data = ALL58951, model = "ph", nboot = 300)

Cure probability model:
              Estimate Std.Error   Z value      Pr(>|Z|)
(Intercept) -0.3710135 0.2423719 -1.530761 1.258285e-01
nci         -1.0174264 0.1669580 -6.093905 1.101891e-09


Failure time distribution model:
                  Estimate Std.Error    Z value  Pr(>|Z|)
nciStandard Risk -0.2910929 0.1957711 -1.486904 0.1370401
```

Note that the printsmcure(MCM.PH.nci) function can be useful if we want to display again these results.

The output clearly distinguishes the two parts of the MCM model with, on the top, the results from the incidence model (here a logistic regression) and below the results from the latency model (here a Cox PH model). The estimated coefficient for our variable in the incidence model is $\hat{\gamma}_{nci} = -1.02$ corresponding to a odds ratio of $\exp(\hat{\gamma}_{nci}) = 0.36$ in favor of the NRS group. To interpret correctly this result, we have to keep in mind that we are actually modeling the probability of being susceptible, see equation (4.4) and this corresponds therefore to a lower risk of event for the NRS group. We can also deduce that the NHR patients have a $\exp(1.02) = 2.77$ increased odd of death compared to the NSR patients. This effect is highly significant (p-value < 0.0001). On the other hand, the estimated coefficient for NCI risk group in the latency model is $\hat{\beta}_{nci} = -0.29$ corresponding to a hazards ratio of $\exp(\hat{\beta}_{nci}) = 0.75$ in favor of the NSR patients. In other words, among the susceptible patients, the NHR patients have a $\exp(0.291) = 1.34$ higher hazard of events. The effect of the NCI risk group on the time to death for the susceptible patients do however not reach statistical significance (p-value = 0.137). The better outcome observed in the SRN patients is therefore mainly due to a higher probability to be cured and only to a less (and non significant) extent to an increased time to death for SNR patients among non-cured patients. We should however acknowledge that given the high percentage of cure resulting in a low number of events, the power to test a significant effect in the latency model is not very high.

When the variable included in the model is a factor, we need to be careful with the parametrization used by R if we want to interpret correctly the intercept term, for example to compute the cure fraction in each group. Indeed, the way smcure handle factors is a bit peculiar, and in fact [55] indicates that the smcure() function can not handle categorical variables with more than 2 levels specified as factor. They therefore advise to either introduced them as numerical values or as dummy variables created outside the call to the function. In the output above, the variable nci is not a dummy variable but actually takes value 1 for NHR patients (reference category, chosen by alphabetical order) and value 2 for NSN patients to find back the estimated cure fraction using equation (4.4):

$$\text{NHR group} \quad : \quad 1 - \frac{\exp(-0.371 + 1 \times (-1.017))}{1 + \exp(-0.371 + 1 \times (-1.017))} = 0.800$$

$$\text{NSR group} \quad : \quad 1 - \frac{\exp(-0.371 + 2 \times (-1.017))}{1 + \exp(-0.371 + 2 \times (-1.017))} = 0.917$$

Note that the values of the estimated coefficient for the intercept and for the variables included in each of the two submodels can be easily obtained from coefsmcure(MCM.PHf). The estimated percentage of cure is therefore 80.0% for SRN patients compared to 92% for HRN patients confirming a strong effect of the NCI risk group on the probability to be cure with a strong advantage for SRN patients.

It is however preferable to include categorical variables either as numerical variable or as dummy variables (depending on whether we are ready to do a linearity assumption or not). In our case, since the variable nci is binary, both solutions are equivalent. With the new variable ncin taking value 0 if the patient belongs to the HRN group and 1 if the patient belongs to the SRN group, we now obtain

```
> MCM.PH.ncin <- smcure(Surv(survt.m,ssurvn)~ncin,cureform=~ncin,
    model="ph",nboot=300,data=ALL58951)
Program is running..be patient... done.
Call:
smcure(formula = Surv(survt.m, ssurvn) ~ ncin, cureform = ~ncin,
    data = ALL58951, model = "ph", nboot = 300)

Cure probability model:
             Estimate   Std.Error    Z value      Pr(>|Z|)
(Intercept) -1.388440  0.07414488  -18.726038  0.000000e+00
ncin        -1.017426  0.16147870   -6.300685  2.963334e-10
```

```
Failure time distribution model:
      Estimate Std.Error   Z value  Pr(>|Z|)
ncin -0.2910929 0.1931755 -1.506883 0.1318406
```

As we can see, the results for the estimated coefficients are, as expected, the same as above and thus relative interpretation of these coefficient is not a problem (this may not be the case for a covariate with more than two levels). It is actually the estimated value of the intercept of the logistic regression which is impacted. The cure rate can now be easily obtained from equation (4.4) with no risk of misinterpretation,

$$\text{NHR group} \quad : \quad 1 - \frac{\exp(-1.388)}{1 + \exp(-1.388)} = 0.800$$

$$\text{NSR group} \quad : \quad 1 - \frac{\exp(-1.388 + 1 \times (-1.017))}{1 + \exp(-1.388 + 1 \times (-1.017))} = 0.917$$

One can also easily obtain these estimated cure rate with the predictsmcure() functions by specifying

```
> Pred.MCM.PH.ncin <- predictsmcure(MCM.PH.ncin,newX=c(0,1), newZ
    =c(0,1),model="ph")
> 1-Pred.MCM.PH.ncin$newuncureprob
          [,1]        [,2]
[1,]  0.8003431 0.9172735
```

where the newX=c(0,1) and newZ=c(0,1) arguments are used to specify the value of the covariates respectively for the latency and incidence submodels for which we want to obtain these estimations.

The resulting object can also be used to plot the predicted population survival curves, using the command

```
> plotpredictsmcure(Pred.MCM.PH.ncin,model="ph")
```

However, it might sometimes be more handy to retrieve directly the predictions from the predictsmcure object (and sorting them to be able to plot a step function). This will allow, for example, to plot on the same graph the KM estimated population survival curves and the model-based estimates of these population survival curves. The result plotted on Figure 4.8 and show a good adequacy of our model-based estimates compared to the non-parametric KM estimates. Note that the non-parametric and model-based curves are nearly indistinguishable.

```
> Time <- Pred.MCM.PH.ncin$prediction[,3]
> PredG1 <- Pred.MCM.PH.ncin$prediction[,1]
> PredG2 <- Pred.MCM.PH.ncin$prediction[,2]
> Time.s <- Time[order(Time)]
> PredG1.s <- PredG1[order(Time)]
> PredG2.s <- PredG2[order(Time)]
> OS.ALL.km.ncin <- survfit(Surv(survt.m,ssurvn)~ncin, conf.type=
    "none",data=ALL58951)
```

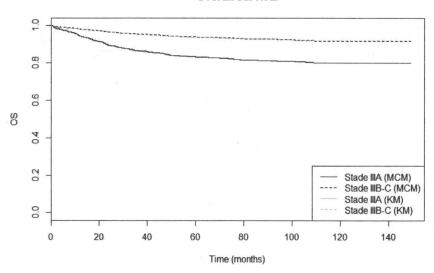

FIGURE 4.8
Children ALL data: Overall survival function by NCI risk group obtained from
the non-parametric Kaplan-Meier estimator (KM, *gray lines*) and predicted
from a logistic/Cox mixture cure model (MCM, *black lines*) with the *smcure*
package.

```
> plot(OS.ALL.km.ncin, lwd=1,ylab="OS",xlab="Time (months)",lty
    =1:2,col=c("darkgray","darkgray"),main="Overall survival")
> lines(Time.s,PredG1.s, type="s")
> lines(Time.s,PredG2.s,type="s",lty=2)
> legend("bottomright",lty=c(1,2,1,2), col=c("black","black","
    darkgray","darkgray"),c("Stade IIIA (MCM)","Stade IIIB-C (MCM)
    ","Stade IIIA (KM)","Stade IIIB-C (KM)"))
```

Furthermore the object created by the smcure() function also contains
the estimated (conditional) baseline survival function of the uncured patients
which is used in the EM algorithm. From these values and based on equation (4.8) we can predict the (conditional) survival function of the uncured
patients for different values of the covariates. Note that these predicted survival curves are forced to be zero beyond the largest observed event time due
to the zero-tail constrain (see Section 4.4), and are obtained assuming proportional hazards (since we used a Cox PH model in the latency). Results
are displayed in Figure 4.9 and confirm that, amongst the uncured patients,
the NSR patients indeed have a better survival than NHR patients. Although
not statistically significant, this difference is however marked with a median

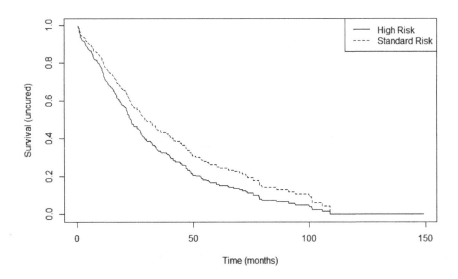

FIGURE 4.9
Children ALL data: Predicted conditional overall survival function by NCI
risk group for the susceptible patients obtained from a logistic/Cox MCM
with the *smcure package*.

(conditional) survival time of about 23 months for the NHR patients versus
about 29 months for the NSR patients.

```
> sOG1 <- MCM.PH.ncin$s
> sOG2 <- MCM.PH.ncin$s^(exp(MCM.PH.ncin$beta))
> Time <- MCM.PH.ncin$Time
> UNC.S <- cbind(Time,sOG1,sOG2)
> UNC.S.s <-UNC.S[order(Time),]
> plot(UNC.S.s[,1],UNC.S.s[,2],type="l",xlab="Time (months)",ylab
    ="Survival (uncured)")
> lines(UNC.S.s[,1],UNC.S.s[,3],lty=2)
> legend("topright",lty=c(1,2), c("High Risk","Standard Risk"))
```

Other optional arguments can be used in the smcure() function, for example the link argument allows to specify the link function to be used in the
incidence model. The default is link=''logit'', corresponding to a logistic
regression model, but a ''probit'' or a ''cloglog'' link can also be specified. One can also specify offset variable which will appear with a coefficient
1 in both the incidence and the latency submodels.

The mixture cure model can also be fitted in SAS with the freely available pspmcm macro [83, 84]. This macro allows to fit parametric and semi-
parametric mixture cure models, allowing for different link functions for the

incidence models and different PH models for the latency. The model for the incidence part is specified via the `incpart` argument and choice can be made among the `logit` (default), `probit`, or `cloglog` link. The model to be used for the latency part is specified via the `survpart` argument as either a parametric model with an exponential (`exp`), a Weibull (`weib`), a log-logistic (`llog`) or a log-normal (`logn`) distribution or as a semi-parametric Cox PH model (`cox`). Further arguments allow (when set to "Y") to estimate the conditional baseline survival function (`baseline`), to plot the estimated conditional and population survival curve for given value of the covariates (to be specified in the argument) (`splot`) and to estimate, for each stratum defined by the specified covariate value, the Kaplan-Meier estimates of the population survival function (`plotfit`). When the latency part of the model is a Cox PH model, other optional arguments are available. In particular, one can specify the type of estimator used for the conditional baseline survival function via the `su0met` argument, using either the Breslow-type estimator (`ch`) or the Kaplan-Meier product-limit estimator (`pl`) which is the default. Also, the `tail` argument specifies the type of constraints to be applied to ensure that the estimated conditional baseline survival function is indeed proper (see Section 4.4). The default is the classical zero-tail constraint (`tail=zero`), which as mentioned before force this estimated conditional survival function to be zero after the largest observed event time. Another possibility available in this macro, is actually to use an exponential or a Weibull completion method, where the tail of the baseline conditional survival curves over the last event time will be completed by a parametric estimation (`tail=etail` or `tail=wtail`). Note that one also has the possibility to not use any such constraint (`tail=none`), but in that case identifiability and convergence problems are to be expected. Arguments linked to the convergence and to the bootstrap are also available, see [84] for all details.

Therefore, we use the following call to the function to fit a logistic/Cox PH model to our data, with the variable `ncin` added to both the incidence and the latency part of the model via the statement `VAR=Stade(IS)`. The zero-tail constraint is imposed and 300 bootstrap samples are used.

```
%pspmcm(DATA= edat58951, ID= seqid, CENSCOD= ssurvn, TIME= survt,
    VAR= ncin(IS,1),
    INCPART= logit,
    SURVPART= Cox,
    TAIL= zero, SUOMET= pl,
    MAXITER= 200, CONVCRIT= 1e-5, ALPHA= 0.05,
    FAST= Y,BOOTSTRAP= Y, NSAMPLE= 300, BOOTMET= pctl,
    GESTIMATE= Y,
    BASELINE=Y,
    SPLOT=Y);
run;
```

The first part of the output provides some general informations about the number of observations, the number of iterations and the value of the convergence criterion as well as the value of the log-likelihood for each part of the model (see equations (4.11) and (4.12) in Section 4.2.2) and recall the number of bootstrap sample used.

```
                        RESULTS FOR DATA edat58951
                       Convergence and Log_likelihood

                                        LogL_      LogL_
N_Obs  N_failed  N_iter     Converg     LOGIT      coxPH    LogTotal  Bootstrap

1941     216       16    9.51055E-06  -683.506   -1003.40  -1686.91     300
```

The second part of the output concerns the results of the incidence model, in our case a logistic regression model with an intercept and the variable NCI risk group. Remember that the `ncin` variable is coded 0 for the HRN group and 1 for the SRN group.

```
              FAST RESULTS FOR THE LOGIT PART (edat58951)
                   Analysis of Maximum Likelihood Estimates

                             Standard     Wald        Pr >     Estimation
   Variable    DF  Estimate   Error    Chi-Square  Chi-Square     Type

   Intercept   1   -1.3943    0.0910    234.6533    <.0001        MLE
   ncin        1   -1.0188    0.1396     53.2481    <.0001        MLE
```

As we can see, the results are very close from the results obtained with the `smcure` package with $\hat{\gamma}_{nci} = -1.02$ and thus a $\exp(\hat{\gamma}_{nci}) = 0.36$ lower odd of not being cured (and thus experiencing the event) for the NSR patients; or a 2.77 higher odd of event for the NHR patients compared to the NSR patients. As in the results obtained previously, this increased risk is highly significant (p-value < 0.0001). We can use exactly the same computation as above to estimate the cure rate in each NCI risk group, leading an estimated cure rate of 80% in the HRN group and 92% in the SRN group as above.

The results for the latency model, here a Cox PH model with the NCI risk group as covariate, are summarized in the third part of the output.

```
             FAST RESULTS FOR THE SURVIVAL PART (edat58951)
                  Analysis of Maximum Likelihood Estimates

                                                95% Lower   95% Upper
                                                Confidence  Confidence
                  Parameter Standard Chi-   Pr >  Hazard Limit for  Limit for
Parameter DF Estimate   Error  Square ChiSq  Ratio Hazard Ratio Hazard
      Ratio

  ncin    1  -0.29035  0.14143 4.2148 0.0401 0.748    0.567       0.987
  lpi     0   1.00000     0       .      .      .        .           .
```

As expected, these results are also similar to those obtained with the `smcure` package with $\hat{\beta}_{nci} = -0.29$ corresponding to a HR of $\exp(\hat{\beta}_{nci}) = 0.75$ in favor of the SRN patients. Note however that the effect of the NCI risk group in the latency has now reached significance, mainly due to a smaller estimated standard error.

Since we have used the `plotfit=Y`, the output also displays for each stratum defined by the value of the covariate `ncin`, an estimated correlation between the non-parametric (Kaplan-Meier) estimates of the population survival function ($\hat{S}_{KM}^{pop}(t \mid X, Z)$) and the corresponding model-based estimator

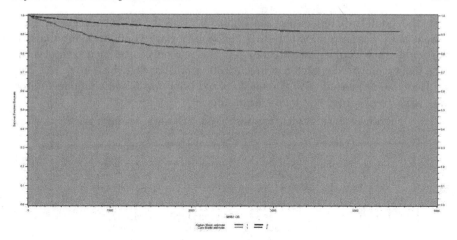

FIGURE 4.10

Children ALL data: Estimated overall survival function by NCI risk group obtained from the non-parametric Kaplan-Meier estimator (KM) and predicted from a logistic/Cox model (MCM) with the **pspmcm SAS** macro.

($\hat{S}^{pop}_{MCM}(t \mid X, Z)$). This correlation coefficient has indeed been proposed as a measure of goodness of fit [244]. A plot of these estimated curves is also provided, as can be seen on Figure 4.10. This plot is similar to Figure 4.8 we have previously obtained in R using the smcure package. As we can see from these results, and as we already suspected from a visual inspection of Figure 4.8, the fit is very good in both groups. A percentile-percentile plot of the KM estimate versus the model-based survival estimate for each strata is also provided.

Correlation statistic between estimated and observed marginal survival
functions

Stratum Number	NCIN	R-squared	Pearson's correlation statistic
1	0	0.99703	0.99851
2	1	0.99167	0.99583

The last part of the output presents bootstrap confidence intervals for the estimated coefficients in the incidence part of the model, as well as for the estimated coefficients and corresponding HR for the latency part of the model. By default (**BOOTMET= all**), different methods are used to compute these confidence intervals. We can however specify one particular method to be used among the percentile (**pctl**), the hybrid method (**hyb**), the normalized bias corrected (**bootn**), the bias corrected (**bc**), the accelerated bias corrected (**bca**) and the jacknife (**jack**) confidence intervals. Note that the **GESTIMATE=Y** argument produces a Q-Q plot and an histogram of the parameters estimates over the bootstrap replicates, see Figure 4.11. A visual inspection of these graphs may be useful for choosing the appropriate confidence intervals; in particular one would probably not use the percentile confidence interval in case our estimates deviates too much from a normal distribution.

Here, we requested 95% percentile based bootsrap based confidence intervals, and we obtained the following results.

```
BOOTSTRAP CONFIDENCE INTERVAL FOR PARAMETERS ESTIMATES
                    Data set= edat58951
        (confidence level=95 %, 300 bootstrap resamples)

                                    Method=         Method=
                       Observed    PCTL Lower      PCTL Upper
       Variable        Statistic   percentile      percentile

       L_Int           -1.39442    -1.61175        -1.20335
       L_NCIN          -1.01883    -1.33029        -0.70713
       S_NCIN          -0.29035    -0.64412         0.04988



               ODDS RATIO FOR THE LOGISTIC PART
                    Data set= edat58951
        (confidence level=95 %, 300 bootstrap resamples)

                         Odds         PCTL           PCTL
       Variable          Ratio      Lower OR       Upper OR

       L_NCIN           0.36102     0.26440        0.49306



               HAZARD RATIO FOR THE SURVIVAL PART
                    Data set= edat58951
        (confidence level=95 %, 300 bootstrap resamples)

                        Hazard        PCTL           PCTL
       Variable         Ratio       Lower RR       Upper RR

       S_NCIN          0.74800      0.52512        1.05114
```

4.5.2   Melanoma data

As introduced in Section 1.3.5 of Chapter 1, the melanoma dataset contains information on the outcome of the 629 patients randomized to the observation arm of the EORTC 18991 phase III clinical trial. Three main outcomes are considered for these patients, relapse-free survival (RFS), distant-metastases free survival (DMFS) and overall survival (OS). Results for these three outcomes can be summarized using the methods discussed in Chapter 2, see Table 4.4 and Figure 4.12.

As we can see, for each of the three endpoints, the estimated survival curves reach a plateau somewhere between 40 and 60 months depending on the endpoint. The largest observed event time and the number of censored observation after this time point are summarized for each endpoint in Table 4.5. Knowing that the maximum observed (censored) time is 3666 days (so about 120 months), we see that we indeed have a long plateau (of more than 1

Event-free survival treatment		Intercept	
CM (coxph / phreg)			0.037 (0.108), p values = 0.731
			HR = 1.038 (95% CI: 0.841 ; 1.281)
PTM (nltm)		−1.544 (0.079)	0.037 (0.108), p values = 0.730
			HR = 1.038 (95% CI: 0.841 ; 1.281)
PTM (miCoPTCM)			
MCM (smcure)	incidence	−1.504 (0.173)	0.060 (0.117), p values = 0.608
	latency		−0.077 (0.127), p values = 0.541
MCM (pspmcm)	incidence	−1.449 (0.082)	0.060 (0.115), p values = 0.604
			OR=1.061 (95% CI: 0.838 ; 1.389)
	latency		−0.077 (0.108), p values = 0.472
			HR = 0.925 (95% CI: 0.689 ; 1.213)

Overall survival treatment		Intercept	
CM (coxph / phreg)			−0.116 (0.136), p values = 0.396
			HR = 0.891 (95% CI: 0.682 ; 1.164)
PTM (nltm)		−1.931 (0.145)	−0.116 (0.136), p values = 0.400
			HR = 0.891 (95% CI: 0.682 ; 1.163)
PTM (miCoPTCM)			
MCM (smcure)	incidence	−1.663 (0.231)	−0.172 (0.156), p values = 0.267
	latency		0.172 (0.192), p values = 0.371
MCM (pspmcm)	incidence	−1.842 (0.093)	−0.171 (0.136), p values = 0.201
			OR = 0.842 (95% CI: 0.642 ; 1.154)
	latency		0.172 (0.138), p values = 0.210
			HR = 1.188 (95% CI: 0.818 ; 1.809)

TABLE 4.2

Children ALL data : Results from different cure models fitted in R (functions coxph, nltm, miCoPTCM, smcure) and in SAS (procedure phreg and macro pspmcm) and including the treatment group as covariate. Results are presented as estimate (standard error) for the intercept term and as estimate (standard error), p-value, hazards ratio (95% confidence intervals) for the treatment effect. For the MCM, confidence intervals are obtained from 300 bootstrap samples based on the percentile method. CM: Cox PH model, PTM: promotion time cure model, MCM: logistic/Cox PH mixture cure model.

		Overall survival		Estimated cure fraction	
		Intercept	Treatment	NHR	NSR
CM (coxph / phreg)			−1.02 (0.14), $p < 0.0001$		
			HR=0.36 (95% CI: [0.27 ; 0.48])		
PTM (nltm)		−1.47 (0.09)	−1.02 (0.14), $p < 0.0001$	79%	92%
			HR=0.36 (95% CI: [0.27 ; 0.48])		
PTM (miCoPTCM)	incidence	−1.46 (0.09)	−1.02 (0.14), $p < 0.0001$	79%	92%
MCM (smcure)	latency	−1.39 (0.07)	1.02 (0.17), $p < 0.0001$	80%	92%
			−0.29 (0.20), $p = 0.137$		
MCM (pspmcm)	incidence	−1.49 (0.09)	−1.02 (0.14), $p < 0.0001$	80%	92%
			OR=0.36 (95% CI: [0.26 ; 0.49])		
	latency		−0.29 (0.14), $p = 0.040$		
			HR=0.75 (95% CI: [0.53 ; 1.05])		

TABLE 4.3

Children ALL data : Results from different cure models fitted in R (functions coxph, nltm, miCoPTCM, smcure) and in SAS (procedure phreg and macro pspmcm) and including the NCI risk group as covariate (ncin). Results are presented as estimate (standard error) for the intercept term and as estimate (standard error), p-value, hazards ratio (95% confidence intervals) for the treatment effect. For the MCM, confidence intervals are obtained from 300 bootstrap samples based on the percentile method. CM: Cox PH model, PTM: promotion time cure model, MCM: logistic/Cox PH mixture cure model.

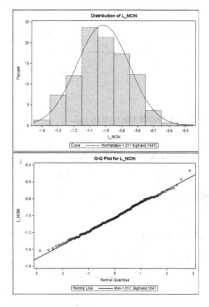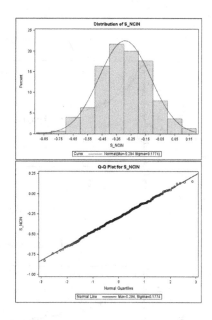

FIGURE 4.11
Children ALL data: Histogram and Q-Q plot of the bootstrap estimators for
the effect of NCI risk group in the incidence (*left*) and latency (*right*) sub-
models as obtained from the `pspmcm SAS` macro.

Outcome	Observation (n=629)
Relapse-free survival (RFS)	
Number of event (%)	399 (63.4%)
Median RFS (months) (95% CI)	28.0 [21.8 ; 34.5]
5-yrs RFS (95% CI)	39.6% [35.7 ; 43.4]
10-yrs RFS (95% CI)	33.6% [28.9 ; 38.5]
Distant metastases-free survival (DMFS)	
Number of event (%)	375 (59.6%)
Median DMFS (months) (95% CI)	38.3 [30.5 ; 47.7]
5-yrs DMFS (95% CI)	43.7% [39.8 ; 47.6]
10-yrs DMFS (95% CI)	38.3% [34.2 ; 42.3]
Overall survival (OFS)	
Number of event (%)	336 (53.4%)
Median OS (months) (95% CI)	66.7 [53.6 ; 85.8]
5-yrs OS (95% CI)	51.6% [47.6 ; 55.5]
10-yrs OS (95% CI)	43.3% [39.0 ; 47.5]

TABLE 4.4
Melanoma data: Results observed for relapse-free survival (RFS), distant-
metastases free survival (DMFS) and overall survival (OS) for the 629 patients
in the observation arm of the EORTC 18991 trial

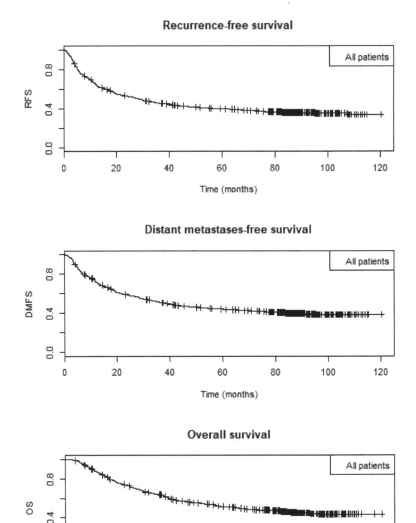

FIGURE 4.12

Melanoma data: Kaplan-Meier estimation of the survival distribution for relapse-free survival (RFS), distant-metastases free survival (DMFS) and overall survival (OS) for the 629 patients in the observation arm of the EORTC 18991 trial.

Outcome	Largest observed event time	Number of censored observation in the plateau (%)
RFS	3275 days (107.6 months)	59 (9.4 %)
DMFS	2896 days (95.1 months)	67 (10.7 %)
OS	2986 days (98.1 months)	74 (11.7 %)

TABLE 4.5
Melanoma data: Observations in the "plateau" of the estimated survival curve for relapse-free survival (RFS), distant-metastases free survival (DMFS) and overall survival (OS) for the 629 patients in the observation arm of the EORTC 18991 trial

year) with a non-negligible proportion of censored observations (about 10%). Furthermore, it is known from a medical point of view that a cure fraction indeed exists among patients treated for melanoma. In the following, we are interested in investigating the prognostic value of three important factors while taking this cure fraction into account. For that, we will mainly consider a Cox PH model, a promotion time cure model (from which we expect the same results) and a mixture cure model. The prognostic factors we consider are the stage of disease (microscopic nodal disease versus clinically palpable disease), the ulceration of the primary (yes versus no) and the presence of only one positive lymph node or more. We will concentrate on OS but results for the other endpoints can be obtained in a similar way.

For this illustration, we will restrict our analysis to the 517 patients with complete information for these three variables. In the following, the variables rndstagen, ulceration2cn, and nblymphnodes are dummy variable with rndstagen=0 for patients with stage N1 (microscopic nodal disease) and rndstagen=1 for patients with stage N2 (clinically palpable nodes), ulceration2cn=0 for patients with no ulceration at the primary and ulceration2cn=1 for patients with ulceration, and nblymphnodes=0 for patients with only one positive lymph node involved and nblymphnodes=1 for patients with more than one positive lymph nodes involved. The variable ostime.m is the same as ostime but measured in months; and the variable osstat has been converted in a numeric variable ostatn (0 = no event, 1 = event).

Results from a univariate analysis for each of these three variables are provided in Table 4.6 and Kaplan-Meier estimates of the population survival functions according to each of these three prognostic factors are presented in Figure 4.13. These results confirm that each of these three variables are indeed prognostic factors, with better outcome for patients with stage N1, no ulceration, and only one positive node involved. Furthermore, we can observe that even for the patients with the value of the covariate associated with the poorest prognostic, there seems to remain a proportion of cure patients.

Variable	n	nb events	median OS (months)	% at 5 years (95% CI)	% at 8 years (95% CI)	coef (s.e.) p-value	HR (95% CI)
Stage							
N1(micro)	254	119	98.1	61.7% [55.4 ; 67.4]	50.4% [43.3 ; 57.0]		
N2(palpable)	263	163	39.8	41.4% [35.3 ; 47.4]	35.5% [29.4 ; 41.5]	0.57 (0.12) $p < 0.0001$	1.76 [1.39 ; 2.23]
Ulceration							
No	336	163	98.1	57.8% [52.3 ; 62.9]	50.2 % [44.5 ; 55.5]		
Yes	181	119	40.2	39.4% [32.1 ; 46.5]	29.3% [21.9 ; 37.0]	0.51 (0.12) $p < 0.0001$	1.66 [1.31 ; 2.11]
Positive lymph nodes							
One	297	140	98.1	57.1% [51.2 ; 62.6]	50.7% [55.4 ; 56.7]		
More than one	220	142	40.0	43.8% [37.1 ; 50.3]	32.0% [25.4 ; 38.8]	0.51 (0.12) $p < 0.0001$	1.66 [1.31 ; 2.10]

TABLE 4.6
Melanoma data: Univariate analysis for each prognostic factor

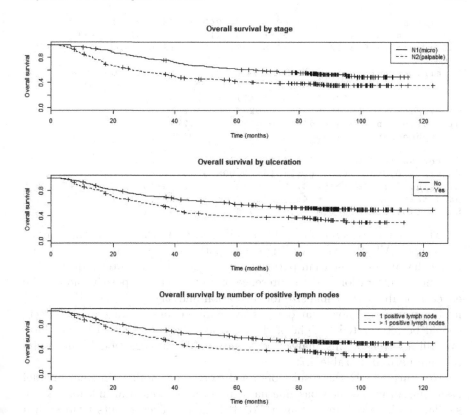

FIGURE 4.13
Melanoma data: Kaplan-Meier estimation of the survival distribution for overall survival (OS) per stage, per presence of ulceration, and per number of positive lymph nodes for the 517 patients with complete information in the observation arm of the EORTC 18991 trial.

We are now interested in studying the prognostic value of each of these factor while taking the two other ones into account. A first idea would be to fit a standard Cox PH model, and the results are summarized in Table 4.7.

```
> OS.mela.ph.all <- coxph(Surv(ostime.m,ostatn)~rndstagen+
    ulceration2cn+nblymphnodesn,data=Dat18991n)
> summary(OS.mela.ph.all)
Call:
coxph(formula = Surv(ostime.m, ostatn) ~ rndstagen +
    ulceration2cn +
    nblymphnodesn, data = Dat18991n)

  n= 517, number of events= 282

              coef exp(coef) se(coef)      z Pr(>|z|)
```

```
rndstagen        0.4707     1.6012    0.1243 3.786 0.000153 ***
ulceration2cn 0.4792        1.6147    0.1210 3.959 7.51e-05 ***
nblymphnodesn 0.3712        1.4495    0.1230 3.019 0.002538 **
---
Signif. codes:  0 '***' 0.001 '**' 0.01 '*' 0.05 '.'. 0.1 ' '  1

                 exp(coef) exp(-coef) lower .95 upper .95
rndstagen            1.601     0.6245     1.255      2.043
ulceration2cn        1.615     0.6193     1.274      2.047
nblymphnodesn        1.450     0.6899     1.139      1.845

Concordance= 0.633  (se = 0.016 )
Rsquare= 0.088    (max possible= 0.998 )
Likelihood ratio test= 47.84  on 3 df,    p=2e-10
Wald test            = 48.42  on 3 df,    p=2e-10
Score (logrank) test = 49.67  on 3 df,    p=9e-11
```

The three factors remain highly significant, even when accounting for the two others. All other things being equal, patients with stage N2 have a 1.60 higher hazard of event than patients with stage N1, even after adjusting for presence of ulceration and the presence of more than one positive node. The effect is of about the same size for ulceration and slightly lower (HR = 1.45) for the presence of more than one positive lymph nodes. However, these effects should be interpreted in light of the presence of a cure fraction in our data. We will now repeat this analysis considering different cure models, all results are summarized in Table 4.7.

Not surprisingly the results obtained from a promotion time cure model assuming an unspecified baseline hazard and an exponential link for θX are similar to those obtained from a Cox PH model. They results from such a promotion time cure model can be obtained with the nltm R package or with the miCoPTCM R. The results from nltm package are obtained as follows:

```
> library(nltm)
> OS.mela.ptm.all <- nltm(Surv(ostime.m,ostatn)~rndstagen+
    ulceration2cn+nblymphnodesn, nlt.model="PHC",data=Dat18991n)
> summary(OS.mela.ptm.all)
Call:
nltm(formula1 = Surv(ostime.m, ostatn) ~ rndstagen +
    ulceration2cn +      nblymphnodesn, data = Dat18991n, nlt.model
    = "PHC")

Non Linear Transformation Model: PHC, fit by maximum likelihood

                 coef exp(coef) se(coef)      z        p
rndstagen       0.470     1.600    0.124   3.78  1.6e-04
ulceration2cn   0.479     1.615    0.121   3.96  7.5e-05
nblymphnodesn   0.371     1.449    0.123   3.02  2.5e-03
cure           -0.706     0.494    0.116  -6.11  1.0e-09

                 exp(coef) exp(-coef) lower .95 upper .95
rndstagen            1.600      0.625     1.254      2.041
ulceration2cn        1.615      0.619     1.274      2.047
nblymphnodesn        1.449      0.690     1.139      1.844
cure                 0.494      2.026     0.394      0.619
```

```
Likelihood ratio test=52.2 on 4 df, p=1.28e-10

n=517
```

As mentioned previously, the line cure actually corresponds to the intercept of the promotion time cure model. These results are (as expected) similar to what we have found with the Cox PH model. These effects take into account both short- and long-term effect All coefficients are positive and therefore when interpreting the results for one covariate (adjusted for the other two), patients with a value 1 of the corresponding covariate will have a larger value of $\theta\mathbf{X}$ (compared to those in the reference category) leading to a lower probability to be cure and shorter event times for the uncured patients. However from this model, we are not able to disentangle the effect of each prognostic factor on the probability to be cure and on the event time for the uncured. Also, this model makes the assumption of proportional hazards at the level of the population, which may not be realistic.

We therefore can fit a mixture cure model. Our first MCM model is fitted in R with the smcure R package, an include our three covariates both in the incidence (specified as a logistic regression model) and in the latency (specified as a Cox PH model).

```
> library(smcure)
> OS.mela.mcm.all <- smcure(Surv(ostime.m,ostatn)~rndstagen+
    ulceration2cn+nblymphnodesn,cureform=~rndstagen+ulceration2cn+
    nblymphnodesn,model="ph",link="logit",nboot=1000,data=
    Dat18991n)
Program is running..be patient... done.
Call:
smcure(formula = Surv(ostime.m, ostatn) ~ rndstagen +
    ulceration2cn +
    nblymphnodesn, cureform = ~rndstagen + ulceration2cn +
        nblymphnodesn,
    data = Dat18991n, model = "ph", link = "logit", nboot = 1000)

Cure probability model:
                Estimate Std.Error   Z value      Pr(>|Z|)
(Intercept)   -0.3476955 0.1626980 -2.137060 0.0325930987
rndstagen      0.3916740 0.2137601  1.832306 0.0669058280
ulceration2cn  0.7458517 0.2196053  3.396328 0.0006829636
nblymphnodesn  0.6265384 0.2154216  2.908429 0.0036324928


Failure time distribution model:
                Estimate Std.Error   Z value     Pr(>|Z|)
rndstagen     0.71072253 0.1628094 4.3653646 1.269109e-05
ulceration2cn 0.26480582 0.1658371 1.5967830 1.103141e-01
nblymphnodesn 0.04528768 0.1554889 0.2912599 7.708525e-01
```

This model allows to disentangle the effect of each prognostic factor for the probability to be cure and on the time-to-event for the uncured patients. In particular, we can observe that the effect of stage (N1 versus N2) is much more pronounced in the latency part of the model, where it is highly significant (p-value < 0.0001) with a $\exp(0.71) = 2.03$ higher hazard of events for patients with N2 stage compared to patients with N1 stage (all other factors being kept equal). In the incidence part of the model, this factor is borderline non significant (p-value $= 0.066$) with an estimated adjusted odds ratio of $\exp(0.39) = 1.48$ also in favor of N1 patients. On the other hand, the presence of ulceration and of more than one positive node are both significant (p-value < 0.001 and p-value $= 0.004$ respectively) in the incidence part of the model but not in the latency (p-value $= 0.110$ and p-value $= 0.771$ respectively). All other things being equal, patients with presence of ulceration have a higher risk of being uncured (and thus experiencing death) with a odds ratio of OR $= \exp(0.75) = 2.12$. However, among the uncured patients, the presence of ulceration is associated only with a HR $= \exp(0.26) = 1.30$ increased hazard. The presence of more than one positive lymph nodes is also associated with an increased risk of being uncured (OR $= \exp(0.63) = 1.88$) but has only very limited impact on the time to death among the uncured patients (HR $= \exp(0.05) = 1.05$). We will see below that the results obtained in SAS are slightly different, mainly with regards to the estimated standard error with an impact on the significance of these factors.

For the sake of sparsity, we may fit a new model removing the stage from the incidence but on the other hand keeping only this covariate in the latency.

```
> OS.mela.mcm.sel <- smcure(Surv(ostime.m,ostatn)~rndstagen,
    cureform=~ulceration2cn+nblymphnodesn,model="ph",link="logit",
    nboot=1000,data=Dat18991n)
Program is running..be patient... done.
Call:
smcure(formula = Surv(ostime.m, ostatn) ~ rndstagen, cureform = ~
    ulceration2cn +
    nblymphnodesn, data = Dat18991n, model = "ph", link = "logit"
    ,
    nboot = 1000)

Cure probability model:
               Estimate Std.Error   Z value       Pr(>|Z|)
(Intercept)  -0.1934029 0.1216850 -1.589373 0.1119761591
ulceration2cn 0.8114271 0.2312476  3.508910 0.0004499467
nblymphnodesn 0.7307096 0.2062689  3.542510 0.0003963385


Failure time distribution model:
          Estimate Std.Error  Z value      Pr(>|Z|)
rndstagen 0.740159 0.1461273 5.065166 4.080441e-07
```

For a given ulceration status, patients with more than one positive nodes have an increase probability to be uncured, with an adjusted estimated OR of OR $= \exp(0.73) = 2.08$. Given the presence or not of more than one positive lymph nodes, patients with ulceration have a higher risk of being uncured, now with an estimated adjusted OR of $\exp(0.81) = 2.25$. According to this model, time-to-event among the uncured patients is only impacted by the stage at randomization, with N2 patients having a HR $= \exp(0.74) = 2.10$ higher hazard of death.

As we have seen before, the mixture cure model can also be fitted in SAS with the macro pspmcm. Using this macro to a logistic/Cox PH model to our data, with all three variables in both part of the model and imposing the zero-tail constraint, is done with following lines of code:

```
%pspmcm(DATA= Dat18991n, ID= seqid, CENSCOD= osstat, TIME= ostime
,
    VAR= rndstagen(IS,1) ulceration2cn(IS,1) nblymphnodesn(IS,1),
    INCPART= logit,
    SURVPART= Cox,
    TAIL= zero, SUOMET= pl,
    MAXITER= 200, CONVCRIT= 1e-5, ALPHA= 0.05,
    FAST= Y,BOOTSTRAP= Y, NSAMPLE= 1000, BOOTMET= Pctl,
    GESTIMATE= Y,
    BASELINE=Y,
    SPLOT=Y,
    PLOTFIT=Y);
run;
```

The results are summarized in Table 4.7 and are slightly different from those obtained in R mainly regarding the estimation of the standard error and this despite the fact that we have increased the number of bootstrap replications in both procedure to 1000. Although the point estimates of the coefficient is very close from what we obtained in R, the stage does now reach significance in the incidence part (but with a lower bound of the confidence interval about equal to 1) such that all three factors remains significant in the incidence submodel. For the latency part of the model, the presence of more than one positive lymph nodes still have a very small effect and is still non significant. On the other hand, while the estimated coefficient for the presence of ulceration is very close from what we obtained in R) the estimated standard error is now smaller explaining that this result now reaches significance (but with a lower bound of the confidence interval very close from 1).

4.6 Further reading

As we have mentioned, the mixture cure model is actually composed of two sub-models, one for the incidence and one for the latency. While in theory any model for binary data could be considered in the incidence, in practice few alternatives to the logistic regression have been proposed and without real implementation in practice. We could however consider another parametric link function, such as the probit link for example. This usually requires only a small modification of the likelihood, and one can then use an EM algorithm. Other proposed ideas consist in considering a more flexible modeling of the incidence, for example using a single-index structure [11]. On the other hand, there have been various proposals for the latency model, for example extending the Cox or the AFT model, considering for example piecewise constant hazard

	Intercept	Stage	Ulceration	Pos. lymph nodes
CM		0.47 (0.12), p < 0.001 HR = 1.60 (95% CI: [1.26; 2.04])	0.48 (0.12), p < 0.001 HR = 1.62 (95% CI: 1.27; 2.05)	0.37 (0.12), p = 0.003 HR = 1.45 (95% CI: 1.14; 1.85)
PTM				
Incidence	−0.71 (0.12)	0.47 (0.12), p < 0.001	0.48 (0.12), p < 0.001	0.37 (0.12), p = 0.003
Latency		HR = 1.60 (95% CI: 1.25; 2.04)	HR = 1.62 (95% CI: 1.27; 2.05)	HR = 1.45 (95% CI: 1.14; 1.84)
MCM (smcure)				
Incidence	−0.35 (0.16)	0.39 (0.21), p = 0.067	0.75 (0.22), p < 0.001	0.63 (0.22), p = 0.004
Latency		0.71 (0.16), p < 0.001	0.26 (0.17), p = 0.110	0.05 (0.16), p = 0.771
MCM* (smcure)				
Incidence	−0.19 (0.12)	-	-	-
Latency		0.75 (0.15), p < 0.001	0.81 (0.23), p < 0.001	0.73 (0.21), p < 0.001
MCM (pspmcm)				
Incidence	−0.37 (0.16)	0.41 (0.19), p = 0.031 OR = 1.50 (95% CI: [1.00; 2.31])	0.75 (0.20), p < 0.001 OR = 2.12 (95% CI: [1.35; 3.42])	0.63 (0.19), p = 0.001 OR = 1.87 (95% CI: [1.24; 2.89])
Latency		0.70 (0.13), p < 0.001 HR = 2.01 (95% CI: [1.44; 2.75])	0.26 (0.12), p=0.036 HR = 1.29 (95% CI: [0.95; 1.78])	0.04 (0.12), p = 0.732 HR = 1.04 (95% CI: [0.75; 1.39])

TABLE 4.7

Melanoma data : Results from different cure models. Results are presented as estimate (standard error) for the intercept term and as estimate (standard error), p-value, hazard ratio (95% confidence intervals) for the treatment effect. For the MCM, confidence intervals are obtained from 1000 bootstrap samples based on the percentile method. CM: Cox PH Model (R function coxph), PTM: Promotion Time cure Model (R function nltm), MCM: Logistic/Cox PH Mixture Cure Model (R function smcure and SAS macro pspmcm).

or approximating the baseline hazard function with splines [82]. It has also been proposed to use another type of survival models for the latency, such as a proportional odds model

$$S_u^{PO}(t \mid \mathbf{Z} = \mathbf{z}, B = 1) = \frac{1}{1 + [S_{u0}(t)^{-1} - 1]\exp(-\beta^t \mathbf{Z})}$$

According to the property of this model, see Section 2.5.3, it assumes that the hazards ratio of the uncured subjects goes to 1 when time goes to infinity [289]. On the other hand, it has also been proposed to consider an *accelerated hazards model* [67, 430], for which

$$S_u^{AH}(t \mid \mathbf{Z} = \mathbf{z}, B = 1) = S_{u0}(\exp(\beta^t \mathbf{Z})t)^{\beta^t \mathbf{Z}}$$

In terms of the hazard function, we have for this model that

$$h_u(t \mid \mathbf{Z} = \mathbf{z}, B = 1) = h_{u0}(\exp(\beta^t \mathbf{Z})t)$$

corresponding to a gradual effect of $\mathbf{Z}$ on the survival time of the uncured subjects. of course, similar to the PH assumption, these assumptions (proportional odds or accelerated hazard) only hold at the level of the latency, and thus for the uncured patients, and not for the whole population as represented by the unconditional survival function $S_{pop}(t)$.

Fully non-parametric estimation of the latency, with or without covariates but still considering a parametric incidence have also been discussed [239, 280]. Lopez-Cheda et al. [235] propose a fully non-parametric model for both the incidence and the latency and including covariates, estimating both parts of the model based on the Beran estimator. However, these less/non parametric models are rarely used in the medical literature. Note that when considering fully non-parametric models, identifibility issue needs to be carefully though of.

As we have already mentioned, the mixture cure models has mainly been studied in a frequentist context. However, Bayesian approach have also been considered and in particular to address more complex data structure. Examples are Zhuang et al. [435] who use Bayesian techniques to estimate the mixture cure models in the presence of missing data in the covariates and Yu et al. [426] who fit a mixture cure model including spatial frailty terms.

Identifiability and estimation of the mixture cure models including a gamma frailty term in the latency (to account for unobserved covariates) have also been studied in a frequentist framework [291, 292]. Peng and Taylor [289] provide an overview of the extension of the mixture cure model to the case of clustered survival data. The most common approach is to include random effects, capturing the latent factors specific to each cluster and thus the intra-cluster correlation, both in the incidence model and in the latency models. These random effects are usually assumed to follow a normal distribution and can be correlated or not, see for example [203, 288, 353, 421].

Contrary to the mixture cure model, the promotion time cure model has been studied mainly in a Bayesian setting, and various alternative estimation approaches have been proposed in this framework for either the standard promotion time cure model as for the extended models discussed in Section 4.3.3, see for example [45, 65, 172, 388, 425]. In most of the proposed approaches, Monte Carlo Markov Chains (MCMC) methods are used to approximate the posterior distribution which often have a too complex form to be handled analytically.

There actually exists a quite important literature on extensions of the promotion time cure models directly inspired from the biological construction of this model, considering for example a different distribution for the number of carcinogenic cells that can metastasize [81]. These extensions mainly find their interest when the objective is indeed the modeling of the latent process leading to tumor progression. Another proposal, based also originally on the biological interpretation of this model, has been made to include a subject specific frailty term to model the association between the activation times of each carcinogenic cell within the same individual [428]. This leads to a new class of models, with the population survival for the ith individual given by

$$S_{pop}(t)(t \mid \mathbf{X}_i = \mathbf{x}_i) = E_{\xi_i}\left[exp(-\theta(\mathbf{x}_i)F(t)\xi_i\right]$$

and different models are obtained based on the distribution assumed for the random effects ξ. To consider clustered survival data, one could also consider that the frailty term ξ_i is shared between the activation times of each carcinogenic cell of all individuals in a same cluster [423], leading to the conditional (on the cluster) population survival function for the ith cluster given now by

$$S_{pop}(t)(t \mid \mathbf{X}_i = \mathbf{x}_i, \xi_i) = \exp\left[-\theta(\mathbf{x}_i)(1 - S(t))_i^{\xi}\right]$$

where $S(t) = 1 - F(t)$ is a proper survival function, and the frailty terms are assumed to follow a one-parameter gamma distribution (see Section 3.4 of Chapter 3).

Acknowledging that promotion time cure models can be seen as an extension of the Cox PH model imposing a bounded cumulative hazard, another way to extend it to clustered data is to include the frailty term accounting for clustered data in a similar way as to extend the Cox PH model to the shared frailty model. We can then write

$$S_{pop}(t)(t \mid \mathbf{X}_i = \mathbf{x}_i, \xi_i) = \exp\left[-\xi_i\theta(\mathbf{x}_i)F(t)\right]$$

and Chen et al. [65] assume a positive stable distribution for the frailty as in this case the resulting marginal model preserve the proportional hazard structure of the condition model. However, other frailty distributions such as the gamma have also been considered [289]. As for the standard promotion time cure model, most of the methods proposed to estimate parameters of promotion time cure models including a frailty terms are in a Bayesian framework.

The issue of measurement errors in the covariates has been investigated in the context of the promotion time cure models, first by Ma and Yin [241] and then by Bertrand et al. [36, 37]. To the best of our knowledge it has not been studied in the framework of the mixture cure model, but the SIMEX procedure [80] could be applied to this models with little adjustment.

Both types of cure models have been studied in the framework of interval-censored data, considering a fully parametric but flexible AFT mixture cure model [351, 352] or a semi-parametric promotion time cure models [234], the latter being implemented in the intercure R package.

In the framework of clinical trial but also in some broader experimental settings, sample size calculation is a crucial issue. Standard procedure for sample size calculation for time-to-event outcome actually rely on the PH assumption and can thus not be applied if the presence of cure leads to a violation of this assumption. Furthermore, ignoring the presence of cure may adversely impact the power of the study since in a survival context it is the number of events which drives the power of the statistical tests. Sample size formula for the case of a logistic/PH mixture cure models have been proposed by Cai et al. [53] and are available through the NPHMC R package [54]. The required sample size for testing a given difference in the proportion of cure and in the conditional survival of the uncured while accounting for different accrual patterns can be obtained. This is to the best of our knowledge, the only publication related to sample size calculation in the context of cure models.

Besides the well know families of mixture cure models and promotion time cure models, other types of models have also been proposed but are clearly much less use in practice and lack implementation in standard software. For example, it has been proposed to extend the proportional odds model to a proportional odds cure model or the additive hazard model to an additive cure hazard model in a same way as the Cox PH model as been extended to the promotion time cure model (so replacing proper baseline distribution/hazard function by improper ones) [148, 228, 295, 425]. Unifying approaches, which embedded both mixture cure models and promotion time cure models as special cases, have been quite extensively discussed in the literature, see [10, 289] for a nice overview. They have been developed mainly following either a mathematical motivation, with models based mainly on a Box-Cox transformation (see for example [425]) or a biological motivation [81, 274, 377], obtaining new classes of unifying models by extending the reasoning of Tsodikov [386]. However, these unifying models are not easily available in standard software and are therefore rarely used in practice. An interesting further development is to use these unifying classes of models to guide the choice of a mixture cure model or a promotion time cure models [290, 370, 425]. However this still require further research.

Using cure models when the time of interest is time to death may seems a bit odd, since typically death will occur for all observations if follow-up is long enough. However, it is typically used when focusing on death due to a given disease. The goal is therefore to distinguish between the individuals who will die early on (and for whom the cause of death is then assumed to be the disease under the study) from the long-term survivors who will die much later on (and for which we will therefore assume that they did of something else). Besides the zero-tailed constrain mentioned in Section 4.4 linked to the idea that no one will die of the cause of interest after the last observed event time, one needs in such a setting to also be careful that death due to other causes can be considered negligible during the follow-up period. When this is not the case and/or if we really want to focus on the death from a given disease, a vast literature has been devoted to the application of cure models to relative survival. So, if we are interested in death from a particular disease and the medical context suggest that a fraction of the population under study will indeed not die of this disease,the idea is to define the occurrence of "statistical cure" when the mortality rate of the diseased cases will have returned to the same general mortality of the population; in other words when the *excess mortality* due to the disease under study reach zero [301]. While both additive and multiplicative hazard models have been studies, the former one seems more common. We then write

$$h_{dis}(t) = h^\star(t) + h_{exc}(t)$$

where $h_{dis}(t)$ is the observed hazard in the diseased group, $h^\star(t)$ is the expected hazard for the general population (and is usually estimated from national life-tables), and $h_{exc}(t)$ is the excess mortality hazard due to the disease under consideration. From this expression we can easily obtain

$$S_{dis}(t) = S^\star(t) S_{exc}(t)$$

or equivalently

$$S_{exc}(t) = \frac{S_{dis}(t)}{S^\star(t)}$$

and $S_{exc}(t)$ is often referred to as the *relative survival*. It can be interpreted as the survival of the diseased patients in an hypothetical world where the patients would not die of any other cause. It is therefore particularly useful if we want to compare the mortality of a given disease between two countries with different other-causes mortality rate. Note that, as mentioned above, this quantity can be estimated without knowing the cause of deaths for the diseased patients in our sample, which is typically the case when the data comes from a registry. The relative survival function is usually an improper function (unless considering a very lethal disease that would kill all patients), and the methods developed in this chapter can be applied in a similar way, see for example amongst many others [19, 208, 209]. Relative survival is typically used when one has no (reliable) information on the cause of death. If such information is available, an alternative is to combine the competing risk approach (see Chapter 5 with cure, see for example the work of [271].

5

Competing Risks

5.1 Introduction

In classical survival analysis, one considers the time from an origin to a single event of interest. However in many applications, and in particular in medical applications, different types of event may occur and the occurrence of one type of event may preclude or modify the risk of occurrence of the other ones. Generally speaking, competing risks data therefore pertain to a situation where each individual may experience failure from K different causes (or event types), but we only observe the time to the first failure, as well as the type of this failure. As in classical survival analysis, the individuals can however be censored before having experienced any event (right-censoring). Note that even if for an individual, we only observe the time to the first event, this also provide some partial information about the other events as we know that they have not occured before. Whether they can still happen after depends on the type of event, e.g. observing the occurrence of distant metastases in a patient does not preclude death to occur (although we may not observe it if the patient goes out of the study) while the opposite is not true.

Although not mandatory, we will most often identify one cause of failure as *the event of interest* and consider the other causes of failure as *competing events*. Considering the possibility for competing events to hinder the occurrence of the event of interest must then be carefully handled in the analysis. A very common example is to consider time to a cause-specific, e.g. cancer, death versus death from another cause. Obviously, these two events are competing since once a patient has died from cancer, he can not die of another cause anymore. However, competing risks will also occur with non-fatal events, as long as the events are mutually exclusive, which is the case as soon as we define the different event types as occuring as first event, e.g. time to progression and time to death in the absence of progression. A general definition is therefore to refer to competing risks data for situations where the subjects under study are at risk for more than one mutually exclusive types of events or causes of failure [382]. Figure 5.1 depicts two general classical examples.

Many examples occur in oncology, where the long follow-up of the patients and the disease history make them particularly prone to the occurrence of different event types. For example, the question of long-term adverse effects is often encountered, e.g. in case of early-stage breast cancer or prostate cancer,

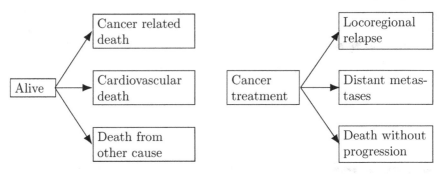

FIGURE 5.1
Competing risks: two classical examples. *Left:* interest lies in time to cause-specific death, distinguishing cancer related death, death due to cardiovascular diseases and death from other cause. *Right:* a typical situation encountered in oncology trials where interest lies in the time to the first event, distinguishing whether it is the occurrence of a locoregional recurrence, the occurrence of distant metastases or death without progression.

and often subjected to competing risks. Evaluating the risk-benefit ratio of treatment is then a complicated task as patients with better prognostic (and thus at lower risk of death as competing event) appear thus at higher risk of experiencing long-term side effects and secondary malignancy [102]. This example (and others) has led to a wide literature and has also led in the past to passionate discussions on which type of analysis to use. For example, the question of the incidence of late toxicity following radiation therapy for carcinoma of the uterine cervix has led to a famous debate in the pages of the International Journal of Radiation Oncology Physics [33, 59, 61, 62, 101]. In retrospect, as we will discuss later, it is now clear that the contention raised around the original publication of [33] was rather on the research question of interest rather than really at the level of the statistical techniques to be used, since each approaches discussed was in fact putting in light one aspect of the data while possibly obscuring the others [103].

Competing risks data are very frequent in oncology but also occur in a wide variety of other situations [194, 211]. Several popular examples have been largely discuss in the literature [132, 186, 260, 300], including, amongst others examples, the study of occurrence of infections or onset of clinical AIDS in HIV infected patients, time to nosocomial infection for hospitalized patients, time to organ rejection for transplanted patients, time to cause-specific deaths in various settings.

For illustrative purpose, let's consider the common example of a study on time to infection during hospital stay [132]. In such a case, the time origin would be the time of hospital admission and the event of interest is the occurrence of an infection during the hospital stay. Obviously, the discharge of the patient without infection is a competing event as such a discharge prevents us from observing infection during the hospital stay. Note that the death of the patient without infection is another type of competing event that might also need to be considered depending on the precise context. As is generally the case, we can see two main goal of collecting and analyzing data on infection during hospital stay: (1) to learn about the etiology of in-hospital infection, and better understanding the causes (e.g. hygienic conditions) and underlying biological process leading to such an event and (2) to improve the prediction (either at the individual or population level) of such an event and gather information about the real burden of such in-hospital infections for example in a specific hospital ward. Obviously, in this later case, it seems important for decision making to take into account that some patients will be discharge before being affected by such an infection.

When faced with competing events, a first intuitive idea is often to apply standard survival analysis techniques for the time to the event of interest while censoring individuals at the time of occurrence of a competing event. In the example above, this would mean to consider the standard techniques of Chapter 2 to study the time to in-hospital infection while censoring the patients discharged or dead without infection at the time of discharge or death.

While this approach is very popular, and still often use in biomedical applications, it has also been strongly criticized. The major problem of such analysis lies in the interpretation of the results. Indeed, in such a situation, the Kaplan-Meier estimator can not be interpreted anymore as a probability to get the event of interest. Denote for any time t, $\hat{S}_k^{naive}(t)$ the naive Kaplan-Meier estimator of the survival function obtained for time-to-event of cause k while censoring individuals at the time of another event type if it occurs before the event of type k. We can also define $\hat{F}_k^{naive}(t) = 1 - \hat{S}_k^{naive}(t)$. In that case, $\hat{F}_k^{naive}(t)$ can not anymore be interpreted as the probability of an event of type k before time t (as would be the case if only one event type) and the sum of the $\hat{F}_k^{naive}(t)$ over all values of k will not be equal the probability of the occurrence of an event of any types obtained from to $\hat{F}(t) = 1 - \hat{S}(t)$ with $\hat{S}(t)$ the Kaplan-Meier estimated survival function for the time to the first event (of any type).

This can be easily illustrated with the following toy example, which for the ease of the explanation consider that the only possible events are in-hospital infection (HI) and discharge without infection (Di) and assume no censoring. A more concrete example, considering censoring, is discussed in Section 5.6. Assume that we have 20 patients admitted to the hospital, and followed for in-hospital infection. For each of these patients, we either observe the time (in days) to the occurrence of in-hospital infection (HI) or to the discharge without infection (Di), the former being the event of interest while the later being considered as a competing risk, see Table 5.1.

As we can see, at the last time-point (29 days), a total of 13 patients (65%) have experienced in-hospital mortality (HI, $k = 1$) while 7 patients (35%) were discharged (Di, $k = 2$) without infection. One can compute the

Time	2	6	6	6	8	11	12	12	15	17
Event	HI	HI	HI	HI	Di	HI	HI	Di	Di	Di
Time	19	20	20	21	23	23	27	27	28	29
Event	Di	HI	HI	Di	Di	HI	HI	HI	HI	HI

TABLE 5.1
Competing risks – Example 1: Time to in-hospital infection in days for 20 patients (HI: in-hospital infection, Di: discharge without infection)

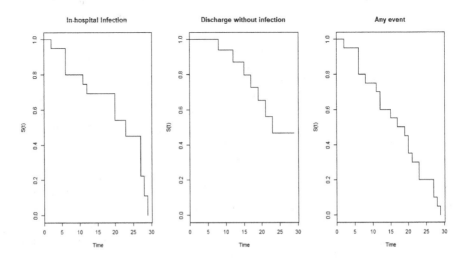

FIGURE 5.2
Competing risks – Example 1: KM estimate of time-to-event for in-hospital infection while censoring for discharge without infection (*left*), time to discharge without infection while censoring for in-hospital infection (*middle*) and time to any event (*left*).

KM estimate of the survival function for time to in-hospital infection while censoring the patients who were discharged without infection, as well as for time to discharge without infection while censoring the patients at the time of in-hospital infection. Combining these two events, we can also compute the KM estimator of the survival function of time to any type of event. Obviously, since we do not consider censoring, 100% of the patients got one event (of any type) at the last time-point (29 days). These KM estimates are displayed respectively on the right, middle, and left panel of Figure 5.2, and the estimator of the distribution function $\hat{F}_k^{naive}(t)$ (obtained from one minus the KM estimator of the survival function) at some fixed time-points for each type of event (while censoring from the other one) are given in Table 5.2.

Time	$\hat{F}(t) = 1 - \hat{S}(t)$ Any	$\hat{F}_1^{naive}(t)$ HI	$\hat{F}_2^{naive}(t)$ Di	CIF HI	CIF Di
1	0.00	0.00	0.00	0.00	0.00
7	0.20	0.20	0.00	0.20	0.00
14	0.40	0.31	0.13	0.30	0.10
21	0.70	0.46	0.44	0.40	0.30
29	1.00	1.00	0.53	0.65	0.35

TABLE 5.2
Competing risks – Example 1: Estimated distribution function for any event (Any), for in-hospital infection (HI), and for discharge without infection (Di) obtained while censoring for the competing event. Estimated cumulative incidence function for in-hospital infection (CIF HI) and for discharge without infection (CIF Di).

Looking at these results, we can observe the following well-known phenomenon. First, the probability of an event of any type at the largest time should obviously be equal to 1 (since we consider no censoring) while the sum of the probabilities give by $1 - KM$ for each event time is actually equal to $1.00 + 0.53 = 1.53$, so clearly above one. Furthermore, if we look at a specific time point, for example 14 days, we directly see that the sum of the probabilities for each type of event as estimated by $\hat{F}_1^{naive}(t)$ (censoring for the event of the other type), so $0.31 + 0.13 = 0.44$ does not equal the probability of the occurrence of an event of any type as estimated by $\hat{F}(t)$, here 0.40. Furthermore, since patients discharged without infection have been censored, there is a strong temptation to interpret the cumulative distribution $\hat{F}_1^{naive}(t)$ for in-hospital infection at a given time, for example here 0.31 at 14 days, as the probability of having an in-hospital infection by 14 days in an *ideal* (or rather *hypothetical*) world where patients would not been discharged from the hospital. However, two important remarks are that (1) we will see that such an interpretation is correct only if the occurrence of the two event types are independent, and (2) such a result, linked to an hypothetical world, is not necessarily of interest.

In fact, the objective of competing risks analysis has been for a long time to draw inference about the distribution of the time to the event of interest, in such an ideal or hypothetical world in which the competing event would not exist. However, such a distribution is not identifiable and can therefore not be estimated from the observed data unless we can make the strong assumption of independence between the distributions of the times to the different types of events [23, 102, 131, 311]. However, information about the dependence between the different event types is generally unknown and can usually not be explored from the data at hand. Indeed, since we usually only have information about the time to first event for each observation, we can not use these data to test the independence assumption between the different event types. [127].

In the early eighties, it has therefore been proposed to palliate this issue with an alternative approach whose idea was to focus on estimable quantities and to formally account for the competing risks [210, 303]. The idea is that if we are not able to estimate the "net" probability of failure from cause k in the absence of other types of failure, we can, on the other hand, estimate the probability of failure of type k in the presence of other event types, i.e. under the study conditions at hand [102]. To do so, one can partition the probability of any event happening into the probability for each type of event while accounting for the presence of the other (competing) events. The concept of *cause-specific cumulative incidence function* (*CIF*) has therefore been introduced. The *CIF* for a given event type can be interpreted as the probability of failure due to this event type event type while taking into account that another type of event may occur before and thus hinder the occurrence of the event type of interest. It has the advantage that at any timepoint, the overall survival function (estimated by $\hat{F}(t)$ calculated for all events) is equal to the sum of the cause-specific CIF for each type of events.

So, while the $\hat{F}_k^{naive}(t)$ approach attempts to estimate the probability of failure of cause k *in the absence of competing risk*, the cumulative incidence estimate this probability *taking into account the presence of competing risk*. As we will discuss, this is a major difference and will translate in a major difference in the definition of our risk sets for the estimation. In the following, we will see how to estimate the cause-specific cumulative incidence function for each type of event. For our example above, the estimated CIF for each event type are displayed on Figure 5.3, together with $\hat{F}_k^{naive}(t)$ and $\hat{F}(t)$ for the sake of comparisons. The value of the estimated CIF at specific time-points are also reported in Table 5.2. These cause-specific cumulative incidence estimates can be interpreted at each time-point as the probability to have experienced an event of type k before that time, given that one may have experienced another type event before (therefore preventing us from experiencing this event). Therefore, at each time-point, the value of the CIF is always lower or equal to the value of the corresponding $\hat{F}_k^{naive}(t)$. Intuitively, this is expected since the CIF take into account the fact that individuals who experienced an event of interest will not be at risk anymore of this event. On the other the $\hat{F}_k^{naive}(t)$ approach, by censoring the individuals who experience another type of events in fact assumes that they are still at risk of an event of type k. Coming back to our example, the CIF for in-hospital infection takes into account the fact that the probability to have an in-hospital infection is "lowered" by the fact that patients may be discharged before, while $\hat{F}_1^{naive}(t)$ actually considers that the patients who are discharged are still at risk (and actually will still experience) in-hospital infection after their censoring time. We can see that the probability to have experienced an in-hospital infection by time 14 days, while acknowledging that we might have been discharged before is only 0.30 (CIF) versus 0.40 ($\hat{F}_1^{naive}(t)$) when not taking into account this competing risk. Considering $\hat{F}_1^{naive}(t)$ does not properly acknowledge that to experience an in-hospital infection, one needs to not have been discharged before. As a consequence,

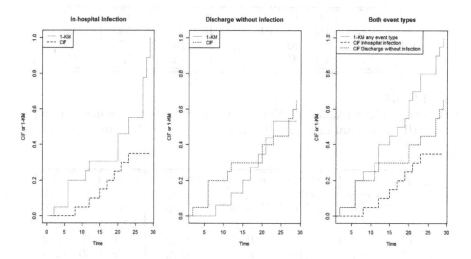

FIGURE 5.3

Competing risks – Example 1: Estimated cumulative incidence function (CIF) and 1-KM estimate $\hat{F}_k^{naive}(t)$ for in-hospital infection (*left*) and for discharge without infection (*middle*). Estimated cumulative incidence function for in-hospital infection and for discharge without infection and 1-KM estimate $\hat{F}(t)$ for event of any type (*right*).

it overestimates the cumulative event-specific probability of experiencing in-hospital infection. If we sum this probability of in-hospital infection (0.10) to the one of having been discharged without having experienced in-hospital infection (0.10), we indeed find back the probability of having experienced any of the event by time 14 days as given by $\hat{F}(t)$ (0.40). At the last event time, we also find back that the probability to have experienced an in-hospital infection or having been discharge without infection over the whole study period are respectively equal to 0.65 and 0.35, summing up to 1, the probability to have one event of any type over the study period.

Note that based on the specific context (i.e. type of hospitalized patients) it may be more realistic in this example to consider a second type of competing events, namely the in-hospital death of the patient without infection. In that case, we will have to estimate three cumulative incidence curves and at each time point, the sum of the estimated CIF for each event type will be equal to one minus the KM estimate of the time to any event. For the sake of the illustration, consider that amongst the 20 patients presented in Table 5.1, 5 of them experience in-hospital death (HD) before in-hospital infection occurs and before being discharged the hospital. Note that for this illustration, these 5 patients were all patients who experienced in-hospital infection in the previous example. The new data are presented in Table 5.3 and the estimated cumulative incidence functions for each event type, as well as the

Time	2	6	6	6	8	11	12	12	15	17
Event	HI	HI	HI	HD	Di	HI	HI	Di	Di	Di
Time	19	20	20	21	23	23	27	27	28	29
Event	Di	HI	HI	Di	Di	HI	HI	HI	HI	HI

TABLE 5.3
Competing risks – Example 2: Time to in-hospital infection in days for 20 patients (HI: in-hospital infection, HD: in-hospital death, Di: discharge without infection)

Time	$\hat{F}(t)$ Any	$\hat{F}_1^{naive}(t)$ HI	$\hat{F}_2^{naive}(t)$ Di	$\hat{F}_3^{naive}(t)$ HD	CIF HI	CIF Di	CIF HD
1	0.0	0.00	0.00	0.00	0.00	0.00	0.00
7	0.2	0.15	0.00	0.05	0.15	0.00	0.05
14	0.4	0.21	0.13	0.12	0.20	0.10	0.10
21	0.7	0.29	0.44	0.22	0.25	0.30	0.15
29	1.0	1.00	0.53	0.67	0.40	0.35	0.25

TABLE 5.4
Competing risks – Example 2: Estimated distribution function for any event (Any), for in-hospital infection (HI), for discharge without infection (Di), and for in-hospital death (HI) obtained while censoring for the competing events. Estimated cumulative incidence function for in-hospital infection (CIF HI), for discharge without infection (CIF Di), and for in-hospital death (CIF Di).

1-KM estimate of $\hat{F}(t)$ for event of any type is plotted on Figure 5.4. Values of these estimates for the same time-points as in Table 5.2 are provided in Table 5.4 and it is interesting to compare these results to those presented previously.

First note that, as expected, $\hat{F}(t)$ for any event type and the $\hat{F}_2^{naive}(t)$ for discharge without infection (Di) have not changed while $\hat{F}_1^{naive}(t)$ for in-hospital infection has obviously changed (since we "removed" 5 HI events to transform them into in-hospital death). Second, as was also expected, the sum of the $\hat{F}_k^{naive}(t)$ for each event type ($k = 1, 2, 3$) is still above one at the last event time while for each time-point, the sum of the estimated CIF values is equal to the global $\hat{F}(t)$, and in this basic example (without censoring), the CIFs estimated at the last event time indeed correspond to the proportion of each event type ($8/20 = 0.40$ for HI, $7/20 = 0.35$ for Di, and $5/20 = 0.25$ for HD). Third, we note that values of the the CIF for Di has not changed, which is due to the fact that we did not modify the occurrence of this event. In this example, some patients died before experiencing in-hospital infection, therefore the estimated CIF for in-hospital infection dramatically decreased. Of course, it would nevertheless be odd to conclude that in-hospital death helps to prevent in-hospital infection.

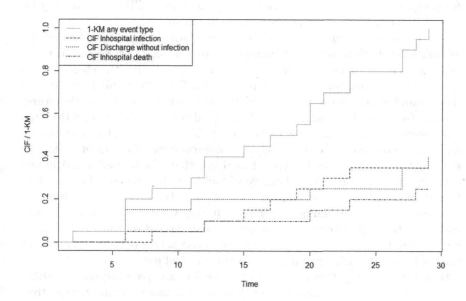

FIGURE 5.4

Competing risks – Example 2: Estimated Cumulative incidence in-hospital infection, discharge without infection, and in-hospital death together with the 1-KM $\hat{F}(t)$ for event of any type.

The apparent discrepancy between the naive $1-KM$ approach ($\hat{F}_k^{naive}(t)$) and CIF estimates has led to a lot of confusion and debate in the biomedical literature, with some authors arguing strongly against one or the other approach. In fact, $\hat{F}_k^{naive}(t)$ and the CIF provide different results simply because they do not estimate the same quantity. Therefore, these two approaches are not to be opposed but simply to be seen as answers to different questions. In the example above, different research questions could be to identify on which factors we can act (e.g. nurse wearing gloves, use of a new antiseptic, ...) independently of the discharge of the patients, to decrease the rate of in-hospital infection or to predict the number of patients who will actually suffer from in-hospital infection for example to ensure enough resources are available to face this or to include this information in a cost-effectiveness analysis. It is however of upmost importance to be able to decide which approach to use when, to be aware of the underlying assumptions and to understand how to interpret the results correctly.

Note that the same confusion and debate also exist with respect to hypothesis testing and modeling of survival data in the presence of competing risks [102, 103]. As we will see, contrary to what we have seen in Chapter 2, in the presence of competing risks there is not anymore a direct link between the (cause-specific) hazard function and the (cause-specific) CIF and two different hazard functions have been studied in the literature.

So, the main difficulty when getting familiar with competing risks and the associated statistical analysis techniques is to not get confused between the different types of questions that we can answer, and with the choice of the quantity that is helpful in which situation [102, 103, 126]. This is made even more complex due to the wide use of different terminology in the literature, and the fact that the terms are not always used consistently between the various references. In the following, we rely as much as possible on the terminology and notations used by Geskus [132]. The approach we follow in this Chapter is to first define three main type of analyzes that can be performed in the presence of competing risks. Then, we will address the question of estimation, hypothesis tests, and modeling for each of these three types of analyzes. A summary of all the techniques discussed in this Chapter is provided at the end of Section 5.2. These techniques will be illustrated on some real data in Section 5.6. For a more in-depth discussion of competing risks, we recommend the books of [40, 132]. Several textbooks on survival data also dedicate a special chapter to competing risks analyzes, see for example Chapter 8 of [192], Chapter 8 of [181] or Chapter 9 of [260] from a more applied perspective. Several review papers have also been published over the last two decades, see for example [311] and [23].

5.2   Basic concepts, notations, and definitions

We consider K possible types of events $(k = 1, ..., K)$ and assume that each subject can experience at most one of these K types of events, in other words the event types are mutually exclusive. One can actually find in the literature two broad approaches for competing risks (see [132] for a detailed description). The first one, sometimes qualified as the *old* one [23], considers K latent failure time variables, one for each possible event type $T_1, T_2, ..., T_K$. Obviously, in a competing risk setting, we only observe the minimum of these latent failures times $T = min(T_1, ..., T_K)$ as well as the failure type. A very important point is that without additional strong assumption (such as the independence of the different latent failure time variables) neither the joint distribution of these latent failure time variables nor the corresponding marginal distribution are identifiable from the data [23, 132, 181, 212, 303, 311, 382]. This should kill any hope to estimate the time to a specific event type in an *hypothetical* world where the other event types do not exist, unless we can assume the independence of the different event types or solve the non-identifiability issue by considering some very specific circumstances [132, 156, 380].

In the second, more common, approach, one considers a single random variable T now representing the time to the first event and the variable E indicating the type of events ($E = 1, ..., K$). The idea is then to rather focus on the joint distribution of the time to the first event T and the type of event E. This approach gave birth to the concept of cause-specific cumulative incidence function and cause-specific hazard function defined below [23, 132, 181, 303, 311, 382].

Note that, since the different event types are mutually exclusive, we have

$$T_k = \begin{cases} T & \text{if } E = k \\ \infty & \text{if } E \neq k \end{cases}$$

and thus $T = \min(T_1, ..., T_K)$.

Similarly to what we discussed in Chapter 2, we will also consider right-censoring and therefore the observed time is in fact $Y = \min(T, C)$ with C the censoring time (for a reason other than a competing risk) and δ the censoring indicator (equal to 1 if an event of any type occurred and to zero otherwise). In some situations, it may be easier to drop the variable C and to extend the possible values of the variable E representing the event type to include censoring, considering $E = 0$ if the subject is censored and $E = 1, ..., K$ if the subject experienced one of the K possible event types.

While the survival function $S(t) = P(T > t)$ is often preferred in classical survival analysis, once dealing with competing risks, the distribution function $F(.)$, often referred to the *cumulative incidence function* in this context, is preferred. Furthermore, we now distinguish the overall cumulative incidence function

$$F(t) = P(T \leq t) \tag{5.1}$$

from the cause-specific cumulative incidence function

$$F_k(t) = P(T_k \leq t) = P(T \leq t, E = k) \tag{5.2}$$

with the corresponding overall and cause-specific survival function $S(t) = \bar{F}(t) = 1 - F(t)$ and $S_k(t) = \bar{F}_k(t) = 1 - F_k(t)$. This cause-specific cumulative incidence function $F_k(t)$ can thus be interpreted as the probability that an individual experiences an event of type k by time t and therefore corresponds to what we loosely call "CIF" in Section 5.1. The sum of all cause-specific cumulative incidences gives the overall cumulative incidence:

$$\sum_{k=1}^{K} F_k(t) = \sum_{k=1}^{K} P(T \leq t, E = k) = P(T \leq t) = F(t) \tag{5.3}$$

We have seen that in classical survival analysis when we are faced with a single type of event, there exists a one-to-one relationship between the hazard function, the cumulative hazard function and the survival function (see equations (1.3)). An immediate consequence is that the effect of a covariate as quantified via a regression model for the hazard translates to a similar effect on the survival function. We will see that in the presence of competing risks, two hazard functions can be defined of which one doesn't have this one-to-one relationship anymore.

As mentioned previously, we can actually do different types of analysis when faced with competing risks. Each of these will involve different quantities and estimation, testing and modeling approaches. It is therefore important to understand the difference between these types of analysis, and to understand that they actually answer different research questions, so to be able to choose the appropriate analysis for a given context. In the following, we shortly introduce them using the example of in-hospital infection as illustration. We will then provide further details with regards to estimation, hypotheses testing and modeling in the next sections.

5.2.1   Combined analysis or time to the first event analysis

The simplest way to analyze competing risks data is to, in a way, forget about the fact that we have different event types and to combine all of them into one *combined event*. The time to this combined event is then defined as the time to the first occurrence of any component of this combined event. Such an approach is obviously equivalent to considering the time to the first event, whatever event type it is.

In the first example of Section 5.1, it corresponds to analyze the time to either in-hospital infection or hospital discharge, whatever comes first. As can be seen from this example, such an analysis does not always make a lot of sense. Indeed, we are often interesting in delaying or even preventing in-hospital infection but probably hoping to shorten time to discharge (which usually means that the patient is doing better).Other situations in which such a combined analysis would be difficult to interpret is when one type of event is rare compared to the other and/or when the gravity of the event types is not of the same magnitude. However, they are some contexts in which such a combined analysis can make sense. A typical example is the analysis of *progression-free survival* in oncology trials, where the event of interest is "either progression or death, whichever comes first", with the hope to delay both event types. We can also see consider overall survival, defined as time to death from any cause, as a combined analysis as opposed to time to cause-specific death in which each type of death (e.g. death due to the disease under study, death due to natural cause, death due to non-natural cause not linked to the disease, ...) is seen as a competing event.

Since, we are left with the time to a single event, the classical survival data analysis methods of Chapter 2 applies. In particular, we will based our analyzes on the overall survival function $S(t)$, the overall cumulative incidence function $F(t) = 1 - S(t)$, and the corresponding overall hazard function $h(t)$. Although such an analysis may also bring some important information, it is usually not considered sufficient when analyzing competing risks data.

5.2.2 Marginal analysis

When faced with competing risks, a somewhat intuitive approach is to focus on one event of interest, e.g. the in-hospital infection, and to quantify the risk to develop such an event, in an *ideal* or *hypothetical* world where the competing event would not exist. The objective is then to quantify a *marginal* or *net* probability of failure from the event of interest, in the absence of any other competing events. A typical research question would then be "What are the factors that would impact the risk of in-hospital infection if patients would stay in the hospital forever"; and answering such a question may be useful to better understand the biological mechanisms behind these in-hospital infection and possibly to identify the factors on which to act to directly prevent such in-hospital infection (and thus not factors that indirectly decrease the risk of infection by shortening the length of in-hospital stay for example). We however have to be aware that such an analysis will obviously overestimate the actual number of in-hospital infections since it does not take into account that some individuals will leave the hospital before developing such an in-hospital infection.

This analysis can be referred to as a *marginal analysis*, and one speaks about the *marginal cumulative incidence* and its corresponding *marginal hazard function*, also sometimes called the "net risk" of the event of interest.

Such an analysis is often performed, *naively* by considering the time to the event of interest while censoring for the other event types. So, in our example a patient who would leave the hospital before developing an in-hospital infection would be censored at the time he/she leaves the hospital. Estimation of the marginal cumulative incidence function and marginal hazard function can then be performed using classical survival methods (since we are back to a single event type). However, it is not always that straightforward. Indeed, such an approach will lead to unbiased estimator of these marginal quantities only under the (strong) assumption of independence of the different event type process. Indeed, standard survival analysis techniques rely on the assumption of non-informative censoring. So, this approach actually assumes that the individuals censored at the time they experience a competing event can be represented by the individuals still in follow-up, which will not be the case anymore of the time to the different event types are correlated [132].

In our example, the question is whether we can consider that patients who are censored because they are discharged from the hospital can be represented by those still in follow-up in the hospital. In other words, if these discharged patients would have stay in the hospital "forever", would they have had the same risk of event (in-hospital infection) after their (true) censoring time as the non-discharged ones. One can probably put this in doubt arguing that they were discharged because they were going better, and thus being stronger against infection than those staying in the hospital. In such a case, the marginal distribution can not be estimated without making additional assumptions [132].

So, while such an analysis seems intuitive, such an independence assumption is often difficult to believe and the interpretation of such an analysis is therefore subject to great caution. For example, in oncology, we may expect a (positive) correlation between, for example the time to locoregional recurrence and distant metastases, with patients with shorter time to locoregional recurrence having also shorter time to distant metastases. Furthermore it is often the case in real-life situations, that we only observe the first event and we do therefore not have enough information to estimate or test the magnitude of the dependence between the different event types [381]. Therefore, we must be very careful with the common habit to interpret the estimates $\hat{F}_k^{naive}(t)$ as a probability of having event k by time t in an hypothetical world where the competing events are eliminated as this is actually only true under the independence of the different causes of failure. Note further, that even in the case of independence, the obtained results would still represent purely hypothetical quantities since in the real-life the presence of competing events indeed do prevent the occurrence of the competing events, and therefore these quantities will overestimate the real-life occurrence of the event k. In our example, it is obvious that patients who are discharged from the hospital are not anymore at risk of in-hospital infection.

Nevertheless, if we can make this independence assumption and are indeed interested by such an hypothetical situation, then we are in fact back to standard analysis techniques. We can indeed work separately on each event type while censoring for the other event types as well as for "real" censoring (as we actually did in Section 5.1). We can then estimate the survival function for the event of interest for example with the Kaplan-Meier estimator, while censoring all the patients who experienced a competing event first. However, a major issue is that we can actually never be sure of this independence assumption, and while it can be possible to show that censoring due to a competing event is informative it is actually not possible to test for non-informative censoring from the data at hand [132].

5.2.3 Competing risk analysis

The idea here is still to focus on one event of interest, e.g. the in-hospital infection, but the objective is now to quantify the risk to develop such an event, taking into account the fact that other types of event may occur first and thus preventing us from observing the one of interest, or modifying the risk of the event of interest to occur. A typical research question would then be "What is the rate of in-hospital infection taking into account the fact that patients may be discharged (or die) before developing such an infection". Answering this question could be used for example to predict the required resources to face the case of in-hospital infection, taking into account that no resources are needed for individuals leaving the hospital before developing such an infection, but could also be of interest if our goal is to evaluate the impact of shortening the length of stay in the hospital on the occurrence of in-hospital infection. In such a situation, we will obviously have to take into account the fact that a subject who has been discharge can not experience an in-hospital infection anymore, and therefore subjects who are discharged do clearly not represent those still in.

During the covid-19 pandemic the world had to face in 2020, a crucial issue which appeared in the course of the pandemic was the availability of mechanical ventilators for all patients who needed it. Patients hospitalized could experience three main types of event as first event: being discharged alive without need for mechanical ventilation, dying (of covid-19 or of another cause) before being put on mechanical ventilation or being put under mechanical ventilation. Obviously, if the objective is to predict the need in mechanical ventilators, a combined analysis of the time to the first event would be useless. Also, a marginal analysis focusing on time to mechanical ventilation while ignoring the competing risks would (1) most probably lead to severely biased estimators as we can really doubt about the independence assumption (as the patients that could be discharged quickly clearly had a somewhat "softer" form of the disease), and (2) be totally useless as the predictions in terms of availability of mechanical ventilators had to be in "our real world" where patients who are discharged or die before being on mechanical ventilators do in fact not need this resource. An appropriate analysis would rather be to consider a competing risk analysis for time to mechanical ventilation, considering discharge from the hospital and death before mechanical ventilation as competing risks. Such an analysis would then provide predictions on the required resources in terms of mechanical ventilators while acknowledging that not all patients will need it.

Numerous papers have therefore considered the estimation of the cumulative incidence probability function for one event type in the presence of other types of events [130, 139, 198, 294]. Different names have been used in the literature, the most common ones are the *cause-specific cumulative incidence function* or the *sub-distribution function*. We will denote $F_k(t)$ the cause-specific cumulative incidence function for the event of interest k, which is defined as

$$F_k(t) = P(T \leq t, E = k) \tag{5.4}$$

Like the overall cumulative distribution function, this function is always non-decreasing, but unlike a proper cumulative distribution function, it does not tend to 1 when t goes to infinity. In fact, the cause-specific cumulative incidence function for event type k tends to the probability of such an event when time goes to infinity

$$\lim_{t \to \infty} F_k(t) = P(E = k)$$

$F_k(.)$ is therefore not a proper distribution function and this explains the terminology "sub-distribution function".

From this cause-specific cumulative incidence function, one can mimic what is done in standard survival analysis and define a hazard function which has a one-to-one relationship with this cumulative incidence function. This hazard is often referred to as the *sub-distribution hazard* and

$$h_k(t) = -\frac{d\log(1 - F_k(t))}{dt}$$

We can show that such a hazard takes the form

$$h_k(t) = \lim_{\Delta t \to 0} \frac{P(t \le T < t + \Delta t, E = k \mid T_k \ge t)}{\Delta t} \tag{5.5}$$

and is based on the fraction of individuals that develops the event of interest at some point, amongst the individuals that either are still at risk for this event of interest or have already experienced a competing event (since in that case $T_k = \infty$).

This sub-distribution hazard therefore has (by construction) a one-to-one link with the cumulative incidence function $S_k(t)$ which is a desirable mathematical property. However, this subdistribution hazard is quite unnatural, as it considers that individuals should survive only to event of type k to still be at risk of this type of event. Indeed, it considers that individuals that experienced of a different type of event before would still be at risk of experiencing the one of interest. It is therefore sometimes seen as a mathematical construction which has the advantage to relate to the cause-specific cumulative incidence function via the usual relationship

$$S_k(t) = 1 - F_k(t) = \bar{F}_k = \exp\left\{-\int_0^t h_k(s)ds\right\}$$

and we can also write

$$h_k(t) = \frac{dF_k(t)/dt}{1 - F_k(t)}$$

This sub-distribution hazard for failure type k can also be seen as the hazard function of a new time variable $\tilde{T}$ defined as $\tilde{T} = T$ if the individual experienced a failure of type k and $\tilde{T} = \infty$ otherwise [122, 145]. Making the link with Chapter 4, this comes back to assuming that an individual who has experience a failure of type k is actually *cured* from the other types of failure [103].

A more intuitive hazard function, actually closer from the concept of the hazard discussed in Chapter 2, can be defined as

$$\lambda_k(t) = \lim_{\Delta t \searrow 0} \frac{P(t \le T < t + \Delta t, E = k \mid T \ge t)}{\Delta t} \tag{5.6}$$

This so-called *cause-specific hazard* quantifies the progression to the event of interest amongst the individuals who are still at risk and who therefore did not experience any event of any type before. This cause-specific hazard is often pointed out as the principal identifiable quantity in a competing risk analysis.

The sum of all the cause-specific hazards for each event types gives the overall hazard, sometimes referred to as the *all-causes hazard* in a competing risks framework

$$\sum_{k=1}^{K} \lambda_k(t) = h(t) \tag{5.7}$$

So, the hazard of an event of any type at time t is equal to the sum of the cause-specific hazards of each of the event types at that time t.

From this cause-specific hazard $\lambda_k(t)$, we can define a cumulative cause-specific hazard $\Lambda_k(t)$, in a similar way as in classical survival analysis, considering

$$\Lambda_k(t) = \int_0^t \lambda_k(s)ds \qquad \text{for } k = 1, ..., K$$

and the cumulative cause-specific cumulative hazards for the k (mutually exclusive) event types sums up to the cumulative hazard function for an event of any type:

$$\sum_{k=1}^{K} \Lambda_k(t) = \Lambda(t)$$

An easy example to fix ideas is to consider death from cancer as the event of interest and death from other causes as the competing event; this translates then to the intuitive idea that at any time the risk of death should be the sum of the risk of death from cancer and of death from other causes.

It follows that the overall cumulative incidence function (and thus the overall survival function) can be written in terms of all cause-specific hazards for each event type

$$
\begin{aligned}
S(t) = 1 - F(t) &= \exp\left\{-\int_0^t h(s)ds\right\} \\
&= \exp\left\{-\int_0^t \sum_{k=1}^{K} \lambda_k(s)ds\right\} \\
&= \prod_{k=1}^{K} \exp\left\{-\int_0^t \lambda_k(s)ds\right\}
\end{aligned}
$$

The cause-specific cumulative incidence and the cause-specific hazard are related by the following relationship [130, 139, 198, 294]:

$$F_k(t) = P(T \le t, E = k) = \int_0^t S(s)\lambda_k(s)ds \qquad (5.8)$$

The intuition behind this formula is that to experience an event of type k at time t, one should have survived all the event types until time t, and that given that we have not experience any other event before, one should experience an event of type k at time t. The cause-specific cumulative incidence function can thus be interpreted as the cumulative probability to have experienced an event of type k by time t in the presence of the other competing events.

An important point is that due to the presence of $S(t)$ in (5.8), we clearly see that the cause-specific cumulative incidence function $F_k(t)$ depends both on the cause-specific hazard of event of type k but also on the cause-specific hazards or all other event types (via $S(t)$). It is thus crucial to realize that there is therefore no one-to-one relationship between the cause-specific hazard and the cause-specific cumulative incidence function. A major implication is that to impact $F_k(t)$ we may either act directly on the event type k or, more indirectly, on the other event types. This comes back to the idea we have mentioned in Section 5.1 that to decrease the incidence of in-hospital infection, we can either act directly on the causes of such infections to lower its incidence, but we can also indirectly lower it by acting on factors that will increase the incidence of hospital discharge ... or even of in-hospital death ! The cumulative incidence function for cause k therefore reflects the rate of event of type k as well as the influence of the competing event types.

So, this cause-specific hazard is close from the concept of hazard in a classical setting, as it is defined based on the fraction of individuals that develops the event of interest at some points amongst the individuals still at risk for this event, and is therefore more intuitive. On the other hand, since there is no one-to-one relationship with the cause-specific cumulative incidence function, the way in which covariates are associated with the cause-specific hazard may not be the same as the way in which these covariates are associated with the cause-specific CI. It is not difficult to construct examples of groups of observations having the same cause-specific hazard for the event of interest but very different cumulative incidence function for this type of event. A covariate that has little effect on the hazard of in-hospital infection can actually have a big effect on the cumulative incidence via its impact on the hazard of discharge from the hospital.

From (5.8), we can also write

$$\lambda_k(t) = \frac{dF_k(t)/dt}{S(t)}$$

Also, we have that at any timepoint, the K cause-specific cumulative incidence functions for each type of event sums up to the probability of failure from any cause,

$$\sum_{k=1}^{K} F_k(t) = \sum_{k=1}^{K} \int_0^t S(s)\lambda_k(s)ds \qquad \text{for each } t$$

$$= \int_0^t S(s) \sum_{k=1}^{K} \lambda_k(s)ds$$

$$= \int_0^t S(s)h(s)ds = \int_0^t f(s)ds = F(t) = 1 - S(t)$$

This is in line with what we have seen in our toy example of Section 5.1.

As discussed by Geskus [132], the cause-specific hazard and the subdistribution hazard are linked by the following relationship:

$$\lambda_k(t)\bar{F}(t^-) = h_k(t)\bar{F}_k(t^-)$$

where $\bar{F}(.) = 1 - F(.)$ and this relation holds both for the theoretical distribution but also for the non-parametric estimators.

From the joint distribution of T and the failure type E, the likelihood function under independent right censoring follows the same idea as in the general case:

$$L \propto \prod_{k=1}^{K}\prod_{i=1}^{n} (\lambda_k(t_i))^{\delta_{ik}} S_k(t_i)$$

$$\propto \prod_{k=1}^{K}\prod_{i=1}^{n} (\lambda_k(t_i))^{\delta_{ik}} \exp\left[-\int_0^{t_i} \lambda_k(t_i)\right] \qquad (5.9)$$

where δ_{ik} is an indicator that take value 1 if subject i failed from cause k and 0 otherwise [23]. As we can see, this likelihood is a function of the cause-specific hazards and the cumulative incidence functions, and these quantities can therefore be estimated from the data without any further assumptions.

As we will discuss below (see Section 5.5), modeling approaches have been based either on the cause-specific hazard or the subdistribution hazards and one has to be aware that the effects of a covariates on each of these two hazards are not necessarily the same. It can even lead to results that differ substantially, and possibly to reversed covariate effect in some extreme situation (see for example [134]). Again, the choice of the modeling approach will mainly be a matter of the research question of interest.

5.2.4 A note on censoring

It is interesting to note that while most papers consider (right-)censoring as a separate issue (which is in fact what we will also do), censoring can actually be seen as a further event type also competing with the other ones [62]. So, the individual are subject to different event types, amongst which the event "is lost to follow-up as first event" or "reaches the end of the study as first event". However, via the assumption of independent censoring, the occurrence of this new type of event will indeed prevent us from observing an other event type but we assume that it does not modify the risk of occurrence of the other event types. Also, in this particular context, since censoring is only related to data collection, it indeed makes sense to be consider an hypothetical world in which such censoring would not occur (which is fact the real world). A "classical" analysis with administrative censoring for patients free of event at the end of the study, could be considered as a marginal analysis of the event of interest (e.g. time to death) with reaching the end of the study as a competing risk. In such a case, it is common to assume administrative censoring as independent and the usual analysis such as the Kaplan-Meier estimates actually estimate correctly the marginal survival (as would be observed in a world where patients would not be censored when reaching the end of the study). This is obviously not the case anymore once censoring is not dependent. The fact that the naive approach to competing risk will lead to unbiased estimate of the marginal risk of event if the competing events are independent is a direct parallel to the fact that the Kaplan-Meier estimator provides an unbiased estimate of the survival curves in the case of independent censoring.

Note that, instead of considering the "usual" right-censoring as a special case of competing risk, we can take the opposite point of view and consider competing event as a special type of right-censoring that would, in most applications, not be non-informative.

5.3 Estimation

Once the type of analysis is identified based on the research question, the analysis of competing risks data usually follows the same flow as classical survival analysis, starting with (non-parametric) estimation of the cause-specific cumulative incidence functions, followed by comparisons of these CIFS and then modeling to investigate the impact of covariates on the outcome.

The overall cumulative incidence function (CIF), so combining all events into one which is equivalent to consider the time to the first event, can be obtained according to the methods presented in Chapter 2, and in particular using the Kaplan-Meier estimate:

$$\hat{F}^{KM} = 1 - \hat{S}^{KM} = 1 - \prod_{j:y_{(j)} \leq t} \left\{ 1 - \frac{d_{(j)}}{R(y_{(j)})} \right\}$$

where the $y_{(j)}, j = 1, ..., r$ are the r distinct observed event type (considering as event the first event, whatever its type), $R(y_{(j)})$ is the number of individ-

	Combined analysis or time to first event	Marginal analysis	Competing risk analysis
Idea:	Ignore that we have different event types and combine them all onto a single event → interest in a composite endpoint	Focus on one event type of interest. Aim to quantify the risk of this event if the competing events would not exist → mainly for etiology: which factors directly impact the risk of the event of interest	Aim to quantify the risk of each event type in the presence of the other (competing) events → mainly for prediction: which factors impact (directly or indirectly) the occurence of an event
Quantity of interest:	↪ Overall survival function $S(t)$ and cdf $F(t) = 1 - S(t)$ ↪ Hazard function $h(t)$ with $S(t) = \exp\left(-\int h(u)du\right)$	↪ Marginal cumulative incidence function ↪ Marginal hazard function ("net" risk of the event of interest)	↪ Cause-specific CIF or subdistribution function $F_k(t)$ ↪ Subdistribution hazard $h_k(t)$ with $S_k(t) = 1 - F_k(t) = \exp\left(-\int h_k(u)du\right)$ ↪ Cause-specific hazard $\lambda_k(t)$ with $F_k(t) = -\int S(u)\lambda_k(u)du$
Methods:	Left with a single event, same methods as in Chapter 2	Naive method (censor other event types), same methods as in Chapter 2 ATTENTION: require independence of the event types to obtain unbiased estimates	Aalen-Johanssen estimator of the CIF, cause-specific hazard logrank and PH model, Gray test and Fine and Gray model for subdistribution hazard

TABLE 5.5
Global overview of the different approaches for dealing with competing risks

ual still at risk at time $y_{(j)}$ (so not having experienced any and not being censored), and $d_{(j)}$ is the number of (first) event (of any type) at time $y_{(j)}$.

To illustrate this, we can use the data of Table 5.1 and compute the estimator of the cumulative incidence function for the time to the first event. The computations are detailed in Table 5.6. The estimated CIF is actually the one displayed as a solid gray line on the right panel of Figure 5.3. This gives us information about the time to the first event, which in some case bring some important information (e.g., progression free survival in oncology trial is often considered as a meaningful endpoint) but not really in this particular situation.

We can also obtain via standard survival analysis technique an estimate of the cumulative incidence function and of the hazard function for each event type while censoring the patients who experienced an event of a different type before. However, these estimates will be unbiased estimator of the marginal cumulative incidence and the marginal hazard only if we can assume that the censoring due to competing risk is non-informative. When this assumption is in doubt, these estimators must be interpreted with great cautious. One should be very careful that such a "naive" approach have been used for a long time without acknowledging the assumption of independent event types processes.

The cause-specific hazard $\lambda_k(t)$, and the functions of it, is actually the principal estimable quantity in a competing risk analysis. The most natural estimator for this cause-specific hazard is an empirical non-parametric estimator obtained simply by considering at each event time the proportion of event of type k amongst the individuals still at risk.

$$\hat{\lambda}_k(y_{(j)}) = \frac{d_k(y_{(j)})}{R(y_{(j)})} \tag{5.10}$$

where $d_k(t_{(j)})$ is the number of event of type k at time $t_{(j)}$. It is important here to point out that $R(y_{(j)})$ is the size of the "classical" risk set $\mathfrak{R}(y_{(i)})$ defined in Chapter 2 and which includes all individuals "who are observed to be at risk", i.e. who have not experienced any event and have not been censored.

An estimator of the cause-specific cumulative incidence function for each event type can be built based on a discrete version of formula (5.8), since in practice the number of observed event times is finite:

$$F_k(t) = P(T \le t, E = k) = \sum_{t_{(j)} \le t} S(t_{(j)}-)\lambda_k(t_{(j)}) \tag{5.11}$$

such that the probability of experiencing an event of type k by time t is the sum over all observed event times up to time t of the probability of surviving all events up to then and experiencing such an event at that time. The Nelson-Aalen estimator of the cause-specific cumulative incidence function is then obtained by replacing in this expression the overall survival function $S(.)$ by its Kaplan-Meier estimator and the cause-specific hazard $\lambda_k(.)$ by its empirical non-parametric estimator (5.10). Based on (5.7), we find back that

$$\sum_{k=1}^{K} \hat{\lambda}_k(y_{(j)}) = \frac{\sum_{k=1}^{K} d_k(y_{(j)})}{R(y_{(j)})} = \frac{d(y_{(j)})}{R(y_{(j)})} = \hat{h}(y_{(j)})$$

From (5.10), we can obtain an estimator of the cumulative cause-specific hasard function, often referred to as the Nelson-Aalen estimator

$$\hat{\Lambda}_k(t) = \sum_{y_{(j)} \leq t} \hat{\lambda}_k(y_{(j)})$$

We therefore obtain the following estimator of the cause-specific cumulative incidence function which is actually a special case of the non-parametric Aalen-Johansen estimator originally developed for transition probabilities in the context of multi-states models [2, 132]

$$\hat{F}_k^{AJ}(t) = \sum_{y_{(j)} \leq t} \hat{S}^{KM}(y_{(j)-}) \hat{\lambda}_k(y_{(j)}) \tag{5.12}$$

Note that in this expression $\hat{S}^{KM}(.)$ can be replaced by any other estimator of the overall survival function.

As we have already mentioned, we have to be careful, especially in the medical literature, that the naive estimator $1 - \hat{S}_k^{KM}(t)$ is still used instead of $\hat{F}_k(t)$ to estimate the cause-specific cumulative incidence function. However this naive estimator will generally overestimate $F_k(t)$ and would only provide a correct estimator of $F_k(t)$ under very strong (and usually unrealistic) conditions, i.e. under independence and in an hypothetical context where the competing event would have been eliminated [23, 130]. Note that the difference between the two estimators can be large, especially when there are a high proportion of individuals experiencing the competing events.

For the sake of illustration, Table 5.6 presents the computation of the cause-specific hazard functions and the cumulative incidence functions for the two event types in the example presented in Table 5.1. The results are the ones we have already discussed on Figure 5.3.

An interesting (although somewhat confusing) remark is that the estimated cause-specific hazard function (5.10) is actually the same as the one we would obtain from standard analysis technique while estimating the hazard function of event type k while censoring all the other event types (see equation (2.10) in Section 2.3.2) of Chapter 2. So, if we are in a situation where we can assume that the occurrence of the competing events is non-informative for the event of interest, the marginal hazard can actually be estimated by the estimated cause-specific hazard. On the other hand, if we can not make this non-informative assumption, then expression 5.10 do not properly estimate the marginal hazard anymore but remains a good estimator of the cause-specific

Time	HI	Di	$\hat{S}^{KM}$	$\hat{F}^{KM}$	$\frac{d_k(y_{(j)})}{R(y_{(j)})}$		$\hat{F}_k^{AJ}(t)=\sum_{y_{(j)}\le t}\hat{S}^{KM}(y_{(j)}-)\hat{\lambda}_k(y_{(j)})$	
			Any	Any	$k=HI$	$k=Di$	$k=HI$	$k=Di$
2	1	0	$(1-\frac{1}{20})=0.95$	0.05	$\frac{1}{20}$	$\frac{0}{20}$	$1\times\frac{1}{20}=0.05$	$1\times 0=0$
6	1	0	$0.95(1-\frac{3}{19})=0.80$	0.20	$\frac{3}{19}$	$\frac{0}{19}$	$0.05+0.95\times\frac{3}{19}=0.20$	$0+0.95\times 0=0$
6	1	0						
6	1	0						
8	0	1	$0.80(1-\frac{1}{16})=0.75$	0.25	$\frac{0}{16}$	$\frac{1}{16}$	$0.20+0.80\times 0=0.20$	$0+0.80\times\frac{1}{16}=0.05$
11	1	0	$0.75(1-\frac{1}{15})=0.70$	0.30	$\frac{1}{15}$	$\frac{0}{15}$	$0.20+0.75\times\frac{1}{15}=0.25$	$0.05+0.75\times 0=0.05$
12	1	0	$0.70(1-\frac{2}{14})=0.60$	0.40	$\frac{1}{14}$	$\frac{1}{14}$	$0.25+0.70\times\frac{1}{14}=0.30$	$0.05+0.70\times\frac{1}{14}=0.10$
12	0	1						
15	0	1	$0.60(1-\frac{1}{12})=0.55$	0.45	$\frac{0}{12}$	$\frac{1}{12}$	$0.30+0.60\times 0=0.30$	$0.10+0.60\times\frac{1}{12}=0.15$
17	0	1	$0.55(1-\frac{1}{11})=0.50$	0.50	$\frac{0}{11}$	$\frac{1}{11}$	$0.30+0.55\times 0=0.30$	$0.15+0.55\times\frac{1}{11}=0.20$
19	0	1	$0.50(1-\frac{1}{10})=0.45$	0.55	$\frac{0}{10}$	$\frac{1}{10}$	$0.30+0.50\times 0=0.30$	$0.20+0.50\times\frac{1}{10}=0.25$
20	1	0	$0.45(1-\frac{2}{9})=0.35$	0.65	$\frac{2}{9}$	$\frac{0}{9}$	$0.30+0.45\times\frac{2}{9}=0.40$	$0.25+0.45\times 0=25$
20	1	0						
21	0	1	$0.35(1-\frac{1}{7})=0.30$	0.70	$\frac{0}{7}$	$\frac{1}{7}$	$0.40+0.35\times 0=0.40$	$0.25+0.35\times\frac{1}{7}=0.30$
23	0	1	$0.30(1-\frac{2}{6})=0.20$	0.80	$\frac{1}{6}$	$\frac{1}{6}$	$0.40+0.30\times\frac{1}{6}=0.45$	$0.30+0.30\times\frac{1}{6}=0.35$
23	1	0						
27	1	0	$0.20(1-\frac{2}{4})=0.10$	0.90	$\frac{2}{4}$	$\frac{0}{4}$	$0.45+0.20\times\frac{2}{4}=0.55$	$0.35+0.20\times 0=0.35$
27	1	0						
28	1	0	$0.10(1-\frac{2}{2})=0$	1.00	$\frac{2}{2}$	$\frac{0}{2}$	$0.55+0.10\times\frac{2}{2}=0.65$	$0.35+0.10\times 0=0.35$
29	1	0						

TABLE 5.6

Competing risks – Example 1: Computation of the overall cumulative incidence function and the cumulative incidence functions for each event type based on the data of Table 5.1

hazard. As raised by [132], the key is that to interpret (5.10) as an estimate of the cause-specific hazard, we do not need to assume that the individuals who are removed from the risk set due to a competing event can be represented by the individuals who are still in the risk set.

We have seen that one can define two hazard functions, the cause-specific hazard function (which is closer from the concept of hazard but do not have a one-to-one relationship with the cause-specific incidence function) and the sub-distribution hazard. The estimation of this sub-distribution hazard is however more complex. The idea behind this sub-distribution hazard is to condition on the individuals who are either still in the risk set or that have already experience a competing event. So, an estimator of this sub-distribution hazard could be

$$\hat{h}_k(y_{(j)}) = \frac{d_k(y_{(j)})}{R^\star((y_{(j)})} \tag{5.13}$$

with $R^\star(t_{(i)})$ the number of individuals still in the extended risk set $\mathfrak{R}^\star(t_{(i)})$, i.e. individuals who did not experience an event of type k and who were not censored (for reason other than a competing event) before $y_{(j)}$. An individual who has experienced another type of event will remain in this extended risk set $\mathfrak{R}^\star(t_{(i)})$ until the time he would have been censored if he would not have experienced a competing event. This obviously raised a difficulty in the estimation of h_k since such an information is usually not available.

This could be done quite easily when the (potential) censoring time is known for everyone (e.g. in case of Type I censoring or administrative censoring), but this is often not the case. Then, we have to rely on an estimator of the censoring distribution. Two main approaches have been proposed to solve this issue. The first one consists in leaving all observations who experienced a competing event in the risk set but to assign them a weight that changes over time according to the estimated probability of remaining uncensored. Fine and Gray [122] proposed to use the inverse probability of censoring weighting (IPCW) technique. The general idea is that the contribution of the ith individual to the risk set at time $y_{(j)}$ for the estimation of the sub-distribution hazard of cause k is:

- one if this individual is still event-free and not censored before time $y_{(j)}$; this individual is therefore still in the "classical" risk set and fully contribute to the extended risk set;

- zero if this individual already experienced an event of type k before time $y_{(j)}$ or was already censored before time $y_{(j)}$; this individual is out of the extended risk set;

- unknown if the individual has experienced another event type at time $y_{(i)}$ before time $y_{(j)}$; the idea is that this individual should contribute to the extended risk set until the time he would be censored and a proposal is to consider as contribution:

$$\frac{1 - \hat{G}(y_{(j)}-)}{1 - \hat{G}(y_{(i)}-)} \tag{5.14}$$

with $\hat{G}(.)$ the estimated distribution function of the censoring process. These weights can actually be seen as a non-parametric estimator of the conditional distribution function of the censoring time given that censoring occur after $y_{(i)}$ (since we know that censoring has not occurred before otherwise the individual would be out of the risk set). As $(1-\hat{G}(.))$ is a decreasing function and $y_{(i)} < y_{(j)}$, we have that this weight is below 1 and decreases to zero when $y_{(j)}$ increases. The contribution of this individual therefore is one when $y_{(j)} = y_{(i)}$ (so if we would compute the risk set at the time of the competing event), and then decreases as further away $y_{(j)}$ is from the time $y_{(i)}$ at which the individual experienced the competing event to go down to zero as time goes by.

A drawback of this approach is the difficulty to implement it in standard software. A second approach, following the same idea but based on a multiple imputation procedure has therefore been proposed [340]. Rather than computing these weights, the proposal is to perform multiple imputation of the unknown censoring times based on random draws from the estimated conditional censoring distribution given that this censoring occur after the failure from the competing event.

Given the one-to-one relationship between this sub-distribution hazard and the CIF for a specific event type, we can use the estimator (5.13) to obtain another estimator of the CIF. Following the same argument as for the KM estimator, we can indeed obtain a product-limit estimator of the cause specific cumulative incidence function as:

$$
\begin{aligned}
\hat{F}_k^{PL}(t) &= 1 - \prod_{y_{(j)} \leq t} \left(1 - \hat{h}_k(y_{(j)})\right) \\
&= 1 - \prod_{y_{(j)} \leq t} \left(1 - \frac{d_k(y_{(j)})}{R^\star(y_{(j)})}\right) \tag{5.15}
\end{aligned}
$$

Comparing this expression with the one of the classical KM estimator (2.2), it appears clearly that since $R^\star(y_{(j)})$ will always be at least equal to $R(y_{(j)})$, the jumps of the 1-KM estimator will always be at least as big as the one from this estimator of the cause-specific cumulative incidence.

Rather than having to first estimate the sub-distribution hazard and then using it to get an estimate of the cumulative incidence function, another possibility is to directly estimate the cause-specific cumulative incidence based on the weighted frequency of observed events of the type of interest [133]. The resulting estimator will have a structure similar to the empirical cumulative distribution function (see Chapter 2) and is thus referred to as $\hat{F}_k^{ECDF}(t)$

$$\hat{F}_k^{ECDF}(t) = \frac{1}{n} \sum_{t_{(j)} < t} \frac{d_k(t_{(j)})}{\hat{G}(t_{(j)})} \qquad (5.16)$$

We therefore have presented three estimators for the cumulative incidence function for each event type, the Aalen-Johansen estimator (5.12), the product-limit estimator (5.15), and the empirical cumulative distribution function (5.16). However, with an appropriate choice of the weights used in the definition of the size of the extended risk set, these estimators are actually algebraically equivalent and will lead to the same results [132]. These weights consist in the weight we have mentioned above (5.14), in which the censoring distribution $G(.)$ is estimated with a Kaplan-Meier estimator while reversing the role of events and censorings. We refer the reader to [132] and the references therein for a detailed discussion on these estimators.

There exists two main approaches for the estimation of the variance of the estimator of the cause-specific cumulative incidence functions $\hat{F}_k(.)$, based on the variance of the estimator of either the cause specific-hazard or the sub-distribution hazard. Several variance estimators have been proposed based on the cause-specific hazards and the Aalen-Johansen estimator $\hat{F}_k^{AJ}(.)$, and the most common ones are reviewed and compared via simulation by [43]. They recommend the estimator developed independently by Gaynor et al. [130] and Betensky and Schoenfeld [39], although this estimator tends to be biased for small samples ($n < 50$). Another possibility is to estimate this variance based on the sub-distribution hazard and the product limit-estimator $\hat{F}_k^{PL}(.)$ in a similar way as to obtain the variance estimator of the Kaplan-Meier estimate of the survival function. We can define an Aalen type or a Greenwood type estimator of the variance of the cumulative sub-distribution hazard and use the delta method to obtain the variance of $\hat{F}_k^{PL}(.)$. We refer the reader to [132] for a detailed description of these estimators. From $v\hat{a}r(\hat{F}_k(.))$, we can use the same ideas as those from standard survival to obtain confidence interval for a given time-point, using for example a log or a $log - log$ transformation.

5.4 Hypotheses testing

There have been several proposals on how to compare groups of observations for the occurrence of events of a given type in the presence of competing events. Most of them are actually comparing the underlying hazard functions using some logrank-like test statistic. The two most popular tests in the context of competing risks are the logrank test on the cause-specific (cumulative) hazards [303] and the Gray test [145] on the sub-distribution hazards. This latter therefore comes back to a test on the cumulative incidence functions, given the one-to-one relationship between the two functions. Given that we don't have this one-to-one relationship between the cause-specific cumulative hazards and the cumulative incidence function, these two tests will usually not lead to the same results (although they may quite often lead to the same conclusion) and one has to decide a priori, based on the research question, which test we want to use given the quantity based on which we want to compare the groups.

A classical logrank test performed while censoring individuals who experience a competing event will be of use to test that the marginal hazards (or the marginal cumulative incidence functions) are similar. Such a test will however only be valid if we can assume that the censoring due to a competing event is uninformative [132].

For each given event type, k, a test for equality of the cause-specific hazards between two groups can be written:

$$\begin{cases} H_0 : \lambda_{k,1}(t) = \lambda_{k,2}(t) & \forall \, t \leq y_{(r)} \\ H_1 : \lambda_{k,1}(t) \neq \lambda_{k,2}(t) & \text{for some } t \leq y_{(r)} \end{cases}$$

and is in fact obtained by applying the classical logrank while censoring individual at the time they experience a competing event. Indeed, remember that the test statistics of the logrank is actually obtained from a collection of 2×2 contingency table built at each event time, comparing the observed failure to the expected ones amongst the individuals still at risk (see Section 2.4 of Chapter 2). Therefore, removing patients from the risk sets because they experience a competing risk of because they are censored will have the same effect on the computation of the logrank test statistic. This can also be deduced from the fact that the non-parametric estimator of the cause-specific hazard is the classical non-parametric hazard estimator. So, this logrank test performed by censoring the individuals who experience a competing events will in general not be a valid test for the comparison of the marginal hazard (unless we can assume independence) but will however be valid to compare the cause-specific hazards.

While this test for cause-specific hazards is equivalent to a logrank test and is therefore easy to compute and can be obtained from any software performing standard survival analysis, it does not have the same interpretation as a classical logrank test and one has to be cautious with how to interpret the results. In particular, one has to keep in mind that there is no one-to-one relationship between the cause-specific hazard and the cause-specific cumulative incidence function and this test is therefore not a test of equality of the cause-specific cumulative incidence function. In particular, one has to be particularly careful when interpreting this test in a situation where the different types of failure are interdependent and/or if the occurrence of the competing events is more likely to occur in one group than in the other. Indeed, for this test to have an easy interpretation, one often actually considers that $\lambda_{k',1}(t) = \lambda_{k',2}(t)$ for $k' \neq k$ such that a difference in the cumulative incidence functions is indeed due to an effect on event type k and not from an indirect effect on another event type. We also have to be careful with the impact of the competing events frequency on the power of the logrank test for a given event type, since this power will depend on the number of observed event of type k.

Another possibility is to directly compare the two groups in terms of their cumulative incidence functions for the event of interest, say for cause k

$$\begin{cases} H_0 : F_{k,1}(t) = F_{k,2}(t) & \forall\, t \le y_{(r)} \\ H_1 : F_{k,1}(t) \ne F_{k,2}(t) & \text{for some } t \le y_{(r)} \end{cases}$$

The Gray test actually compares the CIFs by comparing the underlying sub-distribution hazards [122, 145]

$$\begin{cases} H_0 : h_{k,1}(t) = h_{k,2}(t) & \forall\, t \le y_{(r)} \\ H_1 : h_{k,1}(t) \ne h_{k,2}(t) & \text{for some } t \le y_{(r)} \end{cases}$$

The test statistic of the Gray test for the comparison of two groups is similar to the U test statistic (2.12) seen in Section 2.12 of Chapter 2 except that we have to modify the definition of the risk set

$$U^\star = \sum_{j=1}^{r} \omega(y_{(j)}) \left(d_{kj}^{(1)} - \frac{d_{kj} R_\star^{(1)}(y_{(j)})}{R_\star^{(.)}(y_{(j)})} \right) \tag{5.17}$$

where $d_{kj}^{(1)}$ is the observed number of events of type k in group 1 at time $y_{(j)}$, d_{kj} is the total observed number of events of type k at time $y_{(j)}$ in both groups, $R_\star^{(.)}(y_{(j)}) = R_\star^{(1)}(y_{(j)}) + R_\star^{(2)}(y_{(j)})$ and

$$R_\star^{(g)}(y_{(j)}) = R^{(g)}(y_{(j)}) \frac{1 - \hat{F}_k^{AJ(g)}(y_{(j)-})}{\hat{S}^{KM(g)}(y_{(j)-})} \qquad g = 1,2$$

with $R^{(g)}(y_{(j)})$ the observed number of individuals at risk at time $y_{(j)}$ in group g. The superscript (g) indicates that the corresponding quantity only pertains to group (g). This expression can be re-written as a weighted difference between the group specific estimates of the subdistribution hazards (see [132] for example).

The usual Gray test is obtained for the weight $\omega(t) = 1\ \forall t$. When there is no censoring, the Gray test is equivalent to the logrank test performed on the artificial variable $\tilde{T}$ defined previously ($\tilde{T} = T$ if $E = k$ and ∞ otherwise) [102]. Several options have been proposed to compute the variance of the Gray test statistics [132, 145, 189]. Other tests have been developed for comparing cumulative incidence functions, see for example [199, 226, 229, 294], there are however less often used than the Gray test.

Several simulations studies comparing the performance of the logrank test on the cause-specific hazards and the Gray test on the sub-distribution hazards in various settings have been published [22, 102, 126, 409]. These simulations have studied in particular the impact of the repartition of the competing events and of the correlation between the event of interest and a competing ones on the performance of these tests. Note that in the presence of such a correlation, both tests above may be somehow impacted. Dignam et al. [102] concluded that the logrank test correctly detects differences in cause-specific hazards and is largely unaffected by differences between the two groups in the hazard of the competing events (unless strong dependence). Also, the Gray test correctly detects whether there is the difference between the two groups for a given event, whatever this difference is due to a real difference in the (true) hazards event of interest or due to a difference in the (true) hazards of the competing events. Coming back to our illustrative example, we might have difference in in-hospital infections between two groups of patients (e.g. patients hospitalized in two different hospital wards) either because of a true difference in that endpoint (e.g. because of more hygienic conditions in one of the ward) or simply because patients are discharged earlier in one of the two wards (thus increasing the competing event).

A crucial issue is the power of these tests, which as an in classical survival analysis is linked to the number of events. When designing an experiment for a cause-specific outcome, it is crucial to both decide a priori on the test be used, considering either the difference in the cause-specific hazards (logrank) or the sub-distribution hazards (Gray test), but also to carefully think of the impact of the competing events (in reducing the number of observed events) on the power and type I error of these tests [22, 215].

5.5 Modeling

For "classical survival" analysis with a single endpoint of interest or a "time to the first event" approach of competing risk data, Chapter 2 presents several modeling strategies of which the most popular is certainly the Cox PH model. While this model is built at the level of the hazard function, one can use the one-to-one relationship between this hazard and the survival function to obtain information on the impact of the covariates on the survival function. In the context of competing risks, we have seen that we don't have this one-to-one relationship and an additional challenges is therefore on the choice of the hazard function on which the impact of the covariates will be modeled.

5.5.1 Proportional cause-specific hazards model

A first possible option is to apply a classical survival model, such as the Cox PH model, on one type of event, while censoring the patients experiencing a competing event [97, 260, 311]. For example, if we consider only two types of event such as in-hospital infection (event of interest) and discharge from the hospital (competing risk), the idea is that we can then get the HR quantifying the impact of a variable X, e.g. gender or type of hospital-ward, on in-hospital infection while censoring the patients discharged from the hospital without having had an infection. One can also obtain a second HR for the same variable X by doing the opposite, i.e. considering time to discharge from the hospital while censoring patients who get an in-hospital infection.

This actually corresponds to modeling the impact of the covariates on the cause-specific hazards, and for event type k and a covariate vector $\mathbf{X}$ such a model can be written

$$\lambda_k(t \mid \mathbf{X}_i = \mathbf{x}_i) = \lambda_{k,0}(t) \exp(\beta_k^t \mathbf{x}_i) \tag{5.18}$$

with $\lambda_k(t \mid \mathbf{X}_i = \mathbf{x}_i)$ the cause-specific hazard for event type k for a subject with covariate vector $\mathbf{x}_i$, $\lambda_{k,0}(t)$ the baseline cause-specific hazard for event type k, and $\beta_k = (\beta_{k1}, ...\beta_{kp})$ the p-vector of parameters associated with the vector $\mathbf{X}$. It is therefore important to realize that everything refers to the specific type of event k considered, in particular the parameters β_k quantify the effect of the covariates $\mathbf{X}_i$ on the time-to-event of type k.

Based on the definition of the cause-specific hazard, the individuals who experienced a competing event before the event of interest (k) leave the risk set. Such an analysis can thus be performed via a standard Cox PH model while censoring patients with a competing events. The estimation procedure is exactly the same as for classical survival analysis with one type of events (see Chapter 2) and do not require the independence of the failure times for the different types of event [181, 212].

However, we need, once again to be very careful with the interpretation of the results, taking into account that model 5.18 quantifies the impact of the covariates on the cause-specific hazards. When there is dependence between the different event types, the covariates effets may in fact reflect the influence of the competing event types, and this may lead to some counter-intuitive results. In our example of Section 5.1, acting on the length of in-hospital way with a measure in no way linked to hygiene nor even to the health status of the patient may lead to a reduction of in-hospital infection by shortening to time to discharge or the time to in-hospital death!

As already discussed, this is not equivalent to a marginal analysis, and the β_k can be interpreted as the impact of the covariates on the marginal hazard only if the censoring due to the competing risks is non-informative, i.e. if the different event types are independent. In that case, the results can be interpreted as the impact of the covariates on the hazard of event of type k in an hypothetical world where the other competing events do not exist. However, as already mentioned this independence assumption is often highly suspect and can not be tested from the observed data. It will then be unclear whether the estimated HRs are indeed unbiased estimators of the real (but unobservable) marginal HR. In the case where we don't have independence between the event types, such an approach may lead to odds results and one can even construct a situation when one has an opposite effect of a covariate on the marginal and on the cause-specific hazard. However, if we have about the same amount of censoring due to the competing events in each group, then the relative cause-specific hazards should be comparable to the relative marginal hazards, even though these hazards may differ in absolute value [132].

So, the Cox model can be readily applied to the cause-specific hazard but one has to keep in mind that the results do not pertain to the cumulative incidence of event of a given type. In order to have this point clear, and to misinterpretation, it is advised to refer to model 5.18 as a *proportional cause-specific hazards model* and not a Cox PH model, even though the model is similar in form and the estimation procedure is the same [122, 130, 132].

A simple procedure is to fit a separate model for each event type, using a standard Cox PH procedure while censoring the subjects experiencing a competing event. However, it is also possible to fit simultaneously the cause-specific hazard models for each event type through a data augmentation method [15, 17, 23, 132, 240, 260, 311]. The idea is to first reshape the dataset in a long format, with one line per event type per subject (so K lines per subject), one failure indicator for each event type and creating event type specific covariates (see for example [260] for more practical details). We can then either (i) stratify for the event type (which will lead to identical results to those obtained by fitting each model separately) or (ii) include the event type as a covariate. This latter option assumes proportional baseline hazards between the different event types which may be useful if we want to quantify relative hazards for the different event types by a single summary measure.

As shown in Section 5.6, such an analysis allows to compare and even formally test the equality of the effect of the covariates on the different types of events. Using the corresponding type-specific covariates, one can indeed estimate simultaneously the effect of the covariates on each event type. By further including an interaction term between the type-specific covariates and the event types, one can test whether the covariate effect is indeed the same (so null hypothesis of no interaction term) for the different event types. Rather than including an interaction, another possibility is to create a "compound" variable that will combine the information from the covariate of interest and the endpoint, see Section 5.6. However, a question arises in such a combined analysis with regards to the calculation of the standard errors, since the same observations are replicated to obtained the estimates of the various parameters. Therefore, a robust sandwich-type estimator have been proposed [240]. This will lead to different standard errors and p-values than those obtained in separate analyzes, although the differences will be small [132].

Such a combined analysis offer several advantages. As mentioned above, it allows to test whether the effect of a covariate differs for the different event types. By appropriately defining our model and the different contrasts, one may also force the effect of a covariate to be the same for different event types or to affect only some of the event types. This may be useful for parsimony, for example in situation where one of the event types is actually rare. However, when performing such a combined analysis, one needs to be very careful in the definition of the contrasts as they will determine the interpretation of the parameters.

We have absolutely have to keep in mind that all the estimated parameters from a proportional cause-specific hazards model pertains to the cause-specific hazards, and do not translate directly to an effect on the risk of each event. They can only be interpreted as a quantification of the impact of the covariates on the marginal hazard in case we have independence between the event types and such an analysis do not take into account the presence of competing risks. Also, the results observed at the level of the cause-specific hazards are on an *instantaneous* scale and can not be directly translated to an effect on a *cumulative* scale since there is no one to one relationship between the cause-specific hazards and the cumulative incidence function. While the prediction of the cumulative incidence function from the cause-specific regression hazard model could be achieved from the Aalen-Johassen form of the cause-specific cumulative incidence (5.12) by estimating the cause-specific hazard of each type of events, the variance estimation is much more complex [68].

5.5.2 Fine and Gray model

Models based on the cause-specific hazard can thus not be used to quantify the overall benefit or harm of a covariate to the subjects under study and modeling the the cumulative incidence functions maybe more relevant to clinical practice [23].

To address this issue, and being able to quantify the impact of the covariates directly on the cumulative incidence functions, Fine and Gray [122] proposed to model the impact of the covariates on the sub-distribution hazards. They propose a semi-parametric model which is actually very similar in form to the Cox PH model and can be written:

$$h_k(t \mid \mathbf{X}_i = \mathbf{x}_i) = h_{k,0}(t) \exp(\gamma_k^t \mathbf{x}_i) \tag{5.19}$$

with $h_k(t \mid \mathbf{X}_i = \mathbf{x}_i)$ the sub-distribution hazard for event type k for a subject with covariates value $\mathbf{x}_i$, $h_{k,0}(t)$ the baseline sub-distribution hazard for event type k, and $\gamma k = (\gamma_{k1}, ... \gamma_{kp})$ the p-vector of parameters associated with the vector $\mathbf{X}$.

This model is often referred to as the *Fine and Gray model* or the *competing risks PH model* and inherit his popularity from the one-to-one relationship between the sub-distribution hazard and the cause-specific cumulative incidence. The impact of the covariates are therefore quantified in a "real" world by accounting for the competing events. Furthermore, we can restrict the analysis to a single type of event. However, this does not prevent us from being careful when interpreting the estimates of the regression coefficients. Indeed, we have to keep in mind that the occurrence of an of event type k is impacted by its own baseline risk, the effect of the covariates on this baseline risk but also by the baseline risk and the covariate effects on the competing events.

For example, imagine that we consider the impact of the type of pathology on the occurrence of in-hospital infection. Patients suffering from a disease affecting their immune system will most probably be at higher risk of in-hospital infection. On the other hand, these patients might also have (on average) more serious illness and thus be discharged later which will put them at even higher risk of in-hospital infection. So while impact of this covariate on the sub-distribution hazard of in-hospital infection (increasing the risk for patients with disease linked to their immune system) will translate into an impact of this covariate on the cumulative incidence function of in-hospital infection (and thus the number of cases of in-hospital infections), the estimated coefficient in fact also account for the (indirect) effect of this covariate on time to hospital discharge. Such a model is therefore useful to investigate the impact of a covariate on the number of cases it provides little information about the etiology of in-hospital infection.

A major disadvantage however is that estimation is obviously more complex as we can not directly use the Cox PH estimation procedure. The idea is however to adapt the Cox PH estimation procedure, i.e. maximization of the partial likelihood, while adapting the definition of the risk set to be in accordance with the definition of the sub-distribution hazard. Estimation of the γ coefficients could indeed be based on maximizing a partial likelihood of the form [23, 132]

$$L_{partial}^{FG}(\gamma_k) = \prod_{i=1}^{n} \left(\frac{\exp(\gamma_k^t \mathbf{x}_i)}{\sum_{j \in \mathfrak{R}^\star(y_i)} \exp(\gamma_k^t \mathbf{x}_j)} \right)^{\delta_i I(E=k)=1} \tag{5.20}$$

where the risk set $\mathfrak{R}^\star(y_i)$ includes all subjects who did not fail of cause k and who were not censored before y_i. this expression has the same form as the partial likelihood (2.21) of a classical Cox PH model (see Chapter 2). However we have to take into account that individuals who have actually experienced a competing event in fact leaves this risk set at the time they were supposed to be censored if they would not have experienced this competing event. The parameter estimates for model 5.19 will therefore depend on the right censoring mechanism and we are back to the same issue as for the non-parametric estimation of the cumulative incidence function. As mentioned there, the (hypothetical) censoring time for individuals who failed from a competing event may be known in the case of type I right censoring or in case of administrative censoring at the end of the study. The idea is then for these individuals to replace their event time by the time until the administrative censoring (i.e. the end of the study) and then to treat them as censored (which is clearly different from censoring them at the type they experience an event from another type). One can then fit a standard Cox PH model on the resulting data and obtain parameters estimates for the γ's.

However, things are more complex when we face a more general censoring scheme, and in particular random censoring since in that case we don't know when a subject having experienced a competing event should leave the risk set.

This will for example occurs when, in addition to the administrative censoring at the end of a clinical study, we expect patients to drop out and to be lost-to-follow up in the course of the study. Several approaches have been proposed to handle this case following the same ideas as in Section 5.3. In their seminal paper on the Fine and Gray model, they propose to use inverse probability censoring weights (IPCW) [122]. The idea is to rewrite the likelihood (5.20) as

$$\tilde{L}_{partial}^{FG}(\gamma_k) = \prod_{i=1}^{n} \left(\frac{\exp(\gamma_k^t \mathbf{x}_i)}{\sum_{j \in \tilde{\mathfrak{R}}_i^\star} \omega_{ij} \exp(\gamma_k^t \mathbf{x}_j)} \right)^{\delta_i I(E=k)=1} \tag{5.21}$$

where the risk set $\tilde{\mathfrak{R}}_i^\star$ is the same as $\mathfrak{R}_i^\star$ above except that subjects who experienced a competing event remain in this risk set and it is now the weight ω_{ij} which reduce the influence of these subjects over time according to the censoring distribution. The same weights as those discussed in Section 5.3 can be used. An extension consists in adjusting the weights for the variables included in the model by adjusting the estimation of $G(.)$ for these covariates for example via a Cox PH model. The regression coefficients γ_k can then be estimated by maximizing $\tilde{L}_{partial}^{FG}(\gamma_k)$ and a sandwich variance-covariance matrix of the estimators can be obtained (when weights do not depend on covariates). The alternative approach based on multiple imputations of the censoring time for the individuals who failed from a competing event is also possible in this context with the possibility to extend this to stratified or clustered analysis in a rather straightforward way [340]. The third approach based on a weighted product-limit estimator is also applicable but it requires to fit a survival model with time-dependent weights [132, 133].

Given that the fit of a Fine and Gray model is obviously much simpler under administrative censoring, Bakoyannis and Touloumi [23] have explore via simulations the effect of assuming administrative censoring only (and thus keeping in the risk set all all individuals who failed from another event type under the date of administrative censoring) when in fact a more general censoring at random mechanism is operating. They compare the results with those obtained with the IPCW methods proposed by [122] to handle random censoring. Their conclusions actually depend not only on the censoring distribution, but also on the total duration of the study (and thus the time at which the administrative censoring takes place) and the fraction of competing events (obviously the lower the frequency of competing events, the less this is really an issue). In their simulation setting, they concluded that bias in the covariate effect remain generally relatively small with largest bias however in case of high censoring, long study duration, larger incidence of the competing event and strong and opposite covariate effect on the competing event.

The Fine and Gray model directly quantifies the impact of a covariate on the cumulative incidence function, while taking the other competing events into account. So, in a situation where we are only interested in one specific type of event, we can restrict our modeling to this specific event of interest.

This is obviously a major difference with the modeling of the cause-specific hazard. However, if we are interested in fitting a Fine and Gray model for the different types of event, we can also perform the different analysis at the same time using the same stacked dataset as described for the proportional cause-specific hazards model.

5.5.3   Choice of model

The choice between a proportional cause-specific hazards model and a Fine and Gray model should be based on the research question. We have to keep in mind that since we actually quantify the effect of the covariates on different scales, i.e. the (instantaneous) risk of a specific event or the cumulative probability (incidence) of that event, these can lead to different results for the same data. Both approaches can be correct depending on the objectives, and by interpreting the results appropriately one may actually put in light different aspect of the covariates effects.

When estimating the covariates effects for a given event type with a Cox PH model on the cause-specific hazards, the individuals failing from another event types are removed from the risk set, and thus treated essentially as censored observations. So, in theory, the covariates effects in a proportional cause-specific hazards model only pertains to the event of interest, without considering how the covariates act on the competing events. However, one has to be very careful that the extent to which the estimated covariate effects depict the impact of the covariates solely on the marginal risk of the event of interest actually depends on the independence assumption between the event types. This have been illustrated in different simulations studies, and in particular by Dignam et al. [103]. As expected, their results showed that when generating failure times for two event types from a bivariate distribution while setting the correlation between the failure times to zero, the cause-specific hazard estimated from the available competing risks data (i.e. the time to the first event and the type of this first event) indeed provides valid estimate of the marginal hazard specific to each event time. Fitting a Cox PH model on this cause-specific hazard provides the marginal hazards ratio, which is not influenced by the effect of the covariates on the competing events. Considering in their simulations a positive correlation of 0.6 between the failure times of the two event types, they further show that under moderate dependence, this model still tends to reflect the influence of the covariate on a specific event types, regardless of the competing events. This obviously become less true when considering higher correlation. Unfortunately, we usually have no real information on such a correlation. Indeed, this would require having information on the time to the different event types, and would further require that the context remains the same despite the occurrence of the first event, for example no change in treatment after the occurrence of a loco-regional recurrence, which is clearly rarely the case. Given that these models attempts to recover the "true" or "net" effect on the event of interest, they may be preferred for establishing a treatment or a prognostic biomarker effect on the outcome of interest. However, one has to be careful that they rarely provide the full picture, and can in some cases be misleading, especially if we expect high correlation between the failure times for the different event types [103].

As mentioned previously, modeling the impact of the covariates on the sub-distribution hazards is (qualitatively) equivalent to modeling this impact on the cumulative incidence function. Such a model will therefore identify the impact of a covariate on the event of interest while also reflecting the presence of competing risks. This obviously has to be taken into account when interpreting the hazards ratio resulting from such a model. For example, if we generate data from a setting where a binary covariate X has an effect only on the failure times for the competing event $(k = 2)$ and not for the event of interest $(k = 1)$, the covariate effect as estimated from such a model for the event of interest $(k = 1)$ will also show some effect. Indeed, if such a covariate X increases the rate of the competing events let's say the individuals with $X = 1$, than the individuals with $X = 1$ will somehow be at less risk of the event of interest. Therefore, even if the covariate X has no effect on the event of interest, the estimated coefficient for this covariate will show the indirect effect of the competing event. One therefore always has to be careful when interpreting the HR estimated from a model on the sub-distribution hazards since it may reflects either the direct effect of the covariate on the event of interest (e.g. older age increases the risk of in-hospital mortality because older patients have a weaker immune system), or an indirect effect on the competing event (e.g. older age increases the risk of in-hospital mortality because older patients tends to stay longer in the hospital and thus older age decreases the risk of the competing event of hospital discharge), or a combination of both. An issue pointed out by Dignam et al. [103] in their simulation study is that when a covariate effect is actually "shared" amongst the competing events, it may happen that none of these effects achieve significance when estimated from a model on the sub-distribution hazards. These models, which take into account the presence of competing risks, will be particularly useful when the objective is to predict the number of incident cases, as is for example often required for heath economic evaluation. Indeed, in such a context, one does not need to consider events (e.g. in-hospital infections) which are actually hindered by the occurrence of a competing event (e.g. discharge from the hospital).

Another important issue is the impact of censoring. Indeed in the presence of censoring the assertion that decreasing the occurrence of one type of events will necessarily increase the occurrence of events of another type will not necessarily be true. While the estimates from the Cox PH model on the cause-specific hazards are not influenced by censoring (unless dependence between the event times), the proportion of censored observations can influence the estimates obtained from the Fine and Gray model on the sub-distribution hazard. This could be an issue for example when analyzing long-term outcome (e.g. occurrence of late side effect or cause-specific death) after a successful treatment, as we could then fear a high percentage of censored observations.

Despite the covariate effect in each of these two models can be very different, and even reverse in some cases, several authors have shown that, as long as there is not a strong effect of the covariate on the competing events, the two models are however in general in good agreement [103, 213, 431].

Finally, we should also consider whether the model considered indeed fit the data appropriately. Although it is regularly advised to consider both a cause-specific hazard model and an Fine and Gray model to have a better understanding of the data at hand, the proportional hazards assumption (either at the level of the cause-specific hazard or at the level of the sub-distribution hazard) can in fact not be simultaneously satisfied for both types of models. But several simulations studies have shown a good robustness of these models, and have concluded that hazard ratios from these models will generally provide a reasonably informative summary measure of the covariates effects [41, 142, 213]. Indeed, even when the model are misspecified, we can still, in general, interpret the resulting hazard ratios from both models as time-average hazard ratios.

5.6 Software and examples revisited

As we have seen above, in the presence of competing risk data, the cause-specific hazard ad the cumulative incidence function, together with the hypotheses tests and modeling pertaining to it, actually reveals different aspects of the event histories. It is therefore to be expected that inference on these quantities may lead different results and the choice of the methods to use should, as often the case, be driven by the research questions of interest and certainly not by the results observed. Of course when the competing events are infrequent, such a choice will have less impact. However, it remains important to rely on the correct analysis given the research question.

Since the situations with more than one event type may be complex, it is often advise to add to the results a picture of the cumulative incidence curves. This will indeed provide some further insight into the data. This is particularly true when the competing events are frequent relative to the event of interest or when there is an impact of the covariates on these competing events. These cumulative incidence functions for each event types will be of particular interest when assessing for example treatment or health policy as in that case we are particularly interested in the absolute magnitude of the intervention over time. Displaying the cause-specific cumulative incidence curves will provide a clear information on the estimated probability of actually observing an events of a given type in the presence of competing events. We will for example be interested in the probability to get an in-hospital infection knowing we may be discharged before or to experience long-term adverse effect of a cancer treatment knowing that we may also die of old age before. A common way to display the cause-specific cumulative incidence curves for the different event types is to used a *stacked plot* as we will illustrate below.

When fitting a Cox PH model on the cause-specific hazards of event type k, the exponential of the pth coefficient $\exp(\gamma_{pk})$ can be interpreted as the *cause-specific hazards ratio* for covariate X_p and event type k. On the other hand, if we fit a Fine and Gray model for the same event type k, we assume proportionality at the level of the sub-distribution hazards, and the the exponential of the pth coefficient $\exp(\beta_{pk})$ then corresponds to a sub-distribution hazards ratio. It is important to realize that there is no reason for γ_k to be equal or even close to β_k while it can of course be the case in practice [40]. As mentioned earlier, to have an impact on the the cumulative incidence function of event type k (let's say the event of interest), a covariate may have a direct effect on this cause k or an effect on the competing events. We can think of a covariate which would have an effect on shortening the time to discharge from the hospital, and thus lowering the risk of in-hospital infection while actually not being physiologically linked to the occurrence of infection.

The cause-specific proportional hazards model is actually a Cox PH model, treating individuals with a competing event as censored at the time they experience this competing events and can therefore be fitted within any software allowing for standard survival analysis, see Section 2.6.1 of Chapter 2. The "combined analysis" mentioned in Section 5.5 and allowing to fit simultaneously such a model for each event type requires the creation of a *stacked dataset*. This can be done with any of the two functions crprep and msprep from the mstate R package [98, 310]. The crprep further computes a weighted dataset to be used for estimating the sub-distribution hazards. The event type specific covariates can either be created via the expand.covs function of the same package of by hand which is sometimes easier.

The two main R packages for competing risks analysis are the cmprsk [144] and the mstate [98, 310] package, this later being actually more general as it also allows to fit Multistate models [132]. In the cmprsk package [144], the cuminc and crr functions allows to respectively estimate the cause-specific cumulative incidence function and to fit a Fine and Gray model under random right censoring. In mstate, the equivalent function to estimate a cumulative incidence function is the Cuminc function (with a capital C). On the other hand, the Fine and Gray model is fitted via the usual coxph function from the survival package but after having "prepared" the data with the crprep function.

Note that the cause-specific proportional hazards model, as well as the Fine and Gray model under (known) administrative censoring can be fitted using any software capable of fitting a Cox PH model. The kmi R package [5] for multiple imputations can also be combined with a classical function to fit a Cox PH model (e.g. coxph) to fit a Fine and Gray model in a general random right censoring case with the multiple imputation approach of [6, 340].

Both the cause-specific hazard model and the Fine and Gray model can be fitted in SAS using the phreg procedure [355]. The SAS macro CumInc and CumIncV can be used to obtain cause-specific cumulative incidence curves from the estimates of proportional cause-specific hazard models [336]. The SAS macro CIF [230] provides a non-parametric estimation of the cumulative incidence functions and performs a Gray test for group comparisons.

The Stata software also have commands to estimate cumulative incidence (stcompet, stpm2cif) and fit a Fine and Gray model under random right censoring (sterreh, stcrreg). The sturve plots the cause-specific cumulative incidence function for a given combination of covariable values

5.6.1   Advanced ovarian cancer data

The advanced ovarian cancer dataset introduced in Section 1.3.6 of Chapter 1 contains information on progression free survival (PFS) and overall survival (OS) for 1192 patients randomized between a cyclophosphamide plus cisplatin (CP) arm and a cyclophosphamide plus adriamycin plus cisplatin (SAP) arm. This dataset can be accessed after having load the survival R package.

For the ease of the presentation, we first transform the timescale from years to months, such that the variable timeMonthsS and timeMonthsT now represent respectively the PFS and the OS time in months.

```
timeMonthsT <- timeT*12
timeMonthsS <- timeS*12
```

The PFS as well as the OS Kaplan-Meier estimated curves by treatment group can be obtained from the following code:

```
Ovarian.km.pfs.trt <- survfit(Surv(timeMonthsS, statusS)~trt)
plot(Ovarian.km.pfs.trt, lty=c(1,2),ylab="PFS probability",xlab="
    Time in months")
title("Progression-free survival in ovarian cancer patients by
    treatment group")
legend("topright",lty=c(1,2),c("CP","CAP"))
```

for PFS and

```
Ovarian.km.os.trt <- survfit(Surv(timeMonthsT, statusT)~trt, conf
    .type="log-log")
plot(Ovarian.km.os.trt, lty=c(1,2),ylab="OS probability",xlab="
    Time in months")
```

for OS. The median PFS and OS can be obtained from the Ovarian.km.pfs.trt and Ovarian.km.os.trt objects and are given in Table 5.7 while the estimated curves are displayed in Figure 5.5. The logrank test for the comparison of PFS between the two treatment group is obtained from survdiff(Surv(timeMonthsS, statusS) trt) and lead to a significant p-value (p-value = 0.001). A Cox PH model for PFS (or for OS) can also be fitted with the coxph() function. The estimated β coefficient for the treatment is equal to -0.206 (standard error: 0.064) and is thus in favor of the experimental treatment group (CAP). The corresponding HR is 0.813 (with

Treatment	n	Number of events	Number of deaths	Median PFS [95%CI]	Median OS [95%CI]
CP	606	513	499	2.41 months [2.17; 2.71]	3.56 months [3.15; 41.8]
CAP	586	464	452	3.11 months [2.64; 3.59]	4.24 months [3.65; 5.00]
All	1192	977	951	2.67 months [2.46; 2.98]	3.86 months [3.51; 4.27]

TABLE 5.7
Advanced ovarian cancer data: Summary results for OS and PFS in each treatment group

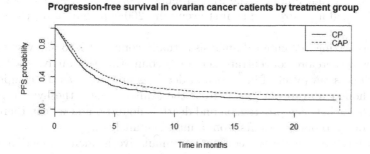

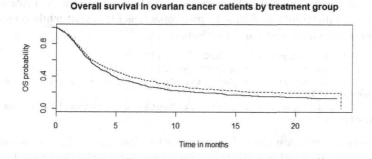

FIGURE 5.5
Advanced ovarian cancer data: Kaplan-Meier estimator of the PFS and OS curves by treatment arm obtained from the *survfit* function in *R*.

95% CI [0.717;0.922]) which can be interpreted as a 1.229 higher risk of events for the patients in the standard groups (CP). As expected, this coefficient is significantly different from 0, with a p-value of 0.001.

For this illustration, we will consider that we are in fact interested in time to progression as first event, rather than in progression-free survival and we will use these data to illustrate the basic concepts of competing risk analysis using the R software.

Therefore, we consider two different types of events: progression of the disease as the first event (type 1) and death as first event (type 2). We start by defining the time to the first event (in months) as well as a new indicator for the type of first event, which is 0 (censored) if the patient is censored for both OS and PFS, 1 (progression as first event) if the patient has a PFS event with a PFS time shorter than the time to death, and 2 (death as first event) if the patient has a PFS event and a PFS time equal to the OS time.

```
timeCR <- pmin(timeS,timeT)
statusCR <- statusS
statusCR[statusS==1 & timeS<timeT] <- 1
statusCR[statusS==1 & timeS==timeT] <- 2
```

We obtain that amongst the 977 patients who experienced a PFS event, in fact 777 had a progression as first event and 200 experienced death as first event.

In this setting, a combined analysis actually comes back to analyzing PFS and we will therefore concentrate here on a competing risk analysis with the progression as our event of interest and death as first event as the competing risk. Although we can not test it from the available data, the hypothesis of independence between progression and death is doubtful and we can therefore not rely on it to obtain results from a marginal analysis.

In order to illustrate the concept of cumulative incidence function, let's first consider all patients together (so not taking the treatment into account). As mentioned in Section 5.1, a first idea is often to compute the KM estimator of the survival distribution of time to progression as first event while censoring the patients who died first (and vice-versa).

```
status.PD <- as.numeric({statusCR == 1})
status.Dt <- as.numeric({statusCR == 2})
Ov.CR.km.PD.all <- survfit(Surv(timeMonthsCR, status.PD)~1, conf.
    type="none")
Ov.CR.km.Dt.all <- survfit(Surv(timeMonthsCR, status.Dt)~1, conf.
    type="none")
```

These two curves are plotted, as cumulative distribution functions, on the top of Figure 5.6 together with the cumulative distribution function for any type of event (as obtained from the combined analysis of PFS). As discussed earlier on in this chapter, we can see for example that 1-KM estimator at 12 months is 73.5% for PD as first event and 27.7% for death as first event, thus summing up to 101.2%, which is obviously bigger than 1-KM for any event (80.9%) (Table 5.8).

The cumulative incidence function for time to progression and for time to death as first event can be estimated using the Cuminc function from the mstate package as follows

```
Ov.CR.ci.all <- Cuminc(time=timeMonthsCR, status=statusCR)
```

Time (months)	$\hat{F}(t) = 1 - \hat{S}(t)$ Any	$\hat{F}_1^{naive}(t)$ PD	$\hat{F}_2^{naive}(t)$ Dt	$\hat{F}_1(t)$ PD	$\hat{F}_2(t)$ Dt
1	0.196	0.152	0.051	0.147	0.049
12	0.809	0.735	0.278	0.659	0.191
18	0.845	0.756	0.365	0.673	0.172

TABLE 5.8
Advanced ovarian cancer data: Time to progression as first event (PD), time to death as first event (Dt) and time to any event (Any) estimated with a naive approach (KM estimator for the event of interest while censoring the competing events) and based on the cumulative incidence function

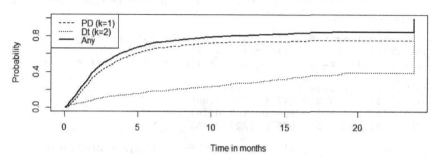

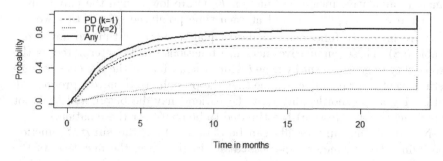

FIGURE 5.6
Advanced ovarian cancer data: (a) Cumulative Distribution of time-to-event estimated from the naive approach (KM estimator for the event of interest while censoring the competing events) (*top*). (b) Cumulative Incidence Functions (dark lines) for time-to-event and naive 1-KM cumulative distribution (gray lines) for time to progression as first event, time to death as first event and cumulative distribution function (1-KM) for any event (*bottom*). PD: progression as first event, Dt: death as first event, Any: any event.

The resulting object contains information for each event time on the global estimated survival curves (for any event), the cumulative incidence function for progression as first event (corresponding to value 1 of the status variable), the cumulative incidence function for death as first event (corresponding to value 2 of the status variable) and the standard error for each point estimate. The first lines are (using the `round()` function to avoid too many decimals):

```
> head(round(Ov.CR.ci.all,3))
   time  Surv  CI.1  CI.2 seSurv seCI.1 seCI.2
1 0.010 0.999 0.001 0.000  0.001  0.001  0.000
2 0.014 0.997 0.001 0.002  0.001  0.001  0.001
3 0.038 0.997 0.001 0.003  0.002  0.001  0.001
4 0.048 0.995 0.001 0.004  0.002  0.001  0.002
5 0.067 0.994 0.001 0.005  0.002  0.001  0.002
6 0.071 0.992 0.001 0.007  0.003  0.001  0.002
```

We can also obtain the estimated value at some specific timepoints using the `summary` function

```
> Ov.CR.ci.all <- Cuminc(time=timeMonthsCR, status=statusCR)
> summary(Ov.CR.ci.all, time=c(1,12,18))
Call: survfit(formula = Surv(time, statuscr) ~ 1, data = tmp)

 time n.risk n.event   P(1)    P(2)   P()
    1    946     232  0.147  0.0488 0.804
   12    197     705  0.659  0.1499 0.191
   18    123      35  0.673  0.1723 0.155
```

The two cumulative incidence estimated functions are plotted on the bottom of Figure 5.6 together with the corresponding naive 1-KM estimates $\hat{F}_k^{naive}(t)$ and the 1-KM estimate for any event $\hat{F}(t)$. As expected, the estimated cumulative incidence function $\hat{F}_k(t)$ are lower than the naive 1-KM estimated curves $\hat{F}_k^{naive}(t)$, and at each time point the sum of the two cumulative incidence functions is indeed equal to $\hat{F}(t)$ for time to any event (Table 5.8). These cumulative incidence functions can be interpreted as the probability to get an event by time t while accounting for the presence of competing events. For example, we see that the probability to have a progression within 1 year (acknowledging that the patient may die before and thus not experiencing a progression) is estimated to be 65.9% for these patients.

Note that the same results can be obtained from the `survfit` function specifying the parameter `type="mstate"`. In this case, the first level of the censoring indicator (here `statusCR`) represents a censored observation while the next values represent the different event types.

```
Ov.CR.ci.all.s <- survfit(Surv(timeMonthsCR,statusCR,type="mstate
    ")~1)
```

The resulting object contains summary information

```
> Ov.CR.ci.all.s
Call: survfit(formula = Surv(timeMonthsCR, statusCR, type = "
    mstate") ~ 1)
```

```
      n nevent    rmean*
1 1192    777 13.982444
2 1192    200  3.329207
  1192      0  6.488348
*mean time in state, restricted (max time = 23.8 )
```

This output provides the estimated τ-restricted mean survival, see Section 1.2.2 from Chapter 2 in "each state". This concept is in fact inherited from multi-states model. In our context it provides information on the tau-restricted mean survival spent in initial state before transition to progression (line 1) and before death as first event (line 2). By default this restricted mean survival is computed until the last censored time (here 23.8 months), however this can be changed for example fixing it in our case to 1 year we obtain

```
> print(Ov.CR.ci.all.s, rmean= 12)
Call: survfit(formula = Surv(timeMonthsCR, statusCR, type = "
    mstate")) ~
    1)

      n nevent   rmean*
1 1192    777 6.088302
2 1192    200 1.325046
  1192      0 4.586652
*mean time in state, restricted (max time = 12 )
```

The estimated value for the cumulative incidence function and standard errors are obtained from `Ov.CR.ci.all.s$pstate[,1]` (PD as first event) and `Ov.CR.ci.all.s$pstate[,2]` (death as first event) and `Ov.CR.ci.all.s$std.err[,1]`). We can also use the summary function as above.

We will now be interested in the effect of the treatment group (CR versus CAP) on the two event types. Main results are summarized in Table 5.9. Results of a naive logrank test for time to progression as first event (censoring patients who died first at the date of death) can be obtained with the usual `survdiff` command

```
> survdiff(Surv(timeMonthsCR, status.PD)~trt)
Call:
survdiff(formula = Surv(timeMonthsCR, status.PD) ~ trt)

          N Observed Expected (O-E)^2/E (O-E)^2/V
trt=0 606      415      369      5.74        11
trt=1 586      362      408      5.19        11

Chisq= 11  on 1 degrees of freedom, p= 9e-04
```

and lead to a highly significant p-value (p= 9e-04) while the same test for time to death as first event lead to a non significant p-value (p= 0.6). A standard Cox PH model including the treatment as covariate could also be fitted for each type of event, each time censoring patients experiencing the competing event, and lead to the same conclusions, with an estimated HR of 0.79 (95% CI: [0.68 ; 0.91]) for progression as first event and 0.92 (95% CI:

[0.70 ; 1.22]) for death as first event (confidence interval values are obtained with the **summary** function)

```
> coxph(Surv(timeMonthsCR, status.PD)~trt)
Call:
coxph(formula = Surv(timeMonthsCR, status.PD) ~ trt)

        coef exp(coef) se(coef)      z       p
trt -0.23780   0.78836  0.07198 -3.304 0.000954

Likelihood ratio test=10.95  on 1 df, p=0.0009366
n= 1192, number of events= 777
```

As mentioned previously, since we don't want to trust the assumption of independence between the two types of events these results should not be interpreted as the level of the marginal hazard, so comparing the risk of events in an hypothetical world where the other event would not exist. However, as discussed in Section 5.5.1, even without this assumption of independent, we can still interpret these results as those from a Cox PH model on the cause-specific hazard. It is however important to realize that this effect will not necessarily translate into similar effect on the cumulative incidence functions.

It is quite common to represent the results of a competing risk analysis as a *stacked plot*. The idea is to represent on the same plot, the estimated cumulative incidence functions for the different event types $\hat{F}_k(.)$ together with the cumulative distribution function $\hat{F}(.)$ for any type of event. Thanks to this plot, we can easily visualize at each time point the probability to observe by that time an event of a given type. On Figure 5.7, we represent such a stacked plot for each of the two treatment groups. This plot has to be interpreted in the light of the relationship $F_1(t) + F_2(t) = F(t)$ at each time point, so that the distance below the first curve represents the (cumulative) probability to get a progression as first event and the distance between the first and the second curve represents the (cumulative) probability to die as first event. We can see that the risk of any event, and the risk of death as first event is higher in the CP group while there seems to be not much difference in the risk of death as first event between the two groups.

We only have two different event types here, nevertheless it could still be convenient to use the **mstate** package to fit simultaneously a Cox PH model on the cause-specific hazard of each event type, with the possibility to compare the treatment effect for each event type. We first have to expand our dataset in a long format, which can be done by creating a transition matrix with the **trans.comprisk** function

```
> tmat <- trans.comprisk(2,names=c("Event-free","PD","Death"))
> tmat
            to
from         Event-free PD Death
  Event-free         NA  1     2
  PD                 NA NA    NA
  Death              NA NA    NA
```

and then using the **msprep** function

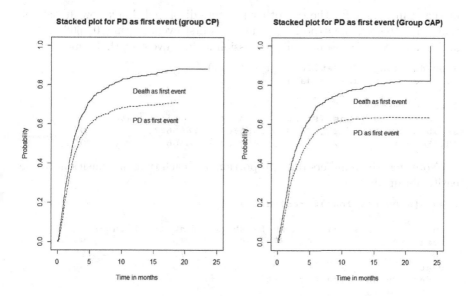

FIGURE 5.7
Advanced ovarian cancer data: Stacked plot for time to progression and time to death as first event for patients in the CP treatment group (*left*) and in the CAP treatment group (*right*).

```
> Ov.dat.long <- msprep(time=cbind(NA,timeMonthsCR,timeMonthsCR),
+                       status=cbind(NA, status.PD, status.Dt),
+                       keep=data.frame(trt),
+                       trans=tmat)
```

As expected, one can check that the resulting dataset indeed have 2 lines per patient (in our case), one for each transition (from event-free to progression as first event and from event-free to death as first event). Note that in a multi-state context, we could also consider the transition from progression as first event to death as second event.

```
> head(Ov.dat.long)
An object of class 'msdata'

Data:
  id from to trans Tstart     Tstop       time status trt
1  1    1  2     1      0  1.261905  1.261905      1   0
2  1    1  3     2      0  1.261905  1.261905      0   0
3  2    1  2     1      0 10.742857 10.742857      1   0
4  2    1  3     2      0 10.742857 10.742857      0   0
5  3    1  2     1      0  0.947619  0.947619      1   0
6  3    1  3     2      0  0.947619  0.947619      0   0
```

For example, the first patient (`id 1`) experienced progression as first event at time 1.261905 (years) and was therefore censored for death as first event at that time; same for the two other patients displayed. Look now at patient textttid 15 below, she experienced death as first event at time 0.2666 (years) and was therefore censored for progression as first event at that time

```
> Ov.dat.long[(Ov.dat.long$id=="15"),]
An object of class 'msdata'

Data:
   id from to trans Tstart    Tstop        time status trt
29 15    1  2     1      0 0.2666667 0.2666667      0   0
30 15    1  3     2      0 0.2666667 0.2666667      1   0
```

Note that the numbers (and proportions) of each type of transition can be easily obtained:

```
> events(Ov.dat.long)$Frequencies
            to
from         Event-free  PD Death no event total entering
  Event-free          0 777   200      215          1192
  PD                  0   0     0      777           777
  Death               0   0     0      200           200
> events(Ov.dat.long)$Proportions
            to
from         Event-free        PD      Death  no event
  Event-free  0.0000000 0.6518456 0.1677852 0.1803691
  PD          0.0000000 0.0000000 0.0000000 1.0000000
  Death       0.0000000 0.0000000 0.0000000 1.0000000
```

The second and third lines are obviously not needed here, but would become interesting if we are modeling multi-state models (see [98, 132] for more details).

By applying a simple Cox PH model for each transition, we obtained exactly the same results as above, for example considering progression as first event:

```
> summary(coxph(Surv(time,status)~trt,data=Ov.dat.long,subset={
      trans==1}))
Call:
coxph(formula = Surv(time, status) ~ trt, data = Ov.dat.long,
    subset = {
        trans == 1
    })

  n= 1192, number of events= 777

        coef exp(coef) se(coef)      z Pr(>|z|)
trt -0.23780   0.78836  0.07198 -3.304 0.000954 ***
---
Signif. codes:  0 '***' 0.001 '**' 0.01 '*' 0.05 '.'. 0.1 ' ' 1

    exp(coef) exp(-coef) lower .95 upper .95
trt    0.7884      1.268    0.6846    0.9078

Concordance= 0.531  (se = 0.01 )
Rsquare= 0.009   (max possible= 1 )
Likelihood ratio test= 10.95  on 1 df,    p=9e-04
```

```
Wald test                 = 10.92  on 1 df,   p=0.001
Score (logrank) test = 10.97  on 1 df,   p=9e-04
```

We can also use this expanded dataset to fit a Cox PH model on cause-specific hazards with the type of transition as stratification factor. This will estimate a single coefficient for the treatment effect whatever the endpoint considered and thus forces the estimated treatment effect to be the same for both endpoint.

```
> Ov.Cox.Strat <- coxph(Surv(time,status)~trt+strata(trans),data=
    Ov.dat.long)
> Ov.Cox.Strat
Call:
coxph(formula = Surv(time, status) ~ trt + strata(trans), data =
    Ov.dat.long)

        coef exp(coef) se(coef)       z      p
trt -0.20639   0.81352  0.06417 -3.216 0.0013

Likelihood ratio test=10.36  on 1 df, p=0.001285
n= 2384, number of events= 977
```

Note that this actually makes little sense in our example, where we have good reasons to believe that the treatment effect is not the same on both types of events. This could however be useful in some specific situations for sparsity reasons, for example if we can indeed believe that the covariate effect is close and if there are very few events for one of the event types.

To formally show that the treatment effect is indeed not the same for both event types, we can add in the model an interaction term between the treatment covariate and the transition type

```
> Ov.Cox.Strat <- coxph(Surv(time,status)~trt+strata(trans),data=
    Ov.dat.long)
> Ov.Cox.Strat
Call:
coxph(formula = Surv(time, status) ~ trt + strata(trans), data =
    Ov.dat.long)

        coef exp(coef) se(coef)       z      p
trt -0.20639   0.81352  0.06417 -3.216 0.0013

Likelihood ratio test=10.36  on 1 df, p=0.001285
n= 2384, number of events= 977
> Ov.Cox.Fact <- coxph(Surv(time,status)~trt*factor(trans),data=
    Ov.dat.long)
> Ov.Cox.Fact
Call:
coxph(formula = Surv(time, status) ~ trt * factor(trans), data =
    Ov.dat.long)

                      coef exp(coef) se(coef)        z        p
trt                -0.24267   0.78453  0.07201  -3.370 0.000751
factor(trans)2     -1.44372   0.23605  0.11231 -12.855   < 2e-16
trt:factor(trans)2  0.17678   1.19336  0.15868   1.114 0.265266
```

```
Likelihood ratio test=375.8   on 3 df,  p=< 2.2e-16
n= 2384, number of events= 977
```

Such a model however assumes proportional hazards for the type of events, i.e. that the ratio of the hazards of time to progression as first event and time to death as first event is constant over time. In our example, this ratio is estimated to be $\exp(1.44) = 0.24$, corresponding to a much lower risk of death as first event compared to the risk of progression as first event. Based on this model the treatment effect for time to progression as first event is estimated to be -0.24, corresponding to a cause-specific HR of $\exp(-0.24) = 0.78$ in favor of the CAP treatment group while the treatment effect for time to death as first event is estimated to be $-0.24 + 0.18 = .06$, corresponding to a cause-specific HR of $\exp(-0.06) = 0.94$ in favor of the CAP treatment group.

Again while the assumption of proportional hazards for the type of events may be useful for sparsity in some specific context, it will usually be more appropriate to relax it by stratifying by transition therefore leaving both hazards functions unspecified and not necessarily proportional

```
> Ov.Cox.Stfa <- coxph(Surv(time,status)~trt*factor(trans)+strata
    (trans),data=Ov.dat.long)
> Ov.Cox.Stfa
Call:
coxph(formula = Surv(time, status) ~ trt * factor(trans) + strata
    (trans),
    data = Ov.dat.long)

                       coef exp(coef) se(coef)      z        p
trt                -0.23780   0.78836  0.07198 -3.304 0.000954
factor(trans)2           NA        NA  0.00000     NA       NA
trt:factor(trans)2  0.15387   1.16634  0.15921  0.967 0.333793

Likelihood ratio test=11.3   on 2 df, p=0.003521
n= 2384, number of events= 977
```

The coefficient for `trt` corresponds to the treatment effect on the first type of event, i.e. progression, and is very close from the results obtained above when considering only this transition (-0.24). The interaction term, `trt:factor(trans)2`, shows us how different is the estimated treatment effect for the second type of event, i.e. death as first event, and is also close to what we obtained with the previous model. As above, we can find back that the HR for time to death as first event according to this model as:

```
> exp(Ov.Cox.Stfa$coefficients[1]+Ov.Cox.Stfa$coefficients[3])
    trt
0.919494
```

As expected, the treatment effect for time to death as first event is much closer to one then for time to progression as first event. However, based on the data at hand, this interaction term do not reach significance, which may be due to the low number of events of the second type. Since

As an alternative to the stacked plot of Figure 5.7, we can also represent the cumulative incidence functions for each type of event per treatment group,

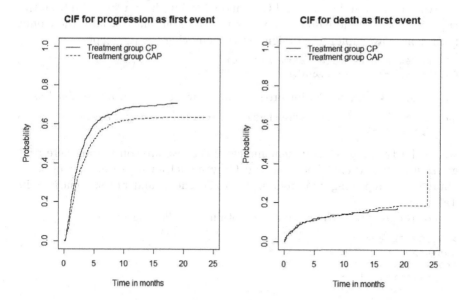

FIGURE 5.8

Advanced ovarian cancer data: Estimated cumulative incidence functions for time to progression as first event (*left*) and for death as first event (*right*) by treatment group.

as is shown on Figure 5.8. This plot highlights more clearly that the estimated cumulative incidence functions for each treatment groups differ for progression as first event but are very close for death as first event.

To confirm the significance of this finding, we can perform a Gray test for these cumulative incidence curves which can be obtained from

```
> cuminc(timeMonthsCR, statusCR, group=trt)$Tests
```

leading to

```
        stat         pv df
1 8.5954507 0.003370038  1
2 0.2346319 0.628110418  1
```

The first line refers to progression as first event (`statusCR=1`) and the second to death as first event (`statusCR=2`). The output displays the value of the test statistics (`stat`), the number of degrees of freedom of the chi-square distribution (`df`) and the p-value (`pv`) of the Gray test. We see that the difference in the cumulative incidence functions for time to progression as first event indeed reaches statistical significance (p-value $= 0.003$) but this is not the case for death as first event (p-value $= 0.628$).

We can also build a Fine and Gray model, using the `crr` function from the cmprsk package. Before doing so, we first have to put all covariates (here only treatment is available) in a design matrix removing the intercept.

```
Ov.cov.matrix <- model.matrix(~trt)
Ov.cov.matr.ni <- Ov.cov.matrix[,-1]
```

The Fine and Gray model for progression as first event can be obtained as:

```
Ov.GM.PD.crr <- crr(timeMonthsCR, statusCR, cov1=Ov.cov.matr.ni,
    failcode=1)
```

where the `failcode=1` argument indicates that we are considering here progression as first event. The Fine and Gray model for death as first event is obtained by replacing `failcode=1` by `failcode=2` and are summarized in Table 5.9.

For progression as first event, we obtain the following results

```
> Ov.GM.PD.crr
convergence:  TRUE
coefficients:
Ov.cov.matr.ni1
        -0.2109
standard errors:
[1] 0.0717
two-sided p-values:
Ov.cov.matr.ni1
         0.0033
```

and more detailed results are obtained with the **summary** function

```
> summary(Ov.GM.PD.crr)
Competing Risks Regression

Call:
crr(ftime = timeMonthsCR, fstatus = statusCR, cov1 = Ov.cov.matr.
    ni,
    failcode = 1)

                  coef exp(coef) se(coef)      z p-value
Ov.cov.matr.ni1 -0.211      0.81   0.0717  -2.94  0.0033

                exp(coef) exp(-coef)  2.5% 97.5%
Ov.cov.matr.ni1      0.81       1.23 0.704 0.932

Num. cases = 1192
Pseudo Log-likelihood = -5128
Pseudo likelihood ratio test = 8.62  on 1 df,
```

The results from the Fine and Gray model are at the level of the sub-distribution hazards and therefore directly translate into effect on the cumulative incidence functions. We have already seen that we have a lower incidence function for progression as first PD of the patients in the CAP treatment group, and this can be found back from the negative estimated coefficient of treatment obtained here. The CAP treatment reduces the risk of progression as first event (with a sub-dstribution HR of 0.81) compared to the CP treatment, and this even when taking into account the fact that patients may die of something else in between. Note that the results obtained here are very similar from those obtained in a cause-specific Cox PH model. This may be explained by the fact that we have only two event types and that the incidence of death without progression is very similar between the two treatment groups.

5.7 Further reading

The literature on competing risk is vast, with of course more methodological and more applied papers, but also several papers published for example in medical journals discussing the different options that exists in a competing risks setting due to the possibility to define different hazards, as well as the interpretation of these different options.

All the methods discussed in this chapter can be accommodated for left truncation [132, 250], see for example [132] for a detailed discussion of the non-parametric estimators of the cause-specific cumulative incidence function of Section 5.3 in the presence of left truncation. This become actually even more obvious when considering competing risk analysis as a special case of multi-state models. On the other, the analysis of competing risk data become more complex in the case of interval-data and only little work is available, mainly in the context of semi-competing risks (when one event type can prevent the occurrence of the other event type but not the opposite) [29, 219].

The Cox PH model for the cause-specific hazard discussed in Section 5.5.1 is certainly the most popular one. However, other parametric and semi-parametric approaches have been proposed, see amongst other [15, 31, 50, 176]. For example [176], propose a fully parametric regression model for the cumulative incidence function based on a two parameters Gompertz distribution.

As an alternative to the Fine and Gray model introduced in Section 5.5.2, [345] propose a broader class of flexible models to model the cumulative incidence functions, which actually include the Fine and Gray model as a special case. This model writes

$$h\left(F_k(t; \mathbf{X}, \mathbf{Z})\right) = \mathbf{X}^t \alpha_k(t) + g(\mathbf{X}, \gamma_k, t)$$

for two known link functions $h(.)$ and $g(.)$ and allows for time dependent effect of covariates. Considering the identify function for $g(.)$ and respectively $h(.) = cloglog(.)$ and $h = -log(.)$ lead to the Fine and Gray and the additive hazards models (allowing for time-dependent effects). Estimation is based on a direct binomial regression approach (which as the original approach of Fine and Gray also depends on IPCW) and a goodness-of-fit test to identify whether time-varying effects are indeed present have also been developed and implemented in the `timereg` R package [341, 345, 346]. This approach can be further extended to the inclusion of random effect for modeling clustered competing risk data [342].

Model	PD as first event	Death as first event	Remarks		
Models for the cause-specific hazards					
Cox PH model	0.238 (0.072) $p < 0.001$ 0.788 [0.685 ; 0.908]	−0.084 (01.42) $p = 0.554$ 0.920 [0.696 ; 0.932]	Any event:	−0.206 (0.064) $p = 0.001$ 0.813 [0.717 ; 0.224]	
Combined Cox PH model strat (same trt coef.)	−0.206 (0.064) p=0.001 0.814 [0.717 ; 0.926]	Idem			
Combined Cox PH model PH (interaction)	−0.243 (0.072) $p < 0.001$ 0.788 [0.681 ; 0.903]	Coef: −0.066 HR: 0.936	Type: Interaction:	−1.443 (0.112) $p < 0.001$ 0.236 [0.189 ; 0.294] 0.177 (0.159) $p = 0.265$ 1.193 [0.874 ; 1.629]	
Combined Cox PH model PH (interaction)	−0.237 (0.072) $p < 0.001$ 0.788 [0.684 ; 0.908]	Coef: −0.084 HR: 0.919	Interaction:	0.154 (0.159) $p = 0.334$ 1.166 [0.854 ; 1.594]	
Models for the sub-distribution hazards					
Fine and Gray	−0.211 (0.072) $p = 0.003$ 0.810 [0.704 ; 0.932]	0.071 (0.141) $p = 0.60$ 1.070 [0.814 ; 1.420]			

TABLE 5.9

Advanced ovarian cancer data: Results from different models including treatment as covariate. Results are presented as estimated coefficient (standard error), p-value, HR, 95% CI for the HR.

The Fine and Gray model (as well as the direct binomial modeling) are based on an IPCW technique, to cope with the fact that individuals who have experience a competing events should remain in the risk set until censoring. However, it is crucial that these weights are estimated without bias, otherwise the estimates of the cumulative incidence functions may also be biased [346]. Scheike et al. [345] therefore propose to replace the Kaplan-Meier estimates of the survival function of the censoring distribution by a Cox PH model to include covariates on which this distribution may depend.

As already discussed, both the Cox PH model for the cause-specific hazard and the Fine and Gray model assume proportional hazards respectively for the cause-specific hazard and the sub-distribution hazard. In case of non-proportional hazards, we can include interaction terms between the covariates and functions of time in a similar way as in a standard Cox PH model. Additive hazards or additive probability models have also been proposed as an alternative to proportional hazards model in a competing risk setting [188, 347]; a flexible Cox-Aalen type model, which allows the inclusion of time-dependent covariate has also been proposed as an alternative to the proportional cause-specific hazards model [343, 344]. As discussed in the "classical" survival context in Chapter 2, summary measures based on the τ-restricted mean survival time (RMST) have been proposed as an alternative to the HR in case of non-proportional hazards. The RMST has been extended to the case of competing risks and in this case, the number of life lost before time τ can be decomposed based on the different event types [14, 58].

Although it has raised debates in the literature in the past, it is now widely recognized that analyzing competing risks data via the cause-specific hazards or the cumulative incidence functions actually reflects different aspects of the underlying competing risk process. A common recommendation is therefore to choose the appropriate type of analysis based on the research question of interest or to perform both types of analysis while acknowledging that they bring different information. Given that these two types of analyzes reflect different dynamics of the process, it has naturally been proposed to analyze jointly the cause-specific hazard and the cumulative incidence function to avoid having these two analyzes to be totally disconnected [214]. For the case of an event of interest and a competing event, Li and Yang [225] propose a two sample joint test for the null hypothesis $H_0 : \lambda_{k,1} = \lambda_{k,2}$ and $S_{k,1}(t) = S_{k,2}(t) \forall t$. Such a joint test is based on the asymptotic joint distribution of the weighted logrank test statistics for the cause-specific hazards $\lambda_{k,i}$ and the Gray test statistic for $S_{k,i}(t)$. Another possibility is to consider a joint test based on the cause-specific hazards and the all-cause hazards. Furthermore, such joint modeling can also be extended to regression analysis. An illustration of the use of these joint tests and regression analyzes on different data is presented in Latouche et al. [214].

Obviously, a further difficulty arise when the type of event is unknown for part of the observations, a typical example being the analysis of cause-specific death with the type of death being unknown or missing for some individuals.

We can define a taxonomy close to the one developed for missing covariates (i.e. Missing Completely At Random, Missing At Random, Missing Not at Random, see for example [257]) and different strategies have been proposed to handle such missing type of events [236, 261]. Some works have been done also in case the type of events is subject to error, again typically in the setting of cause-specific deaths where cause of deaths can be mis-classified for part of the individuals, see for example [396].

Sample size calculation is often a crucial issue in an experimental context, and in particular in clinical trials. This is also the case when considering competing risks, and one then needs to decide upfront whether the sample size will be based on the analysis of the cause-specific hazards, on the analysis of the subdistribution hazards, or on a joint analysis [215, 273, 314, 349, 417].

As already mentioned, a typical setting in which competing risks are present is when analyzing long-term side effects of a treatment. Indeed, by definition these events occur long time after the start of the follow-up leaving the room for other events to occur in the meantime which can, in turn, modify strongly the risk of long-term side effects (e.g. start of a second treatment for another pathology) or even preclude it (e.g. death from another cause). Depending on the context, these long-term side effects may be quite rare, as is the case for example for the occurrence of a second malignancy, and therefore a large dataset is required to appropriately study their occurrence. Typically data from a meta-analysis or from pooling several databases will then be used. The competing risks methodology has thus been extended to situations where we have to deal both with competing risks and clustered data, see among other [149, 192, 434]. For example, an extension of the Fine and Gray model has been used to study the occurrence of a second malignancy following Lenalidomide therapy in a large database of 9 myeloma phase III trials while accounting for heterogeneity across trials [277]. As mentioned above, the broad class of flexible models for the cumulative incidence function developed by Scheike et al. [342] can also handle clustered data.

This also raises the question of the presence of a cure fraction. Actually the definition of "cure" is (even) more complex in the setting of competing risk. We should indeed distinguish situations in which we consider cure from all possible event types from situation where we only consider cure from some selected event types. See for example the work of [73, 116, 271] for different approaches combining cure and competing risks.

It is also interesting to note some work published proposing solutions to include time-dependent covariates, either endogenous or exogenous (see Section 6.2 in Chapter 6) in the framework of competing risks, either in a proportional cause-specific hazard model and in the Fine and Gray model [41, 85, 133].

Note that in some circumstances, we may actually observe the time of different failure types for each individual. For example, in an oncology clinical trial, we typically have information on the date of local recurrence, occurrence of distant metastases and/or death. One however has to be careful that the occurrence of an intermediate event (e.g. local recurrence) will most certainly modify the risk of the other event (either directly, or indirectly for example by changing the treatment protocol). It is therefore strongly advised to either restrict the data to the occurrence of the first event, and thus being back to a competing risks setting, or to also consider in the analysis the impact of intermediate events. Considering the influence of intermediate events on subsequent events can be the main interest, for example to get a better knowledge about the biological mechanisms underlying the course of a disease or to improve the prediction of an event of interest (e.g. cancer death) while accounting for the intermediate events (e.g. occurrence of locoregional recurrence and/or distant metastases). A useful tool in such a setting are multi-state models (see for example [132]), of which standard survival analysis and competing risks can be derived as a special case.

6

Joint Modeling

6.1 Introduction

It is becoming more and more common in longitudinal studies to collect both repeated measurements of a longitudinal marker and information on the time to an event of interest. Most often, these two processes will be somehow linked and a separate analysis of each is obviously not optimal. In the medical field, the two most popular examples are most probably the repeated measurements of CD4 counts and time to AIDS in HIV, and the repeated measurements of PSA level and the time to prostate cancer recurrence. However, other examples can be found in the medical field as well as in other fields.

In the presence of such data, one can raise several questions of interest. Looking at it from a time-to-event perspective, we may be interested in the prognostic value of the longitudinal marker on the risk of event. Indeed, while a lot of work address the evaluation of the prognostic value of a marker measured at baseline, the dynamic nature of these markers is then ignored. When repeated measurements of this marker are available over the course of the disease, it will often be more informative to consider the prognostic value of the whole longitudinal process. For example the prognostic value of repeated measurement of PSA level on the risk of prostate cancer has been extensively studies. An additional difficulties is that we don't know the true full PSA trajectory over time, first because only measurements at discrete time-points are available (most probably following an unbalanced design with different time-points for each patient) and also due to possible (biological) measurement errors. While most standard time-to-event model have been extended to include time-dependent covariates (see Section 6.2), these will often not be appropriate in this context. An alternative approach, *joint modeling*, has therefore been developed over the last decades with a growing popularity. Indeed, we will see that it offers several advantages, and in particular handling of measurement errors and unbalanced deign for the longitudinal outcome as well as informative dropout.

So, when the main interest is on the time-to-event, joint models will offer an elegant solution to account for the effect of an (endogenous) time-dependent covariate. But joint models are also of interest when the main focus is on the longitudinal outcome in itself. They will allow to study the trajectory of the marker while accounting for non-random dropout due to the occurrence of an event. In the example above, we will often not consider the PSA measurements made after the occurrence of prostate cancer recurrence in our analysis, but on the other hand the occurrence of this event is clearly informative on the PSA trajectory.

Finally, the main interest can be in the nature (and the strength) of the association between the longitudinal outcome and the risk of event. Indeed, getting a better view on how the two processes are linked can help grasping a better understanding of the dynamics of the disease or phenomenon under study. As an example, we may want to know whether it is the value of the marker (e.g. PSA) at a given time that impact the risk of the event of interest or whether it is rather the fact that this marker is increasing or decreasing at time t. As another example, the risk to develop lung cancer is much more impacted by some cumulative measure of the cigarettes smoked during life then by the number of cigarettes smoked at the time of diagnosis.

An important aspect of joint modeling is the ability to make prediction, and actually to make dynamic prediction, taking into account the evaluation of the longitudinal outcome to update the prediction on the risk of event. With a growing interest on personalized medicine, being able to use all information collected on the potential prognostic marker, both at baseline but also over time, in order make accurate prediction is obviously highly valuable. Such a prediction could then be used to adapt medical decision about the patient's treatment. In this context of personalized medicine the quest for dynamic models that allow to regularly update the survival prediction based on the evolution of longitudinal biomarkers is an important emergent area of research.

While the examples mentioned above are in the medical field, joint modeling can find applications in very different areas. For example, in engineering, we may collect repeated measurements on a component of a machinery and the time to failure of this machinery. This can for example be used to monitor the various components of a cinema projector (e.g. the temperature of the lamp) to predict the appropriate timing of replacement of the lamp, avoiding extra costs if replaced to early and the unpleasant experience of a black screen for the spectators if not replaced on time (SAS, personal communication).

The basic idea behind the joint model approach is in fact rather simple [141, 306, 320, 379]. It consists in

- defining a model for the repeated measurements of the longitudinal marker; most often a mixed model;

- defining a model for the time-to-event process; most often a proportional hazards model;

- linking both models with a shared latent association structure; two main options exist leading either to a *shared-random effect model* (see Section 6.3) or to a *joint latent class model* (see Section 6.4).

The shared random-effect model (SREM) is inspired from the selection model in missing data problems [320]. The idea is that a summary measure of the longitudinal process is included as a covariate in the time-to-event model. As we will see, several possible summary measure have been considered to capture the dynamics of the marker trajectory. This first approach can thus be seen as an extension of the standard survival models with time-dependent covariates and have lead to numerous publications, applying this model to various situations and extending it in different ways. We will come back to this approach in some more details in Section 6.3.

The joint latent class model (JCLM) is an alternative approaches, whose inspiration is to be found in finite mixture modeling. The general idea is to assume that population of subjects, while heterogeneous, actually consists of latent subgroups of subjects that share the same longitudinal marker trajectory and the same risk of event. As pointed by [306], this approach has received less attention in the literature despite the fact that it provides a computationally attractive alternative. As we will discuss, the two approaches link the two processes in a very different ways, both leading to pro's and con's and the choice between one approach or the other should primarily rely on the research question.

As we will discuss, an important assumption of the joint modeling, whatever the approaches above, is that conditional on the shared latent association structure, the two processes are assumed to be independent. In other words, the latent association structure is assumed to capture all the dependence between the two processes. The field of joint models in survival data analysis is still in its growing phase, with a lot of work being currently done and a lot further research still being performed. We will therefore only give a broad overview here. We refer the reader to the books of Rizopoulos [320] and Elashoof [114] and the review of Tsiatis and Davidian [379], Gould et al. [141] and Papageorgiou et al. [279] and the references therein for a more in-depth treatment of the subject.

6.2 Time-dependent covariates in survival models

In medicine, the identification of biomarkers with a strong prognostic impact on a time-to-event outcome has become a crucial issue. Well know such prognostic factors are for example stage at diagnosis for death of melanoma cancer or HER2 status for progression from breast cancer. These factors are measured at baseline and can be included in standard survival models. However, over last decades, a lot of interest has been put on longitudinal biomarkers and the prognostic capabilities of these biomarkers when considering their evolution over time rather than their value measured at baseline. Well known such biomarkers are the CD4 count in HIV studies, the serum bilirubin level in liver disease, or the prostate specific antigen (PSA) level in prostate cancer studies.

The question of studying the impact of such dynamic factors on a time-to-event outcome is obviously linked to the question of the inclusion of time-dependent covariates in a survival model. Before discuss this, it is important to realize that we can actually distinguish two types of time-dependent covariates: endogenous (or internal) covariates and exogenous (or external) covariates. This distinction is important as it will impact the type of methods that we can use to include them in a survival analysis. While we can use standard extension of survival models to time-dependent covariates for exogenous covariates, more caution are required for the endogenous covariates.

An easy way to distinguish an endogenous (or internal) covariate from an exogenous (or external) one is to see the endogenous covariate as a covariate generated by the patient himself. In simple words, we need the patient to be "alive" to be able to measure the value of the covariate; this is for example the case of forced expiratory volume, blood pressure, PSA level, CD4 count, quality of life ... . Other factors that we may want to take into account in our analysis could be linked to changes in environmental factors, such as the air pollution, or the ozone level. Obviously, we can still collect information on such exposition factors while the patient is dead. In fact, the occurrence of an event for the patient will not impact the value of such external covariates. This description can of course be generalized to other situations.

A more mathematical definition is provided in Rizopoulos [320] and Kalbfleisch and Prentice [181]. This definition states that a time-dependent covariate $X(t)$ is exogenous if it satisfies

$$P(s \leq T_i < s + ds \mid T_i \geq s, \mathcal{X}_i(s)) = P(s \leq T_i < s + ds \mid T_i \geq s, \mathcal{X}_i(t)) \quad (6.1)$$

for all $0 < s \leq t$ and $ds \to 0$ and with $\mathcal{X}_i(t) = \{x_i(s), 0 \leq s \leq t\}$ the covariate history up to time t. A probably more intuitive condition is that

$$P(\mathcal{X}_i(t) \mid \mathcal{X}_i(s), T_i \geq s) = P(\mathcal{X}_i(t) \mid \mathcal{X}_i(s), T_i = s) \quad (6.2)$$

In words, knowing the value of the time-dependent covariate up to time s, the future values up to a time $t > s$ are not impacted by the occurrence of an event at time s. So, typical examples of exogenous variables are time-dependent covariates whose value are actually not impacted by the status of subject under study, such as air pollution, ozone level, weather, ... but also time-dependent variables for which the evolution over time is known or fixed in advance (e.g. age of the patient or treatment dose adjustment based on pre-determined criteria).

On the other hand, endogenous covariates are the ones that do not satisfy (6.1) or equivalently (6.2).

6.2.1 Exogenous time-dependent covariates and extended Cox model

A key issue is that for exogenous covariates, and under condition (6.1) or (6.2), we can use the relationship between the hazard function and the survival function to define the survival function for subject $i, i = 1, ..., n$ conditional on his covariate path [320]:

$$S_i(t \mid \mathcal{X}_i(t)) = P(T_i > t \mid \mathcal{Y}_i(t))$$

$$= \exp\left(-\int_0^t h_i(s \mid \mathcal{Y}_i(s))ds\right)$$

The Cox PH model has been extended to handle exogenous time-dependent covariates. This extension, based on a counting process formulation of the Cox PH model, has been proposed by Andersen and Gill [16] and is therefore sometimes referred to as the Andersen-Gill model. We refer to [13] and [125] for a more detailed (methodological) description, and to [260, 320, 372] for a more applied perspective. Note that this counting process formulation in fact allows several extensions of the Cox PH model, not only to (exogenous) time-dependent covariates, as we will see, but also to other settings such as multiple events or truncated observations (see [372] for example).

The counting process formulation on which this extension is based rely on two following two event-processes for the ith subject:

$$\{N_i(t), R_i(t)\}$$

where $N_i(t)$ count the number of events by time t for individual i (and is therefore either 0 or 1 in a classical survival setting with maximum one event per subject) and $R_i(t)$ is a left-continuous at-risk process (with value 1 if individual i is at risk at time t and 0 otherwise).

In this counting process formulation, the extended Cox model (or Andersen-Gill model) for time-dependent covariates writes for subject $i, i = 1, ..., n$ with $\mathbf{Z}_i$ the vector of time-independent covariates and $\mathbf{X}_i(t)$ the vector of time-dependent covariate at time t, and history $X_i(t)$

$$h_i(t \mid \mathcal{X}_i(t), \mathbf{Z}_i = \mathbf{z}_i) = h_0(t)R_i(t)\exp(\eta^t\mathbf{z}_i + \alpha^t\mathbf{x}_i(t))$$

In this formulation, $h_i(t)$ is called the intensity of the process $N_i(t)$, i.e. the counting process which count the number of events for subject i by time t. This is in line with the intuitive interpretation of the hazard function as the expected number of events per subject per unit of time. $R_i(t)$ is as above the "at-risk" process with value 1 if subject i is still at risk at time t and 0 otherwise. The interpretation of η, the vector of coefficients associated with the time-independent covariates, is exactly the same as in the standard (Cox) PH model (2.14). The interpretation of α is similar, with α_p representing for any particular time t the increase in the log-hazard of an event for an increase of one unit in $x_{pi}(t)$ at the same time point, all the other covariates being fixed. We have a similar interpretation for $\exp(\eta_p)$ and $\exp(\alpha_p)$ in terms of relative increase in the hazard of an event. However, a major difference with the standard (Cox) PH model is that, due to the dependence in time of $\mathbf{X}_i(t)$, we don't anymore have proportional hazards. Based on this counting process formulation, the partial likelihood function can be extended to obtain estimators of β and α, see [13] and [125] for more details.

However, this model also presents some limitations. An major one is that it assumes that the time-dependent covariates remain constant between two measurement time-points. In other words, the evolution of a time-dependent covariate $X_p(t)$ is assumed to be a step-function, with its value changing at measurement time-points. As a consequence, the hazard of an event, at any given time point t is in fact based on a "last-value carried forward" extrapolated value of the covariates from last measurement time. This assumption will be unrealistic for most biomarkers and clinical parameters, especially as measurements can be made at medical visits several weeks apart. More generally, this model assumes that the time-dependent covariates are a predictable process and have their complete path fully specified [320]. Further, it does not account for potential measurement error in the longitudinal biomarker, and adjust the model for the value observed as if it was the real value. For these reasons, this extended Cox model will not be appropriate for endogenous time-dependent covariates which often present these characteristics. Treating an endogenous covariate as exogenous and using this extended Cox model may lead to spurious results [320].

6.2.2 Endogenous time-dependent covariates and joint models

While exogenous covariates are most often representing processes external to the subjects under study, the endogenous covariates on the other hand are typically time-dependent measurements taken on the subject under study and the most obvious examples are biomarkers or clinical parameters (e.g. white blood cells count). As an illustration, if we consider such a biomarker then obviously in case one individual died while under study, the value of the biomarker for this individual after his death simply does not exist anymore. Given that for such a biomarker, a failure of a subject at time s prevent us from observing a value for $x(t)$ at time time $t > s$ for this subject, the condition (6.2) is clearly violated.

A major consequence is that, the hazard function, as defined by

$$h(t \mid \mathcal{X}_i(t)) = \lim_{\Delta t \to 0} \frac{P(t \leq T < t + \Delta t \mid T \geq t, \mathcal{X}_i(t))}{\Delta t}$$

is not anymore directly related to a survival function, i.e we can not obtain anymore the relation $h(t) = \frac{-d}{dt} \log S(t)$, we have seen in Section 1.2.2 of Chapter 1. The functions

$$S_i(t \mid \mathcal{X}_i(t)) = \exp\left(-\int_0^t h_i(s \mid \mathcal{X}_i(s))ds\right)$$

and

$$f(t \mid \mathcal{X}_i(t)) = \frac{h_i(t \mid \mathcal{X}_i(t))}{S_i(t \mid \mathcal{X}_i(t))}$$

do not have the usual survival and density function interpretation [320]. Therefore the usual likelihood function for survival data which is based on the survival and density function, see (2.1) in Chapter 2, is not meaningful for endogenous covariates. The extended Cox model introduced in the previous section and which relies on the standard definition of the hazard function can thus no handle endogenous covariates.

Besides this feature, such endogenous covariates usually also present other typical characteristics. As already mentioned, their values are usually only known at discrete time points (e.g. at the time a blood sample has been taken from the patient), and it is usually not appropriate to consider the value of the covariate as constant between two measurements. Furthermore, the process generating these time points is subject to missing data (e.g. patient not coming at the planned visit for reasons linked or not to his health status), unbalanced design (e.g. not all patients will have the same number of (planned) blood samples), and measurement error due to biological variability or human/technical errors in the measurement process.

Joint modeling has therefore been proposed as an alternative framework for modeling the association between an endogenous time-dependent covariate and a time-to-event outcome [379]. Starting from the idea that we do not have access to the complete true longitudinal marker trajectory but rather to a limited number of observed measurements, probably contaminated with some error, the objective is to use the available data to model the evolution of the true marker trajectory and to then use a summary measure from the modeled true trajectory in our survival model. This has led to the development of joint models for a survival endpoint and a longitudinal (continuous) marker.

So, let's $m_i(t)$ be the true underlying process of our endogenous time-dependent covariate for individual $i = 1, ..., n$. This time-dependent covariate could be the PSA level, the CD4 cell counts, the platelets count, or any other clinical parameter or biomarker. This true process is not observed, instead, we can only observe $X_i(t)$, a version of $m_i(t)$ potentially contaminated with measurement error. Also, we do not observe the complete history $X_i(t)$ for all $t > 0$, but we only have access to a limited number of observed measurements $X_i(t_{ij})$ at specific timepoints $t_{ij}, j = 1, ..., n_i$; the number and timing of these measurements being usually different for each individual. However, these observed measurements $X_{ij} = \{X_i(t_{ij}), j = 1, ..., n_i\}, i = 1, ..., n$ can be used to model the true underlying process $m_i(t)$, typically using mixed model methodology. As mentioned above, the idea is then to "link" our model for $m_i(t)$ with the hazard of event $h_i(t \mid \mathcal{M}_i(t), \mathbf{Z}_i)$ where $\mathcal{M}_i(t) = \{m_i(s), 0 \leq s < t\}$ is the history of the true longitudinal process up to time t, and $\mathbf{Z}_i$ is the vector of time-independent covariates.

Two main approaches have been followed to "link" these models, namely the shared random effect and the joint latent class approach. The main advantages of such joint models is that (i) they do not assume the value of the time-dependent covariate to be constant between two measurement times but rather use all the information available from all patients to model this evolution over time (depending on the model chosen), (ii) they allow for (classical normal additive) measurement error (since we actually model the mean process evolution), and (iii) the longitudinal and survival processes are associated so that informative dropout due to the occurrence of an event is accounted for. However, this comes at the price of a key assumption of conditional independence between the two processes (see next sections for more details).

Note that some endogenous covariates may also present these characteristics, in particular measurements made at discrete time-point and measurement error, as would be the case for example of some marker of air pollution. In that case, it is probably best to handle them using the same approach.

6.3   The shared random effect approach

In this section, we present the shared random effect model (SREM) for the joint analysis of a longitudinal outcome and a time-to-event outcome. For a more detailed description, we refer the reader to the book of Rizopoulos [320] which also presents several applications in R. We present the two-submodels involved in joint modeling, namely the longitudinal model (with an emphasis on the "simpler" case of the linear mixed effect model) and the survival model and discuss possible association structures between these two models. Dynamic predictions for the survival and the longitudinal outcomes are also addressed.

6.3.1   Model for the marker trajectory

We speak about a longitudinal outcome when a given characteristic or marker is measured repeatedly over time. In that case, we can model the evolution of this outcome over time taking into account the fact that repeated measurements taken on the same individual are expected to be (positively) correlated. A common approach for this is the mixed model methodology. Most of the work on SREM consider a continuous longitudinal outcome and use a linear mixed model. However, other types of longitudinal outcome have also been addressed as will be shortly described below. It is important to note that the analysis of longitudinal outcome can be seen as special case of the analysis of correlated or clustered data, which is the subject of a vast literature.

The main idea behind a linear mixed model for a longitudinal continuous outcome is that all individuals have a common marker trajectory which has a specific functional form, and each individual in the population deviates from this common marker trajectory to have his own subject-specific mean marker profile over time. We provide a short overview here, and refer to the literature on mixed models for further details, and in particular to [49, 123, 298, 399, 404].

Let x_{ij} be the observed value of the longitudinal marker process $m_i(t)$ for the subject $i(i = 1, \ldots, n)$ at time $t_{ij}(j = 1, \ldots, n_i)$. Assuming at this stage that the longitudinal marker is continuous, a simple linear model assuming a linear time effect is then given by

$$
\begin{aligned}
x_{ij} &= m_i(t)\epsilon_{ij} \\
&= (\beta_0 + b_{i0}) + (\beta_1 + b_{i1})t_{ij} + \epsilon_{ij}
\end{aligned}
\tag{6.3}
$$

where $\mathbf{b}_i = (b_{i0}, b_{i1})^t$ is a vector of random effects and ϵ_{ij} are the errors terms. It is common to assume that the $\mathbf{b}_i$ are independent from the ϵ_{ij}, and that $\mathbf{b}_i \sim N(0, \mathbf{D})$ and $\epsilon_{ij} \sim N(0, \sigma^2)$. Taking the expectation of (6.3), we see that the fixed effect parameters $\beta = (\beta_0, \beta_1)^t$ represents the averaged (linear) trajectory over all individuals in the population, with β_0 being the average intercept and β_1 being the average slope. The random effect b_{i0} represents the (random) deviation in the intercept β_0 for individual i, while b_{i1} represents the (random) deviation in the slope β_1 for this individual i. See Figure 6.1 for an illustration. On this plot, we have represented as a straight line, the common average (linear) marker trajectory given by $\beta_0 + \beta_1 t$, as well as the subject specific (linear) marker trajectory for three random patients (dotted lines) as given by $(\beta_0 + b_{i0}) + (\beta_1 + b_{i1})t$ for $i = 1, 2, 3$. Finally, we have added the observed values for one of these subject as measured at 10 time-point. It is interesting to see that although these measurements are close from the straight line representing the evolution of the marker for this patient, considering that the value remain constant between two measurements (step function in the bottom part of the figure) would not correctly reflect the value of the marker between two measurements.

We can also easily show that the random effects b_i included in model (6.3) induce a (positive) correlation between measurements made on the same patient

$$
\begin{aligned}
cor(x_{ij}, x_{ij'}) &= \frac{cov(x_{ij}, x_{ij'})}{\sqrt{var(x_{ij})}\sqrt{x_{ij'}}} \quad \text{for } j \neq j' \\
&= \frac{\sigma_d^2}{\sigma_d^2 + \sigma^2}
\end{aligned}
$$

while measurements made on different patients are independent.

This model can be generalized to include additional fixed and random effects. Denoting $\tilde{\mathbf{Z}}_i$ and $\mathbf{W}_i$ the known design matrix for the fixed and random effects respectively, a general expression of the linear mixed models is given

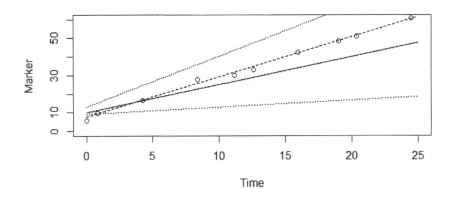

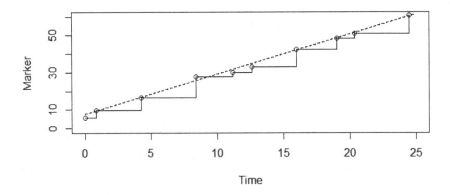

FIGURE 6.1
Linear mixed model – Example 1. *Top:* Linear evolution of a marker over time: common average trajectory (*solid line*), subject-specific trajectory for 3 individuals (*dotted lines*) and marker value measured at 10 timepoint, for a specific individual. *Bottom:* subject-specific trajectory for 1 individual (dotted lines), marker value measured at 10 timepoint, for this individual, and last-value carried forward approach.

by

$$
\begin{aligned}
\mathbf{X}_i &= m_i(t) + \epsilon_i \\
&= \tilde{\mathbf{Z}}_i \beta + \mathbf{W}_i \mathbf{b_i} + \epsilon_i
\end{aligned}
\tag{6.4}
$$

with $\mathbf{b_i} \sim N(0, \mathbf{D})$ and $\epsilon_i \sim N(0, \mathbf{R}_i)$, and one usually assumes that the random effects $\mathbf{b_i}$ are independent of the error terms ϵ_i. It is also common to assume that the error terms are independent and homoskedastic with $\mathbf{R}_i = \sigma^2 Id_{n_i}$ (where Id_{n_i} represent the $n_i \times n_i$ identity matrix. However, we can also consider a more general variance-covariance matrix for the ϵ_i if the random effects considered do not capture all the correlation in the data, e.g. some serial correlation such as an auto-regressive model.

The matrices $\tilde{\mathbf{Z}}$ and $\mathbf{W}$ are known design matrix, respectively for the fixed and the random effects. Usually, the design matrix $\tilde{\mathbf{Z}}$ contains a first column of 1 (for the intercept) and p columns for the covariates included in the model. In that case, the first component of the $(p+1)$ vector of coefficients $\beta = (\beta_0, \beta_1, \ldots, \beta_p)^t$ represents the average intercept while $\beta_l (l = 1, \ldots, p)$ represents the average change in the outcome X_i when the corresponding covariates X_l increases by one unit, all the other covariates being constant. On the other hand, the design matrix $\mathbf{W}$ of the random effects usually do not include an intercept. Random effects can be applied to (a subset of) the regression parameters to capture how the ith subject deviates from the average population parameters, with exactly the same interpretation as in the simple case above. Note that such models are called *mixed effects model* as they include both random and fixed effects. It can easily be shown that model (6.3) is obtained from model (6.4). A key issue is that the b_i's are not parameters but must be seen as realizations of a (normal) distribution. They are therefore usually refer to as "coefficients" and one usually speaks about "predictions" rather than "estimations". The real parameters of interest associated with these random effects are the one of the (normal) distribution which they are assumed to follow, so the parameters in $\mathbf{D}$. Note that this is a considerable advantage of the random effects over fixed effects as the number of parameters does therefore not increase with the sample size.

In case we do not expect the subjects have non-linear profiles, we may gain in flexibility by considering non-linear term in the right hand side of 6.4, or even considering for example polynomials or splines, defining the design matrices $\tilde{\mathbf{Z}}$ and $\mathbf{W}$ appropriately [94, 95].

When applied to a longitudinal outcome, mixed models not only allow to estimate the parameters describing how the mean marker changes in the population (the β's), but also to predict how the individual marker trajectory changes over time based on the estimates of the β's and the prediction of the b's. We can indeed define a population mean function as

$$E(x_{ij}) = \tilde{\mathbf{z}}_{ij}^t \beta$$

whose estimate is obtained by replacing β by their estimates, and a subject-specific mean

$$E(x_{ij} \mid \mathbf{b}_i) = \tilde{\mathbf{z}}_{ij}^t \beta + \mathbf{w}_{ij}^t b_i$$

which required predictions for $\mathbf{b}$.

A major advantage of mixed models is that they are not restricted to balanced design (in which measurements are made at the same time-points for all individuals), but can actually handle any imbalance in the data, either due to the fact that we do not have the same number of measurements for all individuals or due to the fact that the measurements are not taken at the same time interval for all the individuals. This of course reflect a more realistic situation, for example when the biomarker is measured from a blood sample taken when the patients come at the hospital for a visit.

Furthermore, mixed-effects models allow to take into account the correlation between repeated measurements made on the same individual. Indeed, as shown in the simple model (6.3), the measurements made within the ith individual are (marginally) correlated because they share the same random effects b_i. The idea is in fact exactly the same as the one we discussed in Chapter 3 when introducing the shared frailty model which is actually inspired from mixed models. We will often assume a simple diagonal variance-covariance matrix for the subject-specific error components, i.e. $R_i = \sigma^2 I_{n_i}$, which actually assumes that all the correlation between measurements made in the ith patient is captured by the random effects, and that conditional on these, these measurements are independent. However, this may not always be the case and a more general variance-covariance matrix for the subject-specific error components can be considered (covariance-pattern model). In the following, we will consider the case of independent ϵ's.

In a frequentist framework, estimation of model (6.4) can be based on maximum likelihood (ML). This likelihood can be obtained by acknowledging that the observed $\mathbf{X}$ follows a multivariate normal distribution with mean

$$E(\mathbf{X}) = E(\tilde{\mathbf{Z}}\beta + \mathbf{W}\mathbf{b} + \epsilon) = \tilde{\mathbf{z}}\beta$$

and variance

$$\mathbf{V} = Var(\mathbf{X}) = Var(\tilde{\mathbf{Z}}\beta + \mathbf{W}\mathbf{b} + \epsilon) \quad = \quad \mathbf{W}Var(\mathbf{b})\mathbf{W}^t + Var(\epsilon)$$
$$= \quad \mathbf{W}\mathbf{D}\mathbf{W}^t + \mathbf{R}$$

since the individuals are assumed independent.

Based on this normal distribution and the independence of the individuals, the likelihood function is then easily obtained as

$$L(\zeta) = \frac{1}{(2\pi)^{n/2} |\mathbf{V}|^{1/2}} \exp\left[-\frac{1}{2}(\mathbf{X} - \tilde{\mathbf{Z}}\beta)^t \mathbf{V}^{-1}(\mathbf{X} - \tilde{\mathbf{Z}}\beta)\right]$$

where ζ is a vector containing all the model parameters, $\zeta^t = (\beta^t, \gamma_D^t, \gamma_R^t)$ where γ_D^t and γ_R^t are respectively the vectors of the parameters contained in $\mathbf{D}$ and $\mathbf{R}$.

The idea is to first estimate the fixed effect parameters by maximizing (6.5) with respect to β. The following closed form expression can be obtained for $\hat{\beta}$,

$$\hat{\beta} = (\tilde{\mathbf{Z}}\mathbf{V}^{-1}\tilde{\mathbf{Z}})^{-1}\tilde{\mathbf{Z}}^t \mathbf{V}^{-1}\mathbf{X} \tag{6.5}$$

and

$$Var(\beta) = (\tilde{\mathbf{Z}}^t \hat{\mathbf{V}}^{-1} \tilde{\mathbf{Z}})^{-1}.$$

If we can assume $\mathbf{V}$ to be known, then this expression can be used as such and is often referred to as the generalized least square estimator of β. However, in most of the cases, $\mathbf{V}$ is not known and should itself be estimated. This is generally done by plugging the expression (6.5) into (6.5) and to maximize it with respect to the parameters of $\mathbf{V}$. One can then replace $\mathbf{V}$ by $\hat{\mathbf{V}}$ in the expression above.

Nevertheless, it is well known that this may lead, especially in small sample, to biased estimators of $\mathbf{V}$. To tackle this issue, it has been proposed to base the estimation of the variance parameters on a slightly different likelihood called the restricted likelihood, leading to restricted maximum likelihood estimates (REML) [281]. Without entering into details, the main idea is to factorize the likelihood (6.5) as a product of two terms, one based on the residuals $\mathbf{X} - \tilde{\mathbf{Z}}\beta$ and which depends only on the variance parameters and one based on $\hat{\beta}$:

$$L(\beta, \gamma; \mathbf{X}) = L(\gamma; \mathbf{X} - \tilde{\mathbf{Z}}\hat{\beta}) L(\beta; \hat{\beta}, \gamma)$$

where $\gamma = (\gamma_D^t, \gamma_R^t)$ is the vector of all variance parameters and $\hat{\beta}$ is given by (6.5). One can then base the estimation of γ on the maximization of the restricted likelihood or residual likelihood

$$L(\gamma; \mathbf{X} - \tilde{\mathbf{Z}}\hat{\beta}) = \frac{L(\beta, \gamma; \mathbf{X})}{L(\beta; \hat{\beta}, \gamma)}$$

With some calculations, one can easily show that this restricted likelihood is proportional to

$$L(\gamma; \mathbf{X} - \tilde{\mathbf{Z}}\hat{\beta}) \propto \left| \tilde{\mathbf{Z}}^t V^{-1} \tilde{\mathbf{Z}} \right|^{-1/2} |V|^{-1/2} \exp\left[-\frac{1}{2} \left((\mathbf{X} - \tilde{\mathbf{Z}}\hat{\beta})^t V^{-1} (\mathbf{X} - \tilde{\mathbf{Z}}\hat{\beta}) \right) \right]$$
$$(6.6)$$

One can show that this restricted likelihood is actually the one we would have obtained by integrating the likelihood $L(\beta, \gamma; \mathbf{X})$ with respect to β, so *marginalizing* or *averaging* this likelihood with respect to β.

Since this restricted likelihood is a function of γ only, it can be maximized with respect to γ to obtain the REML estimates, which are then plugged-in into (6.5) to obtain estimates of β. Note that the difference between this restricted likelihood (6.6) and the likelihood (6.5) is a factor $|\tilde{\mathbf{Z}}^t V^{-1} \tilde{\mathbf{Z}}|^{-1/2}$ which actually corrects for the fact that the β had to be estimated (see (6.7) below). It is then possible to show that the estimates of the variance parameters obtained in this way are unbiased.

Whatever we consider the maximum likelihood (ML) or the restricted maximum likelihood (REML) approach, the maximization of the (restricted) likelihood with respect to γ lead to non-linear derivatives. There are therefore usually no closed form expression for the estimators of γ which must be obtained numerical optimization. The Newton-Raphson algorithm (implemented in linear-mixed effect models by [204]) and the EM algorithm (implemented in linear-mixed effect models by [233]) are probably the most two common choices.

From the expression (6.5), we can obtain the standard errors of of the estimated fixed effects regression coefficient calculating the variance of the generalized least-square estimator:

$$\hat{Var}(\hat{\beta}) = (\tilde{\mathbf{Z}}^t\hat{\mathbf{V}}^{-1}\tilde{\mathbf{Z}})^{-1} \tag{6.7}$$

in which $\hat{\mathbf{V}}$ is either the ML or the REML estimator. Note that this estimator require $\mathbf{V}$ to be correctly specified. A more robust sandwich estimator can also be used [405].

6.3.2   Model for the time-to-event outcome

Once we have modeled our true underlying longitudinal marker process $m_i(t)$, we need to model the association between this process and the risk of an event $h_i(t \mid \mathcal{M}_i(t), \mathbf{Z}_i)$, while potentially adjusting for time-independent covariates $\mathbf{Z}_i$ which are obviously not necessarily the same as the one included in the longitudinal model for the marker.

A first intuitive approach is to consider a relative risks model of the form

$$h_i(t \mid \mathcal{M}_i(t), \mathbf{Z}_i) = h_0(t) \exp\left(\eta^t\mathbf{Z}_i + \alpha m_i(t)\right) \tag{6.8}$$

in which α quantifies the strength of association between the underlying unobserved longitudinal process and the hazard of an event. The interpretation of η and α is the same as before; in particular α represents the increase risk in log-hazard at time t when $m_i(t)$ increases of one unit at this time t.

While we see from (6.8) that the risk of an event at time t depends only on the current value of the time-dependent longitudinal process $m_i(t)$, it is important to realize that this is not true for the survival function,

$$S_i(t \mid \mathcal{M}_i(t), \mathbf{Z}_i) = \exp\left(-\int_0^t h_0(s) \exp\left(\eta^t\mathbf{Z}_i + \alpha m_i(s)\right) ds\right) \tag{6.9}$$

which on the other hand depends on the whole underlying process $m_i(s)$ until time $s = t$. Therefore, this whole underlying process will have an impact on the estimation of the parameters since this survival function appears in the likelihood function for survival data.

As in a standard Cox PH model, the baseline hazard can either be left unspecified or specified parametrically. This latter option is usually preferred since it has been shown that leaving the baseline unspecified and maximizing the corresponding partial likelihood lead to underestimation of the standard errors of the parameters estimates [168, 320]. A parametric baseline hazard can be obtained by assuming a known parametric distribution for the event times, such as a Weibull or a log-normal, as explained in Section 2.5.1. However, more flexible options are often preferred and common choices assume a piecewise constant baseline hazard or use splines to model the baseline hazard function, see Section 2.5.1 of Chapter 2. In most applications, piecewise constant hazard has been shown to often works satisfactorily.

6.3.3 Estimation

The idea behind joint model is therefore to associate the time-to-event and the longitudinal marker processes and to define a model for their joint distribution. A key assumption is that the random effects actually capture all the dependencies between the two processes.

The *full conditional independence* assumption states that given the random effect

- the time-to-event and the longitudinal marker processes are independent

$$p(X_i, T_i, \delta_i \mid \mathbf{b}_i) = p(X_i \mid \mathbf{b}_i)p(T_i, \delta_i \mid \mathbf{b}_i)$$

- the repeated measurements of the longitudinal marker are independent of each other

$$p(X_i \mid \mathbf{b}_i) = \prod_{j=1}^{n_i} p(X_{ij} \mid \mathbf{b}_i)$$

One however has to be aware that testing for this conditional independence based on the observed data is difficult, if not impossible.

Note that mixed models methodology usually relies on assuming a normal distribution of the random effect. In a joint modeling context, since these random effects need to capture all association, their distribution may play a more prominent role and we may fear that the choice of this distribution is crucial. However, it has been show that the joint model are actually robust with respect to misspecification of the random effect distribution, especially when the number of measurements per subject increases [325].

Another important assumption is that both the censoring and the "visiting" processes are assumed to be non-informative. Rizopoulos [320] refers to the visiting process for the stochastic or deterministic mechanism that generates the time-points at which measurements are made for the longitudinal marker. So, the timing of withdrawal and of measurements of the marker may depend on the observed past history but there should not be additional dependence on latent subject characteristics associated with prognosis.

Under these assumptions, the (marginal) contribution of the ith individual to the likelihood, obtained after integrating out the unobserved random effects, is

$$L_i(\zeta) = \int p(X_i \mid \mathbf{b}_i) p(T_i, \delta_i \mid \mathbf{b}_i) p(\mathbf{b}_i) d\mathbf{b}_i$$

$$= \int \left[\prod_{j=1}^{n_i} p(X_{ij} \mid \mathbf{b}_i) \right] \left[h(T_i \mid \mathbf{b}_i)^{\delta_i} S(T_i \mid \mathbf{b}_i) \right] p(b_i) d\mathbf{b}_i \quad (6.10)$$

where $\mathbf{b}_i$ is the vector of random effects explaining the dependency between the two processes [320].

The (marginal) likelihood is then obtained by considering the product of these contributions over all individuals (since they are assumed to be independent). As can be seen, the likelihood function depends on the survival function which in turns, has shown in (6.9), depends on the whole longitudinal history. One therefore has to be very careful in the specification of the mixed model for this longitudinal history.

Estimation is usually based on the maximization of this (marginal) likelihood function, but Bayesian approaches have also been extensively studied in the literature (see Section 6.7). Indeed, a critical issue is that the likelihood based on the product of the contributions 6.10 contains two integrals, one over the unobserved random effect but also one over time in the survival function $S_i(.)$. These integrals usually can not be solved analytically and both need to be approximated numerically. The integral with respect to the random effect $\mathbf{b}_i$ may be challenging since it increases in dimension with the number of random effects. Standard numerical integration algorithm such as Gaussian quadrature, Laplace approximation, and pseudo-adaptive Gaussian quadrature rules are often used. The likelihood then needs to be maximized for the model parameter using an optimization algorithm such as the Newton-type algorithm. Since the random effects are not observed (latent), a popular alternative approach is to use the EM algorithm [320].

Based on standard theory for maximum likelihood estimators, we can obtain an estimate of the variance of the parameter estimates from the inverse of the observed information matrix. We can also rely on standard asymptotic tests (likelihood ratio tests, score test, Wald test, ...) as well as standard information criteria such as AIC and BIC.

Note that once the joint model has been fitted, it may be useful to obtain the posterior distribution of the random effects which according to the Bayes theorem is given by

$$p(\mathbf{b}_i \mid T_i, \delta_i; \zeta) = \frac{p(T_i, \delta_i \mid \mathbf{b}_i; \zeta) p(\tilde{y}_i \mid \mathbf{b}_i; \zeta) p(\mathbf{b}_i; \zeta)}{p(T_i, \delta_i, X_i; \zeta)}$$

in which ζ is replaced by $\hat{\zeta}$.

6.3.4   Association structure

As we have seen in Section 6.3.2, the standard shared random effect (joint) model (SREM) writes

$$h_i(t \mid \mathcal{M}_i(t), \mathbf{Z}_i) = h_0(t) \exp\left(\eta^t \mathbf{Z}_i + \alpha m_i(t)\right)$$

$$
\begin{aligned}
X_i(t) &= m_i(t) + \epsilon_i(t) \\
&= \tilde{\mathbf{Z}}_i \beta + \mathbf{W}_i \mathbf{b_i} + \epsilon_i
\end{aligned}
$$

and assumes that the risk of an event at time t depends only on the current value of the underlying time-dependent longitudinal process $m_i(t)$. However, this will often be too restrictive. Indeed, one may easily think of situations where the risk of event is more impacted by an increase or decrease in the biomarker rather than its current value. The risk of event could also be impacted by some cumulative summary measured rather than the value at a single time-point; for example the risk of developing lung cancer at a given time t is most certainly more impacted by the cumulative number of cigarettes smoked in the past until that time t rather than by the number of cigarettes smoked on time t.

In the following, we shortly present extensions of the standard shared random effects model (6.8) to other types of associations between the longitudinal marker and the time-to-event. These models differ in the choice of the summary measure of the longitudinal marker trajectory which is incorporated in the survival model. We can of course consider other possible models following the same idea.

Lagged effects: This model assumes that the hazard of an event at time t is associated with the level of the longitudinal marker at a previous time-point for some given lag c

$$h_i(t \mid \mathcal{M}_i(t), \mathbf{Z}_i) = h_0(t) \exp\left(\eta^t \mathbf{Z}_i + \alpha m_i(t_+^c)\right)$$

where $t_+^c = max(t - c, 0)$.

Time-dependent slopes: This model assumes that the hazard of an event at time t is associated both with the current value of the longitudinal marker at time t but also with the slope of the trajectory of the marker at time t

$$h_i(t \mid \mathcal{M}_i(t), \mathbf{Z}_i) = h_0(t) \exp\left(\eta^t \mathbf{Z}_i + \alpha_1 m_i(t) + \alpha_2 m_i'(t)\right)$$

where $m_i'(t) = \frac{d}{dt}(m_i(t))$. This will be particularly helpful when we expect that not only the value of the marker but also an increase (or decrease) in its value is of prognostic value. This will be the case of several blood markers for which a sudden increase may be more informative than the value itself.

Cumulative effects: This model assumes that the hazard of an event at time t is associated with the whole area under the trajectory of the longitudinal marker until time t

$$h_i(t \mid \mathcal{M}_i(t), \mathbf{Z}_i) = h_0(t) \exp\left(\eta^t \mathbf{Z}_i + \alpha \int_0^t m_i(s)ds \right)$$

In such a model, the hazard of an event is not depending on the value of the marker at a given time t but we actually consider a cumulative effect of the marker over time. This will be helpful to assess the impact of a cumulative exposure for example to a drug or to some other product (e.g. alcohol, tobacco or sugar consumption).

Weighted cumulative effects: This model is a refinement of the previous one, and assumes that the hazard of an event at time t is associated with the area under the weighted trajectory of the longitudinal marker until time t, for some appropriately chosen weight function $\omega(t)$.

$$h_i(t \mid \mathcal{M}_i(t), \mathbf{Z}_i) = h_0(t) \exp\left(\eta^t \mathbf{Z}_i + \alpha \int_0^t \omega(t - s)m_i(s)ds \right)$$

These weights can be used to consider the cumulative effect of the marker while giving some more importance to some time period, for example to the more recent values. Common choices are to consider for $\omega(.)$, a Gaussian or Student density.

Random effects: This model assumes that the hazard of an event at time t is associated only with the random effects of the longitudinal marker model

$$h_i(t \mid \mathcal{M}_i(t), \mathbf{Z}_i) = h_0(t) \exp\left(\eta^t \mathbf{Z}_i + \alpha^t \mathbf{b}_i \right)$$

While this model is a priori, more difficult to interpret, it is a popular option probably due to its easier mathematical tractability. Indeed, since the random effects $\mathbf{b}_i$ do not depend on time, it avoids the numerical integration for the survival function. However, the interpretation may be more difficult, especially when the dimension of the random effects vector increases. In the simple case where the random effects represent for each subject, the deviation in intercept and slope from an average trajectory (6.3); the idea is that what impact the hazard of an event is actually the magnitude of the deviation of the subject-specific trajectory from the average trajectory. A positive value of the parameter α could then be interpreted as a higher risk of event for subject who are further away from the average value.

6.4   The joint latent class approach

A nice and clear description of the JLCM is provided in Proust et al. [305, 306], on which this section is mainly based. The main idea behind the JLCM approach is to assume that the (heterogeneous) population is actually composed of a number of homogeneous subpopulations (classes) in such a way that given the class membership the survival and the longitudinal process are independent. The latent structure linking the longitudinal marker process and the time-to-event process is therefore a latent class membership, which is modeled via a multinomial logistic model.

A JLCM is therefore composed of a multinomial logistic regression model for the latent class membership probability, a model for the class-specific marker trajectory (usually a standard linear mixed model), and a class-specific survival model for the risk of events (usually a PH model). Therefore, each latent class is characterized by its own class-specific marker trajectory and its own class-specific risk of the event of interest. The key assumption is the conditional independence, i.e. the independence of the longitudinal marker measurements and the time-to event given the latent class.

6.4.1 Model for the latent class membership probability

We assume that the population can be divided into a finite number, say G, of latent homogeneous subgroups and we define the latent categorical variable $C_i = 1, \ldots, G$ representing the latent class membership of the ith individual. The probability of individual i to belong to the latent class $g, g = 1, \ldots, G$ is denoted π_{ig}. Considering a vector $\mathbf{Z}$ of time-independent covariates, a multinomial logistic regression model for π_{ig} is given by

$$\pi_{ig} = P(c_i = g \mid \mathbf{Z}_i) = \frac{\exp(\xi_{0g} + \mathbf{Z}_i^t \xi_{1g})}{\sum_{l=1}^{G} \exp(\xi_{0l} + \mathbf{Z}_i^t \xi_{1l})} \tag{6.11}$$

with ξ_{0g} is the intercept for class g, and ξ_{1g} the vector of class-specific parameter associated with $\mathbf{Z}$. For identifiability purposes, it is common to set $\xi_{0G} = \xi_{1G} = 0$.

6.4.2 Model for the class-specific marker trajectory

The longitudinal marker measurements $X_i = (X_i(t_1), \ldots, X_i(t_{ij}), \ldots, X_i(t_{in_i}))$ are actually modeled in a similar way as what is done in the SMER, so usually considering a standard linear mixed effect model, with the difference that the model is now class specific. Using the same notation as in Section 6.3, and considering first a simple linear mixed model with a random slope and a random intercept we therefore have for the latent class g

$$\begin{aligned} X_{ij} \mid_{c_i=g} &= m_{gi}(t) + \epsilon_{ij} \\ &= (\beta_{g0} + b_{gi0}) + (\beta_{g1} + b_{gi1})t_{ij} + \epsilon_{ij} \end{aligned} \tag{6.12}$$

with $\mathbf{b}_{ig} = (b_{gi0}, b_{gi1})^t = \mathbf{b}_{ig} \mid_{c_i=g}$ the vector of class-specific random effects, and it is common to assume that $\mathbf{b}_{ig} \sim N(0, \mathbf{D}_g)$. The errors terms ϵ_{ij} are also assumed to follow a normal distribution $N(0, \sigma_i^2)$.

This model can be extended to a more general formulation in the same way as for SREM with the only difference that we now have a class specific model

$$
\begin{aligned}
\mathbf{X}_i \mid_{c_i=g} &= m_{gi}(t) + \epsilon_i \\
&= \tilde{\mathbf{Z}}_i \beta_g + \mathbf{W}_i \mathbf{b}_{ig} + \epsilon_i
\end{aligned}
\tag{6.13}
$$

with $\mathbf{b}_{ig} \sim N(0, \mathbf{D}_g)$. The variance-covariance matrix $\mathbf{D}_g$ can be common to all classes or class-specific, but in this later case, Proust et al. [306] advise to limit the number of parameters by considering $\mathbf{D}_g = \omega_g^2 \mathbf{D}$ with $\mathbf{D}$ unstructured and $\omega_G = 1$ for identifiability. Also, the variance-covariance matrix Σ_i of the error terms is usually restricted to a diagonal matrix $\sigma^2 I_{n_i}$ for homescedastic individual errors but inclusion of covariance patterns could also be considered. As in Section 6.3, $\mathbf{b}_{ig}$ is the vector of random effects associated with the random effect design matrix $\mathbf{W}_i$ and β_g is the vector of fixed effects parameters associated with the design matrix $\tilde{\mathbf{Z}}_i$. Both the vector of random effects and the vector of fixed effect parameters are now class-specific, and are thus indexed by g. We have to be careful that this will obviously lead to a larger number of parameters to be estimated and this will have to be kept in mind when fitting such a model.

6.4.3   Model for the class-specific risk of event

While any standard survival model could be used, the PH model is most certainly the most commonly used. As for the longitudinal marker, the time-to-event model is class-specific. Considering a Cox PH model and a vector $X_e(t)$ of (possibly time-dependent) covariates, we have for the latent class g

$$
h_i(t \mid c_i = g; \eta_{\mathbf{g}}) = h_{0g}(t) exp(\eta_{\mathbf{g}}{}^t \mathbf{Z}_i(t))
\tag{6.14}
$$

where $\eta_{\mathbf{g}}$ is the class-specific vector of parameters associated with the (possibly time-dependent exogenous) covariates $\mathbf{Z}_i(t)$. If the baseline hazard $h_{0g}(.)$ is fully parametric then its associated parameters are also class-specific. This baseline hazard can also be either be stratified for the latent class structure or specified as proportional baseline hazards in each latent class with $h_{0g}(t) = h_0(t)e^{\xi_g}$ (with $\xi_G = 0$ for identifiability). In order to be able to estimate the JCLM via likelihoood maximization, it is common to assume a parametric hazard function, such as a Weibull baseline hazard or some more flexible options such as considering a piecewise constant hazard or using M-Splines to model it [305].

6.4.4   Estimation

Assuming a parametric baseline hazard in the class-specific models for the risk of events, the estimation of a JLCM for a fixed number of latent classes G can be performed via maximum likelihood.

Based on the conditional independence assumption and assuming a fixed number of classes G, the contribution of the $i^t h$ individual to the likelihood can be obtained as :

$$
\begin{aligned}
L_i(\zeta_G) &= \sum_{g=1}^{G} \pi_{ig} f_M(X_i \mid c_i = g; \zeta_G) f_T(T_i \mid c_i = g; \zeta_G) \\
&= \sum_{g=1}^{G} \pi_{ig} f(X_i \mid c_i = g; \zeta_G) h_i(T_i \mid c_i = g; \zeta_G)^{\delta_i} S_i(T_i \mid c_i = g; \zeta)
\end{aligned}
$$

where the vector ζ_G contains all the parameters for the JLCM with G classes, π_{ig} is the probability for this individual to belong to class g, $f_M(. \mid c_i = g; \zeta_G)$ is the class-specific density function for the marker, and $f_T(. \mid c_i = g; \zeta_G)$ is the class-specific density function for the event time. Given the usual relationship (1.3), this density for the time-to-event can be re-written based on the conditional hazard and survival function. Assuming model (6.13) for the longitudinal marker, the density function $f(X_i \mid c_i = g; \theta_G)$ in class g is a multivariate normal $N(\tilde{\mathbf{Z}}_i \beta_g + \mathbf{W}_i \mathbf{b}_{ig}, \tilde{\mathbf{Z}}_i \mathbf{D}_g \tilde{\mathbf{Z}}_i^t + \Sigma_i)$.

The log-likelihood for a fixed number of latent classes G is the given by

$$
l(\zeta_G) = \sum_{i=1}^{N} \log\left(L_i(\zeta_G)\right)
$$

and can be maximized using an optimization algorithm such as the (modified) Marquardt algorithm [247]. Variances of the estimated parameters can be obtained from the inverse of the Hessian matrix.

Although the maximum likelihood estimation approach is quite straightforward for the JLCM, Proust et al. [306] discuss several issues inherent to mixture models that may be problematic for the estimation of a JLCM. A well known phenomenon encountered when estimating a mixture model is the problem of "label switching". However, it has been shown that while this may be an issue with Bayesian estimation techniques [361] this is not a problem for maximum likelihood estimation [316]. Another difficulty which may arise when trying to fit a mixture model is that this estimation becomes in some contexts problematic due to a lack of information in the data. This is however less a concern in the context of JLCM for which the latent class structure is based on more information with observations for both the longitudinal marker and the time-to-event. A more problematic issue is that likelihood of mixture models often have multiple local maxima. It is therefore highly recommended when fitting a JLCM to ensure that the global maximum is indeed reached. A practical option is to run the maximization algorithm several times with different starting values. Besides these issues, we refer to [305] for a validation of the JCLM estimation procedure via an extensive simulation study.

From a more conceptual point of view, it is important to keep in mind that estimation of the models parameters is made assuming a fixed number of classes. The model will therefore typically needs to be fitted for different values of G and selection of the appropriate number of classes will be a key issue. This optimal number of classes is most often determined using the BIC, which is defined as

$$BIC(G) = -2l(\theta_G) + n_\theta \log(N)$$

where n_ζ is the number of estimated parameters. The BIC has indeed been shown to be more appropriate in the context of mixture models [155]. Other criteria are discussed by [151] in the context of JLCM. Note however, that the selection of the optimal number of classes should not be based only on such an information criterion. A key point should also be how well the conditional independence assumption is fulfilled; a model with a better BIC but for which the conditional independence assumption is not met should not be preferred to a model with a higher BIC but for which this assumption is better verified (see [306] for an example). Other criteria to be taken into account are the quality of predictions and of the discrimination between the classes as well, if possible, whether meaningful latent classes are obtained.

6.5   JCLM versus SREM

While we have seen that the SREM require to precisely define the type of link between the longitudinal markers and the time-to-event processes, this is not the case for the JLCM in which the link between the two processed remain unobserved. Depending on the research question of interest, this may be seen either as an advantage of a disadvantage. Obviously, the JLCM will not be the method of choice if our goal is to evaluate a specific assumption regarding the type and strength of association between the two processes; contrary to the SREM, the JLCM does not include any association parameters to interpret. On the other hand, if our objective lies in the construction of a predictive joint model, with no real interest on the association itself, then the JLCM will prevent us from having to appropriately specify the type of association. If the JCLM approach does not provide any information on the association structure, we can on the other easily obtain from this model the posterior class-membership probabilities given all the observations for the markers and the occurence of the event. Such probabilities may be useful if there is an interest in buidling a posterior classification of the individuals under study.

It has been argued that a disadvantage of the JCLM is that it requires multiple fits to find the optimal number of classes, which is typically done comparing the model fit for different number of classes with an information criteria such as the BIC. This is obviously not necessary for the SREM, but without a good a priori information on the type of link between the longitudinal markers and the time-to-event processes, we may have to fit several models with different association structure to choose the one with the best fit or use some other model selection strategy [20].

The fact that the marker trajectory are modeled via a class-specific model in the JCLM approach rather than with a global model for all individuals in the SREM also has pro's and con's. On one hand, with sufficient sample size we can probably achieve a better fit when considering class-specific model but it obviously requires the estimation of the more parameters and we may have to "give up" some flexibility in the modeling by adding some constraints if the sample size does not allow an appropriate estimation of all the parameters.

From a computational point of views, the JCLM approach avoids the need for (high-dimensional) numerical integration but on the other hand maximization of the likelihood may raise some issue such as falling into a local maximum.

Both approaches allows to perform individual dynamic predictions [305, 306, 309, 320]. Both appraoches have been extended to a categorical longitudinal marker and both approaches have been extended to multiple longitudinal markers (see Section 6.7). Finally, as we will see in the next section, both approaches have been implemented in R packages and can therefore be readily used.

6.6   Software

The extended Cox (or Andersen-Gill) model can be fitted in R using the start/stop specifications in the coxph function of the survival package. The data however needs to be in a long format, see [260, 320].

Joint models can be used either with a focus on the time-to-event outcome, and offers than the possibility to capture the impact of a endogenous time-dependent covariates possibly measured with error or with a focus on the longitudinal marker while correcting for non-random dropout due to the occurence of the event. We have introduced the two main families of joint models described in the literature: the SREM and the JCLM. Both approaches can be implemented in the R software using existing packages.

The SREM for a longitudinal marker and a time-to-event outcome can be fitted either with the JM package [321], which rely mainly on frequentist methods or with JMbayes [322] for a Bayesian approach. The JM package allows to fit different SREM for a normal longitudinal continuous marker with different choice for the survival model. One can specify for the latter, a Cox PH model, a parametric Weibull model either under the PH or the AFT formulation (see Section 2.5.2 of Chapter 2) or a flexible parametric PH model in which the baseline hazard function is modeled as piecewise constant or approximated via B-splines (see Section 2.5.1 of Chapter 2). For all these models, the Gauss-Hermite quadrature or a pseudo Gauss-Hermite integration rule can be used to approximate the required integrals [319]. In addition, an additive log-cumulative hazard model, in which the log-cumulative baseline hazard is approximated with B-splines is also available [324]. Regarding the association structure, we can include in the survival model, the current value $m(t)$ or the slope $m'(t)$ of the longitudinal process or both and each can be computed at the actual time t or with some lag effect $(t - k)$ to be specified. The model is then fitted based on the maximization of the algorithm based on the EM algorithm or on a combination of the EM and the Newton-Raphson algorithm. The JM is based on nlme R package [298, 299] and on the survival package for the specification of the longitudinal and survival model respectively. The nlme package allows to fit a wide range of linear and non-linear mixed models for a continuous longitudinal marker. Of note, the lme4 package [30] can also be used to fit a mixed models for a longitudinal markers but also fit generalized linear mixed models for categorical markers.

Besides these two popular R packages, SREM for a time-to-event and a longitudinal outcome can also be fitted with the joineR R package [297]. The longitudinal outcome is modeled using a linear mixed effects model while the time-to-event model is a Cox PH model with time varying covariate and including a log-normal frailty. Contrary to the package JM the association here is modeled by allowing the normal random effects of the linear mixed model to be correlated with the frailty term from the survival model [158, 411]. The model is estimated using an EM algorithm. This package further extends the SREM approach to the case of competing risks considering then a proportional cause-specific hazards model (see Section 5.5.1 of Chapter 5).

The JLCM approach is implemented in the lcmm R package [307, 308]. This package allows to fit joint latent class models for either a continuous (Gaussian or not) or a discrete or categorical longitudinal outcome. The baseline hazard function of the survival PH model can be specified as a parametric Weibull baseline hazard, as piecewise constant or approximated via cubic M-splines [309]. All models are fitted based on the maximization of the likelihood (using a modified Marquadt algorithm [247]). Note that this package actually allows to fit other extensions of the mixed models not covered in this book.

While SAS has a long history in fitting (generalized) linear mixed models with several build-in functions (see for example [363, 364]), the estimation of a joint model for a longitudinal and a time-to-event endpoint has to be performed via specific macros, such as the %JM [1, 128] and the %JMFit macros. The %JM macro allows to fit a wide range for SREM models considering a continuous marker but allowing also for a binary, binomial or Poisson longitudinal marker, with a trajectory modeled as a linear function or via more flexible functions approximated via splines. The time-to-event model is a parametric PH model (possibly stratified) with an exponential, Weibull, piecewise exponential baseline hazard but also allows generalizations of the Weibull and the Gompertz models based on splines. Also, one has the possibility to choose between different structures of association among the current-value-dependent and slope-dependent shared parameters, lagging effects, cumulative effects, random effects coefficients as shared parameters and interaction effects. The estimation procedure is performed via the `SAS proc nlmixed` function which allows to approximate the marginal likelihood using adaptive or non-adaptive Gauss-Hermite quadrature and to maximize it using different optimization techniques (the default being a dual Quasi-Newton algorithm).

6.7 Further reading

Extensive material on the SREM and available packages can be accessed on Dimitris Rizopoulos website (www.drizopoulos.com). More details and extensive real data analyses (using mainly `JM` and `JMbayes` R packages) are also presented in his book [320]. Note that a lot of work on SREM has been done also in a Bayesian context, in particular relying on an MCMC algorithm appears to be very popular in this situation (see for example [120]). Several of the references given in this section are actually based on Bayesian estimation procedure.

Several extension of the SREM, and probably to a lesser extent of the JLCM, have been proposed to tackle various encountered issue either regarding the longitudinal process (non-normally distributed longitudinal marker, multiple longitudinal marker) or the time-to-event process (multivariate survival data [69], competing risks [267, 113, 112], presence of a cure fraction [28, 66, 357], ...). The key point in all these extensions is to properly states the conditional independence assumption and in the case of the SREM to handle the numerical integration required to obtain the likelihood function to be maximized. The joint modeling of a recurrent event and possibly a terminal event [200, 332] can also be seen as an extension of these models.

The SREM discussed in Section 6.3 has been originally developed for a single continuous longitudinal marker. However, the SREM can be extended to other types of marker by replacing the (linear) mixed model by a generalized (linear) mixed model (GLMM) [1, 401]. Such a model assumes that the longitudinal marker follows a distribution from the exponential family with mean

$$m_i(t) = E(X_{ij}(t)) = g^{-1}(\mathbf{Z}_i\beta + \mathbf{W}_i\mathbf{b}_i)$$

were $g(.)$ is an appropriate link function (see for example [258]). While the idea remains the same, we may face some additional computational issues. Having in mind that the normal distribution is part of the family of exponential family, the standard SREM can be seen as a particular case of this model.

The SREM have been extended to take into account multiple longitudinal markers, possibly of different types (see for example [162, 251, 323, 408, 427]).

Indeed, while have considered a single longitudinal marker, we may face situation where we actually have information on several longitudinal markers, of which some can be continuous and some categorical. In this case, the standard SREM can be extended by considering a generalized (linear) mixed model for each longitudinal marker. The correlation between the different longitudinal markers is obtained from assuming a multivariate normal distribution for the random effects involved in the longitudinal model of each marker. One can then incorporate the impact of each of these longitudinal marker as multiple linear predictor in the survival model. Such an extension to multiple longitudinal markers is straightforward as long as we assume full conditional independence, which assumes that conditional on the random effects:

- the repeated measurements for each longitudinal markers are independent;

- the longitudinal markers are independent of each other;

- the longitudinal markers are independent of the time-to-event outcome.

In other words, we assume that the random effects (which are allowed to be correlated) capture all the dependencies between the different measurements of the different outcome. Again, this assumption is crucial but difficult to ascertain. Also, while this extension to multiple outcome is in theory straightforward, it can quickly become very computational intensive due to the high-dimensional numerical integration over the random effects.

While SREM are usually based on a relative risks model, this may not always be appropriate. The extended Cox model used in the standard SREM can actually be replaced by any survival models for which an extension to time-dependent covariate exists. For example, one may consider the extension of the AFT model to time-dependent covariates proposed by [91]. This leads to a SREM similar to our standard SREM in which the model for the hazard is replaced by

$$h_i(t \mid \mathcal{M}_i(t), \mathbf{Z}_i) = h_0 \left(\int_0^t \exp(\eta^t \mathbf{Z}_i + \alpha m_i(s)) ds \right) \exp\left(\eta^t \mathbf{Z}_i + \alpha m_i(t)\right)$$

Over the last decade, there has been a huge interest on the SREM and various extensions have been presented in the literature. The JLCM, although probably a bit less popular, has also led to several applications and most of the extensions discussed above are also valid for the JLCM. The success of SREM is certainly due to the possibility to easily extend it to more than two outcomes (of possibly different types), the (relatively easy) implementation and the simplicity of the interpretation. However, this comes at the price of the conditional independence assumptions, which can usually not be tested with data at hand. One also has to keep in mind that extending the SREM in a way that increase the number of random effects will require more computer intensive algorithms for the resolution of the integrals in the definition of the algorithms.

Bibliography

[1] A. Garcia-Hernandez and D. Rizopoulos. %JM: A SAS macro to fit jointly generalized mixed models for longitudinal data and time-to-event responses. *Journal of Statistical Software, Articles*, 84:1–29, 2018.

[2] O.O. Aalen. Nonparametric inference for a family of counting processes. *The Annals of Statistics*, 6:701–726, 1978.

[3] O.O. Aalen. Heterogeneity in survival analysis. *Statistics in Medicine*, 7:1121–1137, 1988.

[4] O.O. Aalen. Modelling heterogeneity in survival analysis by the compound Poisson distribution. *Annals of Applied Probability*, 2:951–972, 1992.

[5] A. Allignol. *Kmi: Kaplan-Meier multiple imputation for the analysis of cumulative incidence functions in the competing risks setting*, 2019. version 0.5.5.

[6] A. Allignol and J. Beyersmann. Software for fitting nonstandard proportional subdistribution hazards models. *Biostatistics*, 11:674–675, 2010.

[7] A. Allignol and A. Latouche. CRAN Task View: Survival Analysis. 2020.

[8] P.D. Allison. *Survival Analysis Using SAS: A Practical Guide. Second Edition*. SAS Press, Cary North Carolina, 2010.

[9] B. Altshuler. Theory for the measurement of competing risks in animal experiments. *Mathematical Biosciences*, 6:1–11, 1970.

[10] M. Amico and I. Van Keilegom. Cure models in survival analysis. *Annual Review of Statistics and Its Application*, 5:311–342, 2018.

[11] M. Amico, I. Van Keilegom, and C. Legrand. The single-index/Cox mixture cure model. *Biometrics*, doi: 10.1111/biom.12999. [Epub ahead of print], 2018b.

[12] E.W. Andersen. Statistical models based on counting process. *Lifetime Data Analysis*, 11:333–350, 2005.

[13] P. Andersen, O. Borgan, R. Gill, and N. Keiding. *Statistical Models Based on Counting Processes*. New-York: Springer-Verlag, 1993.

[14] P.K. Andersen. Decomposition of number of life years lost according to causes of death. *Statistics in Medicine*, 32:5278–5285, 2013.

[15] P.K. Andersen and O. Borgan. Counting process models for life history data: a review. *Scandinavian Journal of Statistics*, 12:97–158, 1985.

[16] P.K. Andersen and R.D. Gill. Cox's regression model for counting processes: a large sample study. *The Annals of Statistics*, 10:1100–1120, 1982.

[17] P.K. Andersen, L.S. Hansen, and N. Keiding. Nonparametric and semi-parametric estimation of transition-probabilities from censored observation of a nonhomogeneous Markov process. *Scandinavian Journal of Statistics*, 18:153–167, 1985.

[18] J.E. Anderson and T.A. Louis. Survival analysis using a Scale Change Random Effect Model. *Journal of the American Statistical Association*, 90:669–679, 1995.

[19] T.M.L. Andersson and P.C. Lambert. Fitting and modeling cure in population-based cancer studies within the framework of flexible parametric survival models. *The Stata Journal*, 12:623–638, 2012.

[20] E.R. Andrinopoulou and D. Rizopoulos. Bayesian shrinkage approach for a joint model of longitudinal and survival outcomes assuming different association structures. *Statistics in Medicine*, 35:4813–4823, 2016.

[21] K.E. Atkinson. *An Introduction to Numerical Analysis*. John Wiley & Sons, Inc., Second Edition. Wiley & Sons. New York, 1989.

[22] R. Bajorunaite and J.P. Klein. Comparison of failure probabilities in the presence of competing risks. *Journal of Statistical Computation and Simulation*, 78:951–966, 2008.

[23] G. Bakoyannis and G. Touloumi. Practical methods for competing risks data: a review. *Statistical Methods in Medical Research*, 21:257–272, 2010.

[24] T.A. Balan and H. Putter. *FrailtyEM: Fitting frailty models with the EM algorithm*, 2017. version 0.8.2.

[25] T.A. Balan and H. Putter. FrailtyEM: an R package for estimating semi-parametric shared frailty models. *Journal of Statistical Software*, 90:1–29, 2019.

[26] T.A. Balan and H. Putter. Non-proportional hazards and unobserved heterogeneity in clustered survival data: When can we tell the difference? *Statistics in Medicine*, 38:3405–3420, 2019.

[27] T.A. Balan and H. Putter. A tutorial on frailty models. *Statistical Methods in Medical Research*, 29: 3424–3454, 2020.

[28] A. Barbieri and C. Legrand. Joint longitudinal and time-to-event cure models for the assessment of being cured. *Statistical Methods in Medical research*, 29:1256–1270, 2019.

[29] J.K. Barrett, F. Siannis, and V.T. Farewell. A semi-competing risks model for data with interval-censoring and informative observation: An application to the MRC cognitive function and ageing study. *Statistics in Medicine*, 30:1–10, 2010.

[30] D. Bates, M. Maechler, B. Bolker, and S. Walker. *Lme4: Linear mixed-effects models using 'Eigen' and S4*, 2020. version 1.1-23.

[31] J. Benichou and M.H. Gail. Estimates of absolute cause-specific risk in cohort studies. *Biometrics*, 46:813–826, 1990.

[32] S. Bennett. Analysis of survival data by the proportional odds model. *Statistics in Medicine*, 2:273–277, 1983.

[33] S.M. Bentzen, M. Vaeth, D.E. Pedersen, and J. Overgaard. Why actu-arial estimates should be used in reporting late normal-tissue effects of cancer treatment. *International Journal of Radiation Oncology, Biology, Physics*, 32:1531–1534, 1995.

[34] R. Beran. Nonparametric regression with randomly censored survival data. *Technical Report, University of California, Berkley*, 1981.

[35] J. Berkson and R. Gage. Survival curve for cancer patients following treatment. *Journal of the American Statistical Association*, 47:501–515, 1952.

[36] A. Bertrand, C. Legrand, R.J. Carroll, C. De Meester, and I. Van Kei-legom. Inference in a survival cure model with mismeasured covariates. *Biometrika*, 104:31–50, 2017.

[37] A. Bertrand, C. Legrand, D. Leonrad, and I. Van Keilegom. Robust-ness of estimation methods in a survival cure model with mismeasured covariates. *Computational Statistics and Data Analysis*, 113:3–18, 2017.

[38] A. Bertrand, C. Legrand, and I. Van Keilegom. *MiCoPTCM: Promotion time cure model with mis-measured covariates*, 2016. version 1.0.

[39] R.A. Betensky and D.A. Schoenfeld. Nonparametric estimation in a cure model with random cure times. *Biometrics*, 57:282–286, 2001.

[40] J. Beyersmann, A. Allignol, and M. Schumacher. *Competing Risks ad Multistate models with R, use R! First Edition*. New-York: Springer-Verlag, 2012.

[41] J. Beyersmann and Schumacher M. Time-dependent covariates in the proportional subdistribution hazards model for competing risks. *Biostatistics*, 9:765–776, 2008.

[42] K. Bogaerts, A. Komarek, and E. Lesaffre. *Survival Analysis with Interval-Censored Data: A Practical Approach with Examples in R, SAS, and BUGS*. Chapman & Hall/CRC Interdisciplinary Statistics Series, 2017.

[43] T.M. Braun and Yuan Z. Comparing the small sample performance of several variance estimators under competing risks. *Statistics in Medicine*, 26:1170–1180, 2007.

[44] V. Bremhorst, M. Kreyenfeld, and P. Lambert. Fertility progression in Germany: An analysis using flexible nonparametric cure survival models. *Demographic Research*, 35(18):505–534, 2016.

[45] V. Bremhorst and P. Lambert. Flexible estimation in cure survival models using Bayesian P-splines. *Computational Statistics and Data Analysis*, 93:270–284, 2016.

[46] N.E. Breslow. Contribution to the discussion of a paper by D.R. Cox. *Journal of the Royal Statistical Society, Series B*, 34:216–217, 1972.

[47] J. Bretagnolle and C. Huber-Carol. Effects of omitting covariates in cox's model for survival data. *Scandinavian Journal of Statistics*, 15:125–138, 1988.

[48] B.M. Brown and Y.G. Wang. Induced smoothing for rank regression with censored survival times. *Statistics in Medicine*, 26:828–836, 2006.

[49] H. Brown and R. Prescott. *Applied Mixed Models in Medicine, Second Edition*. John Wiley & Sons, Ltd, 2006.

[50] J. Bryant and J.J. Dignam. Semiparametric models for cumulative incidence function. *Biometrics*, 60:182–190, 2004.

[51] A. Buja, T. Hastie, and R Tibshirani. Linear smoothers and additive models. *The Annals of Statistics*, 17:453–555, 1989.

[52] B. Cai. Bayesian semiparametric frailty selection in multivariate event time data. *Biometrical Journal*, 52:171–85, 2010.

[53] C. Cai, S. Wang, W. Lu, and J. Zhang. NPHMC: An R-package for estimating sample size of proportional hazards mixture cure models. *Computer Methods and Programs in Biomedicine*, 113:290–300, 2012.

[54] C. Cai, S. Wang, W. Lu, and J. Zhang. *NPHMC*, 2013. version 2.2.

[55] C. Cai, Y. Zou, Y. Peng, and J. Zhang. Smcure: An R-package for estimating semiparametric mixture cure models. *Computer Methods and Programs in Biomedicine*, 108:1255–1260, 2012.

[56] C. Cai, Y. Zou, Y. Peng, and J. Zhang. *Smcure: Fit semiparametric mixture cure models*, 2012. version 2.0.

[57] K.C. Cain and N.T. Lange. Approximate case influence for the proportional hazards regression model with censored data. *Biometrics*, 40:493–499, 1984.

[58] K.L. Calkins, C.E. Canan, C.R. Moore, R.D. an Lesko, and B. Lau. An application of restricted mean survival time in a competing risks setting: comparing time to ART initiation by injection rug use. *BMC Medical Research Methodology*, 18, 2018.

[59] R.J. Caplan, T.F. Pajak, Cox, J.D. In response to Benzen et al., IJROBP 32: 1531–1534, 1995. *International Journal of Radiation Oncology, Biology, Physics*, 32: 1547, 1995.

[60] S.H. Chang. Estimating marginal effects in accelerated failure time models for serial sojurn times among repeated events. *Lifetime Data Analysis*, 10:175–190, 2004.

[61] R. Chappell. RE: Caplan et al. and Bentzen et al. *Int J Radiat Oncol Biol Phys*, 36:988–989, 1996.

[62] R. Chappell. Competing risk analyses: how are they different and why should you care. *Clinical Cancer Research*, 18:2127–2129, 2012.

[63] D.G. Chen, Peace K.E., and P. Zhang. *Clinical Trial Data Analysis Using R and SAS*. Chapman & Hall/CRC Biostatistics Series, 2017.

[64] D.G. Chen, J. Sun, and Peace K.E. *Interval-Censored Time-to-Event Data: Methods and Applications*. Chapman & Hall/CRC Biostatistics Series, 2012.

[65] M.H. Chen, J.G. Ibrahim, and D. Sinha. A new bayesian model for survival data with a surviving fraction. *Journal of the American Statistical Association*, 94:909–919, 1999.

[66] M.H. Chen, J.G. Ibrahim, and D. Sinha. Journal of Multivariate Analysis. A new joint model for longitudinal and survival data with a cure fraction. *Journal of Multivariate Analysis*, 91:18–34, 2004.

[67] Y.Q. Chen and M.C. Wang. Analysis of accelerated hazards models. *Journal of the American Statistical Association*, 95:608–618, 2000.

[68] S.C. Cheng, J.P. Fine, and L.J. Wei. Prediction of the cumulative incidence function under the proportional hazards model. *Biometrics*, 54:219–228, 1998.

[69] Y.Y. Chi and G. Ibrahim. Joint models for multivariate longitudinal and multivariate survival data. *Biometrics*, 62:432–445, 2006.

[70] S. Chiou, S. Kang, and J. Yan. Fitting accelerated failure time model in routine survival analysis with R package aftgee. *Journal of Statistical Software*, 61:1–23, 2014.

[71] S. Chiou, S. Kang, and J. Yan. Rank-based estimating equations with general weight for accelerated failure time models: an induced smoothing approach. *Statistics in Medicine*, 34:1495–1510, 2015.

[72] S.H. Chiou, S. Kang, and J. Yan. *Aftgee: Accelerated failure time model with generalized estimating equations*, 2020. version 1.1.5.

[73] S. Choi, L. Zhu, and X. Huang. Semiparametric accelerated failure time cure rate mixture models with competing risks. *Statistics in Medicine*, 37:48–59, 2018.

[74] G. Claeskens, R. Nguti, and P. Janssen. One-sided tests in shared frailty models. *TEST*, 17:69–82, 2008.

[75] D. Clayton. A model for association in bivariate life tables and its application in epidemiological studies of familial tendency in chronic diseasde incidence. *Biometrika*, 65:141–151, 1978.

[76] W.S. Cleveland. Robust locally weighted regression and smoothing scatterplots. *Journal of the American Statistical Association*, 74:829–836, 1979.

[77] M. Cleves, W.W. Gould, and Y.V. Marchenko. *An Introduction to Survival Analysis Using STATA. Revised Third Edition*. Stata Press, 2016.

[78] D. Collett. *Modelling Survival Data in Medical Research. Third Edition*. Chapman & Hall/CRC Press, 2014.

[79] D. Commenges and P.K. Andersen. Score test of homogeneity for survival data. *Lifetime Data Analysis*, 1:145–156, 1995.

[80] J.R. Cook and L.A. Stefanski. Simulation-extrapolation in parametric measurement error models. *Journal of the American Statistical Association*, 89:1314–1328, 1994.

[81] F Cooner, S Banerjee, B. Carlin, and D. Sinha. Flexible cure rate modeling under latent activation scheme. *Journal of the American Statistical Association*, 102:560–572, 2017.

[82] F. Corbière, D. Commenges, J. Taylor, and P. Joly. A penalized likelihood approach for mixture cure models. *Statistics in Medicine*, 28:510–524, 2009.

[83] F. Corbiére and P. Joly. Pspmcm a sas macro for survival models with a cured fraction (mixture cure models).

[84] F. Corbière and P. Joly. A SAS macro for parametric and semi-parametric mixture cure models. *Computer Methods and Programs in Biomedicine*, 85:173–180, 2007.

[85] G. Cortese and P.K. Andersen. Competing risks and time-dependent covariates. *Biometrical Journal*, 51:138–158, 2009.

[86] J. Cortinas-Abrahantes and T. Burzykowski. A version of the EM algorithm for proportional hasards model with random effects. *Biometrical Journal*, 47:847–862, 2005.

[87] J. Cortinas-Abrahantes, C Legrand., T. Burzykowski, P. Janssen, V. Ducrocq, and L. Duchateau. Comparison of different estimation procedures for proportional hazards model with random effects. *Computational Statistics and Data Analysis*, 51:3913–3930, 2007.

[88] C. Cox, H. Chu, M.F. Schneider, and A. Munoz. Parametric survival analysis and taxonomy of hazard functions for the generalized gamma distribution. *Statistic in Medicine*, 26:4352–4374, 2007.

[89] D. Cox. Regression models and life tables (with discussion). *Journal of the Royal Statistical Society, Series B*, 74:187–220, 1972.

[90] D. Cox. Partial Likelihood. *Biometrika*, 62:269–276, 1975.

[91] D. Cox and D. Oakes. *Analysis of Survival Data*. London: Chapman & Hall, 1984.

[92] D.R Cox and E.J. Snell. A general definition of residuals (with discussion). *Journal of the Royal Statistical Society, Series A*, 30:248–275, 1968.

[93] M.J. Crowder. *Multivariate Survival Analysis and Competing Risks*. Chapman & Hall/CRC Press, New-York, 2012.

[94] M. Davidian. Longitudinal data analysis. In *Non-linear Mixed-effects Models. Eds. G. Fitzmaurice, M. Davidian, G. Verbeke, G. Molenberghs. Boca Raton: Chapman & Hall/CRC Press*, 2009.

[95] M. Davidian and D.M. Giltinan. Nonlinear models for repreated measurement data: an overview and update. *JABES*, 8:387–419, 2003.

[96] B. De Moerloose, S Suciu, and et al. Bertrand, Y. Improved outcome with pulses of vincristine and corticosteroids in continuation therapy of children with average risk acute lymphoblastic leukaemia (ALL) and lymphoblastic non-Hodgkin lymphoma (NHL): report of the EORTC randomized phase 3 trial 58951. *Blood*, 116:36–44, 2010.

[97] L.C. de Wreede, M. Fiocco, and H. Putter. mstate: An R package for the analysis of competing risks and multi-state models. *Journal of Statistical Software*, 38:1–30, 2011.

[98] L.C. de Wreede, M. Fiocco, and H. Putter. The mstate package for estimation and prediction in non- and semi-parametric multi-state and competing risks models. *Computer Methods and Programs in Biomedicine*, 99:261–274, 2011.

[99] C. Delbaldo, M. Ychou, J.Y. Douillard, T. André, V. Guerin-Meyer, P. Rougier, O. Dupuis, R. Faroux, A. Jouhaud, E. Quinaux, M. Buyse, P. Piedbois, AERO, GERCOR, FNLCC, and FFCD. Postoperative irinotecan in resected stage II-III rectal cancer: final analysis of the French R98 Intergoup trial. *Annals of Oncology*, 26:1208–1215, 2015.

[100] A.P. Dempster, N.M. Laird, and D.B. Rubin. Maximum likelihood from incomplete data with the EM algorithm (with discussion). *Journal of the Royal Statistical Society, Serie B*, 39:1–38, 1977.

[101] J.W. Denham, C.S Hamilton, and P. O'Brien. Regarding actuarial late effect analyses: Bentzen et al. IJROBP 32: 1531-1534; 1995 and Caplan et al. IJROBP 32: 1547; 1995. *Int J Radiat Oncol Biol Phys*, 35:197, 1996.

[102] J.J. Dignam and M.N. Kocherginsky. Choice and interpetation of statistical tests used when competing risks are present. *Journal of Clinical Oncoloy*, 26:4027–4034, 2008.

[103] J.J. Dignam, Q. Zhang, and M.N. Kocherginsky. The use and interpretation of competing risks regression models. *Clinical Cancer Research*, 18:2301–2308, 2012.

[104] C. Domenech, S Suciu, and et al. De Moerloose, B. Dexamethasone (6 $mg/m^2/day$) and prednisolone ($60mg/m^2/day$) were equally effective as induction therapy for childhood acute lymphoblastic leukemia in the EORTC CLG 58951 randomized trial. *Haematologica*, 99:1220–1227, 2014.

[105] D.M. dos Santos, R.B. Davies, and B. Francis. Nonparametric hazard versus nonparametric frailty distribution in modelling recurrence of breast cancer. *Journal of Statistical Planning and Inference*, 47:111–127, 1995.

[106] L. Duchateau and P. Janssen. Understanding heterogeneity in generalized mixed and frailty models. *The American Statistician*, 59:143–146, 2005.

[107] L. Duchateau and P. Janssen. *The Frailty Model*. Springer, New York 2008.

[108] B. Efron. The efficiency of Cox's likelihood function for censored data. *Journal of the American Statistical Association*, 72:557–565, 2005.

[109] A.M. Eggermont, S. Suciu, and M. Santinami, et al Adjuvant therapy with pegylated interferon alfa-2b versus observation alone in resected stage III melanoma: Final results of EORTC 18991, a randomised phase III trial. *Lancet*, 372:117–126, 2008.

[110] A.M. Eggermont, S. Suciu, and A. Testori, et al. Long-term results of the randomized phase III trial EORTC 18991 of adjuvant therapy with pegylated interferon alfa-2b versus observation alone in resected stage III melanoma. *Journal of Clinical Oncology*, 30:3810–3818, 2012.

[111] A.M. Eggermont, S. Suciu, and A. Testori, et al. Ulceration and stage are predictive of interferon efficacy in melanoma: Results of the phase III adjuvant trials EORTC 18952 and EORTC 18991. *European Journal of Cancer*, 48:218–225, 2012.

[112] R. Elashoff, G. Li, and Li N. A joint model for longitudinal measurements and survival data in the presence of multiple failure types. *Biometrics*, 64:762–771, 1982.

[113] R. Elashoff, G. Li, and N. LI. An approach to joint analysis of longitudinal measurements and competing risks failure time data. *Statistics in Medicine*, 26:2813–2835, 1982.

[114] R. Elashoff, G. Li, and N. LI. *Joint Modeling of Longitudinal and Time-to-Event Data*. Chapman & Hall/CRC Press, Boca Raton 2012.

[115] C. Elbers and G. Ridder. True and spurious duration dependence: the identifiability of the proportional hazard model. *Rev. Economic Studies*, 49:403–409, 1982.

[116] S. Eloranta, C. Lambert, T.M. Andersson, M. Bjorkholm, and P.W. Dickman. The application of cure models in the presence of competing risks: a tool for improved risk communication in population-based cancer patient survival. *Epidemiology*, 25:742–748, 1982.

[117] H.B. Fang, G. Li, and J. Sun. Maximum likelihood estimation in a semi-parametric logistic/proportional-hazards mixture model. *Scandinavian Journal of Statistics*, 32:59–75, 2005.

[118] V.T. Farewell. A model for a binary variable with time-censored observations. *Biometrika*, 64:43–46, 1977.

[119] V.T. Farewell. The use of a mixture model for the analysis of survival data with long-term survivors. *Biometrics*, 38:1041–1046, 1982.

[120] C.L. Faucett and D.C. Thomas. Simultaneously modelling censored survival data and repeatedly measured covariates: a Gibbs sampling approach. *Statistics in Medicine*, 15:1663–1685, 1996.

[121] W. Feller. *An Introduction to Probability Theory and Applications, Volume 2*. New York: Wiley, 1971.

[122] J.P. Fine and R.J. Gray. A proportional hazards model for the subdistribution of a competing risk. *Journal of the American Statistical Association*, 94:496–509, 1999.

[123] G.M. Fitzmaurice, N.M. Laird, and J.H. Ware. *Appied Longitudinal Analysis*. Hoboken, NJ: Wiley, 2004.

[124] T.R. Fleming and D.P. Harrington. Nonparametric estimation of the survival distribution in censored data. *Communications in Statistics - Theory and Methods*, 13(20):2469–2486, 1984.

[125] T.R. Fleming and D.P. Harrington. *Counting Processes and Survival Analysis*. New York: Wiley, 1991.

[126] B. Freidlin and E.L. Korn. Testing treatment effects in the presence of competing risks. *Statistics in Medicine*, 24:1703–1712, 2005.

[127] M.H. Gail. A review ad critique of some models used in competing risk analysis. *Biometrics*, 31:209–222, 2012.

[128] A. Garcia-Hernandez and D. Rizopoulos. %jm macro website.

[129] G. Garibotti, A. Tsodikov, and M. Clements. *Nltm: Non-linear transformation model*, 2019. version 1.4.2.

[130] J.J. Gaynor, E.J. Feuer, C.C. Tan, Wu D.H., C.R. Little, D.J. Straus, B.D. Clarkson, and M.F. Brennan. On the use of cause-specific failure and conditional failure probabilities: Examples from clinical oncology data. *Journal of the American Statistical Association*, 88:400–409, 1993.

[131] G. Gelman, R. Gelber, and I.C. et al. Henderson. Improved methodology for analyzing local and distant recurrence. *Journal of Clinical Oncology*, 8:548–555, 1990.

[132] R. Geskus. *Data Analysis with Competing Risks and Intermediate States*. Chapman & Hall/CRC Press, Boca Raton 2016.

[133] R.B. Geskus. Cause-specific cumulative incidence estimation and the Fine and Gray model under both left truncation and right censoring. *Biometrics*, 67:39–49, 2011.

[134] R.B. Geskus. Censoring strategies when using competing risks with time-dependent covariates. Letter to the editor. *Journal of Acquired Immune Deficiency Syndrome*, 46:512, 2011.

[135] Y.K. Getachew, P. Janssen, D.Y. Gebre, N. Speybroek, and L. Duchateau. Coping with time and space in modelling malaria incidence: a comparison of survival and count regression models. *Statistics in Medicine*, 32:3224–3233, 2013.

[136] M.E. Ghitany, R.A. Maller, and S. Zhou. Exponential mixture models with long term survivors and covariates. *Journal of Multivariate Analysis*, 49:218–241, 1994.

[137] D.V. Glidden and E. Vittinghoff. Modelling clustered survival data from multicentre clinical trials. *Statistics in Medicine*, 23:369–388, 2004.

[138] K. Goethals, P. Janssen, and L. Duchateau. Frailty models and copulas: similarities and differences. *Journal of Applied Statistics*, 35:1071–1079, 2008.

[139] T.A. Gooley, W. Leisenring, J. Crowley, and B.E. Storer. Estimation of failure probabilities in the presence of competing risks: New representations of old estimators. *Statistics in Medicine*, 18:695–706, 1999.

[140] M. Gorfine, D.M. Zucker, and L. Hsu. Prospective survival analysis with a general semiparametric shared frailty model: a pseudo full likelihood approach. *Biometrika*, 93:735–741, 2016.

[141] A.L. Gould, M.E. Boye, M.J. Crowther, J.G. Ibrahim, G. Quartey, S. Micallef, and F.Y. Bois. Joint modelling of survival and longitudinal non-survival data: current methods and issues. report of the DIA Bayesian joint modeling working group. *Statistics in Medicine*, 34:2181–2195, 2015.

[142] N. Grambauer, M. Schumacher, and J. Beyersmann. Proportional subdistribution hazards modeling offers a summary analysis, even if misspecified. *Statistics in Medicine*, 29:875–884, 2010.

[143] P.M. Grambsch and T.M. Therneau. Proportional hazards tests and diagnostics based on weighted residuals. *Biometrika*, 81:515–526, 1994.

[144] B. Gray. *Cmprsk: Subdistribution analysis of competing risks*, 2020. version 2.2.10.

[145] R.J. Gray. A class of K-sample tests for comparing the cumulative incidence of a competing risk. *Annals of Statistics*, 16:1141–1154, 1988.

[146] R.J. Gray. Flexible methods for analysing survival data using splines, with applications to breast cancer prognosis. *Journal of the American Statistical Association*, 87:942–951, 1992.

[147] R.J. Gray. cmprsk: Subdistribution analysis of competing risks. R package version 2.2-1. 2010.

[148] Y. Gu, D. Sinha, and S. Banerjee. Analysis of cure rate survival data under proportional odds model. *Lifetime Data Analysis*, 17:123–134, 2011.

[149] I.D. Ha, N.J. Christian, J.H. Jeong, J. Park, and Y. Lee. Analysis of clustered competing risks data using subdistribution hazard models with multivariate frailties. *Statistical Methods in Medical Research*, 25:2488–2505, 2016.

[150] I.D. Ha, R. Sylvester, C. Legrand, and G. MacKenzie. Frailty modelling for survival data from multi-centre clinical trials. *Statistics in Medicine*, 30:2144–2159, 2011.

[151] J. Han, E.H. Slate, and E.A Pena. Parametric latent class joint modelling of longitudinal and time-to-event data. *Statistics in Medicine*, 26:5285–5302, 2007.

[152] D.D. Hanagal. *Modeling Survival Data Using Frailty Models*. Chapman & Hall/CRC, 2010.

[153] F.E. Harrell. *Regression Modeling Strategies: With Applications to Linear Models, Logistic Refression, and Survival Analysis. Second Edition.* New York: Springer, 2015.

[154] D.P. Harrington and T.R. Fleming. A class of rank test procedures for censored survival data. *Biometrika*, 69:553–566, 1982.

[155] D.S. Hawkins, D.M. Allen, and A.J. Stromberg. Determining the number of components in mixtures of linear models. *Computational Statistics and Data Analysis*, 38:15–48, 2001.

[156] J.J. Heckman and B.E. Honoré. The identifiability of the competing risk model. *Biometrika*, 76:325–330, 1989.

[157] J.J. Heckman and B. Singer. Population heterogeneity in demographic models. In *Multidimensional Mathematical Demography. Eds. K. Land and A. Rogers.* New York: Academic Press, 1982.

[158] R. Henderson, P.J. Diggle, and A. Dobson. Joint modelling of longitudinal measurements and event time data. *Biostatistics*, 1:465–480, 2000.

[159] J. Herndon and F. Harrell. The restricted cubic spline hazard model. *Communication in Statistics - Theory and Methods*, 19:639–663, 1996.

[160] K. Hess and R. Gentleman. *Muhaz: Hazard function estimation in survival analysis*, 2019. version 1.2.6.1.

[161] K.R. Hess and B. Brown. Hazard function estimators: a simulation study. *Statistics in Medicine*, 18:3075–3088, 1999.

[162] G.L. Hickey, P. Philipson, and A. Jorgensen. Joint modelling of time-to-event and multivariate longitudinal outcomes: recent developments and issues. *BMC Medical Rsearch Methodology*, 16:117–132, 2016.

[163] K. Hirsch and A. Wienke. Software for Semiparametric Shared Gamma and Log-Normal Frailty Models: An Overview. *Computer Methods and Programs in Biomedicine*, 107:582–597, 2012.

[164] P. Hougaard. Life table methods for heterogeneous population. *Biometrika*, 71:75–83, 1984.

[165] P. Hougaard. A class of multivariate failure time distributions. *Biometrika*, 73:671–678, 1986.

[166] P. Hougaard. Survival models for heterogeneous populations derived from stable distributions. *Biometrika*, 73:387–396, 1986.

[167] P. Hougaard. *Analysis of Multivariate Survival Data*. New York: Springer-Verlag, 2000.

[168] F. Hsieh, Y.K. Tseng, and J.L. Wang. Joint modelling of survival and longitudinal data: likelihood approach revisited. *Biometrics*, 62:1037–43, 2007.

[169] W. Hsu, D. Todem, and K. Kim. A sup-score test for the cure fraction in mixture models for long-term survivors. *Biometrics*, 76:1348–1357, 2016.

[170] P Schnell (https://stats.stackexchange.com/users/41260/p schnell). The positive stable distribution in r. Cross Validated. URL:https://stats.stackexchange.com/q/89026 (version: 2014-03-06).

[171] R. Huster, R. Brookmeyer, and G. Self. Modelling paired survival data with covariates. *Biometrics*, 45:145–156, 1989.

[172] J. G. Ibrahim, M.-H. Chen, and D. Sinha. Bayesian semiparametric models for survival data with a cure fraction. *Biometrics*, 57:444–452, 2001.

[173] J.G. Ibrahim, M.H. Chen, and D. Sinha. *Bayesian survival analysis*. Springer-Verlag, New York 2001.

[174] SAS Institute Inc. Sas/stat software, version 9.4, 2003. Cary, NC.

[175] Boag J. Maximum likelihood estimates of the proportion of patients cured by cancer therapy. *Journal of the Royal Statistical Society, Series B*, 11:15–53, 1949.

[176] J.H. Jeong and J.P. Fine. Parametric regression on cumulative incidence function. *Biostatistics*, 8:184–196, 2007.

[177] Z. Jin. M-estimation in regression model for censored data. *Journal of Statistical Planning and Inference*, 137:3894–3903, 2007.

[178] Z. Jin, D.Y. Lin, L.J. Wei, and Z. Jing. Rank-based inference for the accelerated failure time model. *Biometrika*, 90:341–353, 2003.

[179] P. Joly, D. Commenges, and L. Letenneur. A penalized likelihood approach for arbitrarily censored and truncated data: application to age-specific incidence of dementia. *Biometrics*, 54:185–194, 1998.

[180] J. Kalbfleisch and R. Prentice. Marginal likelihoods based on Cox's regression and life model. *Biometrika*, 60:267–278, 1958.

[181] J. Kalbfleisch and R. Prentice. *The Statistical Analysis of Failure Time Data, Second Edition*. New York: Wiley, 2002.

[182] E.L. Kaplan and P. Meier. Nonparametric estimation from incomplete observations. *Journal of the American Statistical Association*, 53:457–481, 1958.

[183] N. Keiding, P.K. Andersen, and J.P. Klein. The role of frailty models and accelerated failure time models in describing heterogeneity due to omitted covariates. *Statistics in Medicine*, 16:215–224, 1997.

[184] M.G. Kendall. A new measure of rank correlation. *Biometrika*, 30:81–93, 1938.

[185] S. Kim, M. Chen, D. Dey, and D. Gamerman. Bayesian dynamic models for survival data with a cure fraction. *Lifetime Data Analysis*, 13:17–35, 2007.

[186] J. Klein and M. Moeschberger. *Survival Analysis - Techniques for Censored and Truncated Data*. New York: Springer-Verlag, 2003.

[187] J.P. Klein. Semiparametric estimation of random effects using the Cox model based on the EM algorithm. *Biometrics*, 48:795–806, 1992.

[188] J.P. Klein. Modelling competing risks in cancer studies. *Statistics in Medicine*, 25:1015–1034, 2006.

[189] J.P. Klein and R. Bajorunaite. Inference for competing risks. In *Handbook of Statistics*. Eds. N. Balakrishnan and C.R. Rao, volume 23. Elsevier Science, Amsterdam, 2004.

[190] J.P. Klein, M.L. Moeschberger, Y.H. Li, and S.T. Wang. Estimating random effects in the Framingham heart study. *Survival Analysis: State of the Art*, Boston: Kluwer Academic, 99–120, 1992.

[191] J.P. Klein, C. Pelz, and M.J. Zhang. Random effects for censored data by a multivariate normal regression model. *Biometrics*, 55:497–506, 1999.

[192] J.P. Klein, H.C. van Houwelingen, J.G. Ibrahim, and T.H. Scheike. *Handbook of Survival Analysis.* Chapman & Hall/CRC Press. Boca Raton 2013.

[193] D.G. Kleinbaum and M. Klein. *Survival Analysis: A Self-Learning Text. Second Edition.* Springer, New York 2005.

[194] M.T. Koller, H. Raatz, E.W. Steyerberg, and M. Wolbers. Competing risks and the clinical community: irrelevance or ignorance? *Statistics in Medicine,* 31:1089–1097, 2012.

[195] A. Komarek, E. Lesaffre, and J.F. Hilton. Accelerated failure time model for arbitrarily censored data with smoothed error distribution. *Journal of Computational and Graphical Statistics,* 14:726–745, 2007.

[196] A. Komarek, E. Lesaffre, and C. Legrand. Baseline and treatment effect heterogeneity for survival times between centers using a random effects accelerated failure time model with flexible error distribution. *Statistics in Medicine,* 26:5457–5472, 2007.

[197] C. Kooperberg. *Polspline: Polynomial spline routines,* 2020. version 1.1.19.

[198] E.L. Korn and F.J. Dorey. Applications of crude incidence curves. *Statistics in Medicine,* 11:813–829, 1992.

[199] D. Kraus. Adaptive Neyman's smooth tests of homogeneity of two samples of survival data. *Journal of Statistical Planning and Inference,* 139:3559–3569, 2009.

[200] A. Krol, A. Mauguen, Y. Mazroui, A. Laurent, S. Michiels, and V. Rondeau. Tutorial in joint modeling and prediction: a statistical software for correlated longitudinal outcome, recurrent events and a terminal event. *Journal of Statistical Software,* 81, 1992.

[201] A. Kuk and C. Chen. A mixture model combining logistic regression with proportional hazards regression. *Biometrika,* 79:531–541, 1992.

[202] S.W. Lagakos. General right censoring and its impact in the analysis of survival data. *Biometrics,* 35:139–56, 1979.

[203] X. Lai and K.K.W. Yau. Long-term survivor model with bivariate random effects: Applications to bone marrow transplant and carcinoma study data. *Statistics in Medicine,* 27:5692–5708, 2008.

[204] N.M. Laird and J.H. Ware. Random-effects models for longitudinal data. *Biometrics,* 38:963–974, 1979.

[205] K.F. Lam and Y.W. Lee. Merits of modelling multivariate survival data using random effects proportional odds model. *Biometrical Journal,* 46:331–342, 2002.

[206] K.F. Lam, Y.W. Lee, and T.L. Leung Modeling multivariate survival data by a semiparametric random effects proportional odds model. *Biometrics*, 58:316–323, 2002.

[207] P.C. Lambert. Modeling the cure fraction in survival studies. *The Stata Journal*, 7:1–25, 2007.

[208] P.C. Lambert, P.W. Dickman, C.L. Weston, and J.R. Thompson. Estimating the cure fraction in population-based cancer studies by using finite mixture models. *Journal of the Royal Statistical Society, Series C*, 59:35–55, 2010.

[209] P.C. Lambert, J.R. Thompson, C.L. Weston, and P.W. Dickman. Estimating and modeling the cure fraction in population-based cancer survival analysis. *Biostatistics*, 8:576–594, 2007.

[210] M.G. Larson and G.E. Dinse. A mixture model for the regression analysis of competing risks data. *Journal of he Royal Statistical Society, Series C, Applied Statistics*, 34:201–211, 1985.

[211] A. Latouche, A. Allignol, J. Beyersmann, M. Labopin, and J.P. Fine. A competing risks analysis should report results on all cause-specific and cumulative incidence functions. *Journal of Clinical Epidemiology*, 66:648–653, 2013.

[212] A. Latouche, J. Beyersmann, and J.P. Fine Leter to the editor: Comments on analysing and interpreting competing risks data. *Statistics in Medicine*, 26:3676–3680, 2007.

[213] A. Latouche, V. Boisson, S. Chevret, and R. Porcher. Misspecified regression model for the subdistribution hazard of a competing risk. *Statistics in Medicine*, 26:965–974, 2007.

[214] A. Latouche, G. Li, and Q. Yang. Competing risks. In *Textbook of Clinical Trials in Oncology: A Statistical Perspective*. Eds. S. Halabi and S. Michiels. Chapman & Hall/CRC Press, Boca Raton 2019.

[215] A. Latouche and R. Porcher. Sample size calculations in the presence of competing risks. *Statistics in Medicine*, 26:5370–5380, 2007.

[216] J.A. Laurie, C.G. Moertel, T.R. Fleming, et al. Surgical adjuvant therapy of large-bowel carcinoma: an evaluation of levamisole and the combination of levamisole and fluorouracil: The North Central Cancer Treatment Group and the Mayo Clinic. *Journal of Clinical Oncology*, 7:1447–1456, 1989.

[217] J.F. Lawless. *Statistical Models and Methods for Lifetime Data. Second Edition.* New York: Wiley, 2002.

[218] E.W. Lee, L.J. Wei, and D. Amato. Cox-type regression analysis for large number of small groups of correlated failure time observations. In Survival *Analysis, State of the Art*. Eds. J. P. Klein and P. K. Goel. Netherlands: Kluwer, 1992.

[219] K. Leffondré, C. Touraine, C. Helmer, and P. Joly. Interval-censored time-to-event and competing risk with death: is the illness-death model more accurate than the Cox model? *International Journal of Epidemiology*, 42:1177–1186, 2013.

[220] C. Legrand and A. Bertrand. Cure models in cancer clinical trials. In *Textbook of Clinical Trials in Oncology. A Statistical Perspective*. Eds. S. Halabi and S. Michiels. CRC Press, Chapman & Hall/CRC Press. Boca Raton. 2019.

[221] C. Legrand, L. Duchateau, P. Janssen, V. Ducrocq, and R. Sylvester. Validation of prognostic indices using the frailty model. *Lifetime Data Analysis*, 15:59–78, 2009.

[222] C. Legrand, L. Duchateau, R. Sylvester, P. Janssen, van der Hagen J.A., C.J.H. van de Velde, and P. Therasse. Heterogeneity in disease free survival between centers: lessons learned from an EORTC breast cancer trial. *Clinical Trials*, 3:10–18, 2006.

[223] C. Legrand, V. Ducrocq, P. Janssen, R. Sylvester, and L. Duchateau. A Bayesian approach to jointly estimate center and treatment by center interaction heterogeneity in a proportional hazards model. *Statistics in Medicine*, 24:3789–3804, 2005.

[224] C.-S. Li and J.M.G. Taylor. A semi-parametric accelerated failure time cure model. *Statistics in Medicine*, 21:3235–3247, 2002.

[225] G. Li and Q. Yang. Joint inference for competing risks survival data. *Journal of the American Statistical Association*, 111:1289–1300, 2016.

[226] J. Li, J. Le-Rademacher, and J. Zhang. Weighted comparison of two cumulative incidence functions with R-CIFsmry package. *Computer Methods and Programs in Biomedicine*, 116:205–2014, 2014.

[227] Y. Li and L. Ryan. Modeling spatial survival data using semiparametric frailty models. *Biometrics*, 58:287–297, 2002.

[228] D.Y. Lin. Cox regression analysis of multivariate failure time data: the marginal approach. *Statistics in Medicine*, 13:2233–2247, 1994.

[229] D.Y. Lin. Non-parametric inference for cumulative incidence functions in competing risks studies. *Statistics in Medicine*, 16:901–910, 1997.

[230] G. Lin, Y. So, and G. Johnston. *Analyzing survival data with competing risk using SAS software*, 2012. SAS Global Forum.

[231] N.X. Lin, S. Logan, and W.E. Henley. Bias and sensitivity analysis when estimating treatment effects from the Cox model with omitted covariates. *Biometrics*, 69:850–860, 2013.

[232] D.P. Lindstrom. Economic opportunity in Mexico and return migration from the United States. *Demography*, 33:357–374, 2009.

[233] M.J. Lindstrom and D.M Bates. Newton-Raphson and EM algorithms for linear mixed-effects models for repeated-measures data. *Journal of the American Statistical Association*, 83:1014–1022, 1988.

[234] H. Liu and Y. Shen. A semiparametric regression cure model for interval-censored data. *Journal of the American Statistical Association*, 104:1168–1178, 2009.

[235] A. Lopez-Cheda, R. Car, M. Jácome, and I. Van Keilegom. Nonparametric incidence estimation and bootsrap bandwidth selection in mixture cure models. *Computational Statistics and Data Analysis*, 105:144–165, 2017.

[236] K. Lu and A.A. Tsiatis. Multiple imputation methods for estimating regression coefficients in the competing risks model with missing cause of failure. *Biometrics*, 57:1191–1197, 2001.

[237] W. Lu. Maximum likelihood estimation in the proportional hazards cure model. *Annals of the Institute of Statistical Mathematics*, 60:545–574, 2008.

[238] W. Lu. Efficient estimation for an accelerated failure time model with a cure fraction. *Statistica Sinica*, 20:661–674, 2010.

[239] W. Lu and Z. Ying. On semiparametric transformation cure models. *Biometrika*, 91:331–343, 2004.

[240] M. Lunn and D. McNeil. Applying Cox regression to competing risks. *Biometrics*, 51:524–532, 1995.

[241] Y. Ma and G. Yin. Cure rate model with mismeasured covariates under transformation. *Journal of the American Statistical Association*, 103:743–756, 2008.

[242] A.S. Macdonald. Modeling the impact of genetics on insurance. *North American Actuarial Journal*, 3:83–105, 1999.

[243] S. Maetani and W. Gamel. Parametric cure model versus proportional hazards model in survival analysis of breast cancer and other malignancies. *Advances in Breast Cancer Research*, 2:119–125, 2013.

[244] R.A. Maller and X. Zhou. *Survival Analysis with Long-Term Survivors*. Wiley, John Wiley & Sons Ltd, Chichester, England 1997.

[245] S.O. Manda and R. Meyer. Bayesian inference for recurrent events data using time-dependent frailty. *Statistics in Medicine*, 24:1263–1274, 2005.

[246] N. Mantel and W. Haenszel. Statistical aspect of the analysis of data from retrospective studies of disease. *Journal of the National Cancer Institute*, 22:719–748, 1999.

[247] D. Marquardt. An algorithm for least-squares estimation of nonlinear parameters. *SIAM Journal of Applied Mathematics*, 11:431–441, 1963.

[248] T. Martinussen and T.H. Scheike. *Dynamic Regression Models for Survival Data*. Springer, New York 2006.

[249] E. Marubini and G. Valsecchi. *Analysing Survival Data from Clinical Trials and Observational Studies*. Wiley, 2004.

[250] M. Matsuura and S. Eguchi. Modeling late entry bias in survival analysis. *Biometrics*, 61:559–566, 2005.

[251] K. Mauff, E. Steyerberg, I. Kardys, E. Boersma, and D. Rizopoulos. Joint models with multiple longitudinal outcomes and a time-to-event outcome: a corrected two-stage approach. *Statistics and Computing*, 30:999–1014, 2020.

[252] A. Mauguen, S. Collette, J.P. Pignon, and V. Rondeau. Concordance measures in shared frailty models: application to clustered data in cancer prognosis. *Statistics in Medicine*, 32:4803–4820, 2013.

[253] C.A McGilchrist. REML estimation for survival models with frailty. *Biometrics*, 49:221–225, 1993.

[254] C.A McGilchrist and C.W. Aisbett. Regression with frailty in survival analysis. *Biometrics*, 47:461–466, 1991.

[255] C.G. Moertel, T.R. Fleming, J.S. MacDonald, D.G. Haller, J.A. Laurie, P.J. Goodman, J.S. Ungerleider, W.A. Emerson, D.C. Tormey, J.H. Glick, M.H. Veeder, and J.A. Maillard. Levamisole and fluorouracil for adjuvant therapy of resected colon carcinoma. *New England Journal of Medicine*, 332:352–358, 1990.

[256] C.G. Moertel, T.R. Fleming, J.S. MacDonald, D.G. Haller, J.A. Laurie, C.M. Tangen, J.S. Ungerleider, W.A. Emerson, D.C. Tormey, J.H. Glick, M.H. Veeder, and J.A. Maillard. Fluorouracil plus Levamisole as an effective adjuvant therapy after resection of stage II colon carcinoma: a final report. *Annals of Internal Medicine*, 122:321–326, 1995.

[257] G. Molenberghs and M.G. Kenward. *Missing Data in Clinical Studies*. Wiley, John Wiley & Sons, Ltd, Chichester, England 2007.

[258] G. Molenberghs and G. Verbeke. *Models for Discrete Longitudinal Data*. Springer Verlag, 2005.

[259] V. Mondelaers, S Suciu, and De Moerloose, B, et al. Prolonged versus standard native E. coli asparaginase therapy in childhood acute lymphoblastic leukemia and non-Hodgkin lymphoma: final results of the EORTC-CLG randomized phase III trial 58951. *Haematologica*, 102:1727–1738, 2017.

[260] D.F. Moore. *Applied Survival Analysis Using R*. Springer, 2016.

[261] M. Moreno-Betancur and A. latouche. Regression modeling of the cumulative incidence function with missing causes of failures using pseudo-values. *Statistics in Medicine*, 32:3206–3223, 2013.

[262] H.G. Muller and J.L. Wang. Hazard rate estimation under random censoring with varying kernels and bandwidths. *Biometrics*, 50:61–76, 1994.

[263] M. Munda and C. Legrand. Adjusting for centre heterogeneity in multicentre clinical trials with a time-to-event outcome. *Pharmaceutical Statistics*, 13:145–152, 2014.

[264] M. Munda, C. Legrand, L. Duchateau, and P. Janssen. Testing for decreasing heterogeneity in a new time-varying frailty model. *Test*, 25:591–606, 2016.

[265] M. Munda, F. Rotolo, and C. Legrand. parfm: Parametric Frailty Models in R. *Journal of Statistical Software*, 51, 2012.

[266] S.A. Murphy, A. Rossini, and A.W. van der Vaart. Maximum likelihood estimation in the proportional odds model. *Journal of the American Statistical Association*, 92:968–976, 1997.

[267] J.Z. Musoro, R.B. Geskus, and A.H. Zwinderman. A joint model for repeated events of different types and multiple longitudinal outcomes with application to a follow-up study of patients after kidney transplant. *Biometrical Journal*, 57:185–200, 1997.

[268] N. J. D. Negelkerke. A note on a general definition of the coefficient of determination. *Biometrika*, 78:691–692, 1991.

[269] R.B. Nelsen. *An Introduction to Copulas*. New York: Springer-Verlag, 2006.

[270] W. Nelson. Theory and applications of hazard plotting for censored failure data. *Technometrics*, 14:945–966, 1972.

[271] M.A. Nicolaie, J.M.G. Taylor, and C. Legrand. Vertical modeling: analysis of competing risks data with a cure fraction. *Lifetime Data Analysis*, 25:1–25, 2019.

[272] G.G. Nielsen, R.D. Gill, P.K. Andersen, and T.I.A.A. Sorensen. A counting process approach to maximum likelihood estimation in frailty models. *Scandinavian Journal of Statistics*, 19:25–43, 1992.

[273] K. Ohneberg and M. Schumacher. Sample size calculations for clinical trials. In *Handbook of Survival Analysis*. Eds. J. Klein, H. van Houwelingen, J.G. Ibrahim, and T.H. Scheike. Chapman & Hall/CRC Press, 2014.

[274] E.M.M. Ortega, G.D.C. Barriga, V.G. Hashimoto, and G.M. Cordeiro. A new class of survival regression models with cure fraction. *Journal of Data Science*, 12:107–136, 2014.

[275] F. O'Sullivan. Fast computation of fully automated log-density and log-hazard estimators. *SIAM Journal of Science and Statistical Computation*, 9:363–379, 1988.

[276] M. Othus, M. Barlogie, M.L. LeBlanc, and J.J. Crowley. Cure models as a useful tool for analysing survival. *Statistics in Clinical Cancer Research*, 18:3731–3736, 2012.

[277] A. Palumbo, S. Bringhen, and S.K. et al. Kumar. Second primary malignancies with lenalidomide therapy for newly diagnosed myeloma: a meta-analysis of individual patient data. *The Lancet Oncology*, 15:333–342, 2014.

[278] X. Paoletti and Asselain B. Survival analysis on clinical trials: Old tools or new techniques. *Surgical Oncology*, 19:55–58, 2010.

[279] G. Papageorgiou, K. Mauff, A. Tomer, and D. Rizopoulos. An overview of joint modeling of time-to-event and longitudinal outcomes. *Annual Review of Statistics and Its Application*, 6:223–240, 2019.

[280] V. Patilea and I. Van Keilegom. A general approach for cure models in survival analysis. Annals of Statistics, 48:2323–2346, 2020.

[281] H.D. Patterson and R. Thompson. Recovery of inter-block information when block sizes are unequal. *Biometrika*, 58:545, 1971.

[282] K.E. Peace. *Design and Analysis of Clinical Trials with Time-to-Event Endpoints*. Boca Raton: Chapman & Hall/CRC Press, 2009.

[283] Y. Peng. Estimating baseline distribution in proportional hazards cure models. *Computational Statistics and Data Analysis*, 42:187–201, 2003.

[284] Y. Peng. *Gfcure: Parametric Accelerated Failure Time Mixture Cure Model*, 2017. version 2.0.

[285] Y. Peng and K. Dear. A nonparametric mixture model for cure rate estimation. *Biometrics*, 56:237–243, 2000.

[286] Y. Peng, K. B.G. Dear, and J. W. Denham. A generalized f mixture model for cure rate estimation. *Statistics in Medicine*, 17:813–830, 1998.

[287] Y. Peng and J. Taylor. Residual-based model diagnosis methods for mixture cure models. *Biometrics*, 73:495–505, 2017.

[288] Y. Peng and J.M.G. Taylor. Mixture cure model with random effects for the analysis of a multicentre tonsil cancer study. *Statistics in Medicine*, 30:211–223, 2011.

[289] Y. Peng and J.M.G. Taylor. Cure models. In *Handbook of Survival Analysis*. Eds. J. Klein, H. van Houwelingen, J.G. Ibrahim, and T.H. Scheike. Chapman and Hall/CRC Press, Boca Raton 2014.

[290] Y. Peng and J. Xu. An extended cure model and model selection. *Lifetime Data Analysis*, 18:215–233, 2012.

[291] Y. Peng and J. Zhang. Estimation method of the semiparametric mixture cure gamma frailty model. *Statistics in Medicine*, 27:5177–5194, 2008.

[292] Y. Peng and J. Zhang. Identifiability of mixture cure frailty model. *Statistics & probability Letters*, 78:2604–2608, 2008.

[293] M.L. Pennell and D.B. Dunson. Bayesian semiparametric dynamic frailty models for multiple event time data. *Biometrics*, 62:1044–1052, 2006.

[294] M.S. Pepe and M. Mori. Kaplan-Meier, marginal, or conditional probability curves in summarizing competing risks failure time data. *Statistics in Medicine*, 12:737–751, 1993.

[295] A.N. Pettitt. Proportional Odds Models for Survival Data and Estimates Using Ranks. *Journal of the Royal Statistical Society, Series C*, 33:169–175, 1984.

[296] A.N. Pettitt and I. Bin Daud. Case-weighted measures of influence for proportional hazards regression. *Applied Statistics*, 38:51–67, 1989.

[297] P. Philipson, I. Sousa, P.J. Diggle, P. Williamson, R. Kolamunnage-Dona, R. Henderson, and G.L. Hickey. *JoineR: Joint modelling of repeated measurements and time-to-event data*, 2020. version 1.2.5.

[298] J. Pinheiro and D. Bates. *Mixed-Effects Models in S and S-Plus*. Springer, New York 2000.

[299] J. Pinheiro and D. Bates. *Nlme: Linear and Nonlinear mixed effects models*, 2020. version 3.1-148.

[300] M. Pintilie. *Competing Risks: A Practical Perspective*. Wiley, John Wiley & Sons, Ltd Chichester, England 2006.

[301] M. Pohar and J. Stare. Relative survival analysis in R. *Computer Methods and Programs in Biomedicine*, 81:272–278, 2017.

[302] F. Portier, A. El Ghouch, and I. Van Keilegom. Efficiency and bootstrap in the promotion time cure model. *Bernoulli*, 23:3437–3468, 2017.

[303] R.L. Prentice, J.D. Kalbfleisch, A.V. Peterson, N. Flournoy, V.T. Farwell, and N.E. Breslow. The analysis of failure time in the presence of competing risks. *Biometrics*, 34:541–554, 1978.

[304] D.L. Price and A.K. Manatunga. Modelling survival data with a cured fraction using frailty models. *Statistics in Medicine*, 20:1515–1527, 2001.

[305] C. Proust-Lima, P. Joly, and H. Jacqmin-Gadda. Joint modelling of multivariate longitudinal outcomes and a time-to-event: a nonlinear latent class approach. *Computational Statistics and Data Analysis*, 53:1142–1154, 2009.

[306] C. Proust-Lima, S Mbery, J.M.G Taylor, and H. Jacqmin-Gadda. Joint latent class models for longitudinal and time-to-event data: a review. *Statistical Methods in Medical Research*, 23:74–90, 2014.

[307] C. Proust-Lima, V. Philippes, A. Diakite, and B. Liquet. *Lcmm: Extended mixed models using laten classes and latent processes*, 2020. version 1.9.2.

[308] C. Proust-Lima, V. Philipps, and B. Liquet. Estimation of extended mixed models using latent classes and latent processes: The R package lcmm. *Journal of Statistical Software*, 78:1–56, 2014.

[309] C. Proust-Lima and J. Taylor. Development and validation of a dynamic prognostic tool for prostate cancer recurrence using repeated measures of posttreatment PSA: A joint modeling approach. *Biostatistics*, 10:535–549, 2009.

[310] H. Putter, L. de Wreede, M. Fiocco, and R. Geskus. *Mstate: Data preparation, estimation and prediction in multi-state models*, 2019. version 0.2.12.

[311] H. Putter, M. Fiocco, and R.B. Geskus. Tutorial in biostatistics: competing risks and multi-state models. *Statistics in Medicine*, 26:2389–2430, 2007.

[312] H. Ramlau-Hansen. Smoothing counting process intensities by means of kernel functions. *The Annals of Statistics*, 11:453–466, 1983.

[313] J.O. Ramsey. Monotone regression splines in action. *Statistical Science*, 3:425–461, 1988.

[314] G. Rauch and J. Beuersmann. Planning and evaluating clinical trials with composite time-to-first-event endpoints in a competing risk framework. *Statistics in Medicine*, 32:3595–3608, 2013.

[315] P. Rebora, A. Salim, and M. Reilly. *Bshazard: Nonparametric smoothing of the hazard function*, 2018. version 1.1.

[316] R.A. Redner and Walker F.H. Mixture densities, maximum likelihood and the EM algorithm. *SIAM Review*, 26:195–239, 1984.

[317] S. Ripatti, K. Larsen, and J. Palgrem. Maximum likelihood inference for multivariate frailty models using an automated Monte-Carlo EM algorithm. *Lifetime Data Analysis*, 8:349–360, 2000.

[318] S. Ripatti and J. Palgrem. Estimation of multivariate frailty models using penalized partial likelihood. *Biometrics*, 56:1016–1022, 2000.

[319] D. Rizopoulos. Fast fitting of joint models for longitudinal and even time data using a pseudo-adaptive Gaussian quadrature rule. *Computational Statistics and Data Analysis*, 56:491–501, 2012.

[320] D. Rizopoulos. *Joint Models for Longitudinal and Time-to-Event Data*. Chapman & Hall/CRC Press, Boca Raton 2012.

[321] D. Rizopoulos. *JM: Joint Modeling of Longitudinal and survival data*, 2018. version 1.4.8.

[322] D. Rizopoulos. *JMbayes: Joint modeling of longitudibal and time-to-event data under a Bayesian approach*, 2020. version 0.8-85.

[323] D. Rizopoulos and P. Ghosh. A Bayesian semiparametric multivariate joint model for multiple longitudinal outcomes and a time-to-event. *Statistics in Medicine*, 30:1366–1380, 2011.

[324] D. Rizopoulos, G. Verbeke, and E. Lesaffre. Fully exponential Laplace approximation for the joint modeling of survival and longitudinal data. *Journal of the Royal Statitsical Society, Series B*, 71:637–654, 2009.

[325] D. Rizopoulos, G. Verbeke, and G. Molenberghs. Shared parameter models under random effects misspecification. *Biometrika*, 95:63–74, 2008.

[326] C.S. Rocha. Survival models for heterogeneity using the non-central chi-square distribution with zero degrees of freedom. In *Lifetime Data: Models in Reliability and Survival Analysis*. Eds. N. Jewell et al. Dordrecht: Kluwer Academic Publishers, 1996.

[327] V. Rondeau, D. Commenges, and P. Joly. Maximum penalized likelihood estimation in a gamma frailty model. *Lifetime Data Analysis*, 9:139–153, 2003.

[328] V. Rondeau, L. Filleul, and P. Joly. Nested frailty models using maximum penalized likelihood estimation. *Statistics in Medicine*, 25:4036–4052, 2005.

[329] V. Rondeau, J.R. Gonzales, Y. Mazroui, A. Mauguen, A. Diakite, A. Laurent, M. Lopez, A. Krol, C.S. Sofeu, J. Dumerc, and D. Rustand. *Frailtypack: General Frailty Models: Shared, joint and nested frailty models with prediction; Evaluation of Failure-time surrogate endpoints*, 2020. version 3.3.0.

[330] V. Rondeau and J.R. Gonzalez. frailtypack: A computer program for the analysis of correlated failure time data using penalized likelihood estimation. *Computer Methods and Programs in Biomedicine*, 80:154–164, 2005.

[331] V. Rondeau, J.R. Gonzalez, Y. Mazroui, A. Mauguen, A. Diakite, and A. Laurent. frailtypack:General Frailty Models Using a Semi-Parametrical Penalized Likelihood Estimation or a Parametrical Estimation. R package version 2.2-26. 2012.

[332] V. Rondeau, S. Mathoulin-Pelissier, H. Jacqmin-Gadda, V. Brouste, and P. Soubeyran. Joint frailty models for recurring events and death using maximum penalized likelihood estimation: application on cancer events. *Biostatistics*, 8:708–721, 2007.

[333] V. Rondeau, Y. Mazroui, and J.R. Gonzalez. Frailtypack: An R package for the analysis of correlated survival data with frailty models using penalized likelihood estimation or parametrical estimation. *Journal of Statistical Software*, 47:1–28, 2012.

[334] V. Rondeau, S. Michiels, B. Liquet, and J.P. Pignon. Investigating trial and treatment heterogeneity in an individual patient data meta-analysis of survival data by means of the penalized maximum likelihood approach. *Statistics in Medicine*, 27:1894–1910, 2007.

[335] P. Rosenberg. Hazard function estimation using B-splines. *Biometrics*, 51:874–887, 1995.

[336] S. Rosthoj, P.K. Andersen, and S.Z. Abidstrom. SAS macros for estimation of the cumulative incidence functions based on a Cox regression model for competing risks survival data. *Computer Method and Programs in Biomedicine*, 74:69–75, 2004.

[337] F. Rotolo, M. Munda, and A. Callegaro. *Parfm: Parametric frailty models*, 2018. version 2.7.6.

[338] P. Royston and M.K.B. Parmar. Flexible parametric proportional-hazards and proportional-odds models for censored survival data, with application to prognostic modelling and estimation of treatment effects. *Statistics in Medicine*, 21:2175–2197, 2012.

[339] P. Royston and M.K.B. Parmar. Restricted mean survival time: an alternative to the hazard ratio for the design and analysis of randomized trials with a time-to-event outcome. *BMC Medical Research Methodology*, 13:152, 2013.

[340] P.K. Ruan and R.J. Gray. Analyses of cumulative incidence functions via non-parametric multiple imputation. *Statistics in Medicine*, 27:5709–5724, 2012.

[341] T. Scheike, T. Martinussen, J. Silver, and K. Holst. *Timereg: Flexible regression models for survival data*, 2020. version 1.9.6.

[342] T.H. Scheike, Y. Sun, M.J. Zhang, and T.K. Jensen. A semiparametric random effects model for multivariate competing risks data. *Biometrika*, 97:133–145, 2010.

[343] T.H. Scheike and M.J. Zhang. An additive-multiplicative Cox-Aalen Model. *Scandinavian Journal of Statistics in Medicine*, 28:75–88, 2002.

[344] T.H. Scheike and M.J. Zhang. Extensions and applications of the Cox-Aalen survival models. *Biometrics*, 59:1033–1045, 2003.

[345] T.H. Scheike and M.J. Zhang. Flexible competing risks regression modelling and goodness-of-fit. *Lifetime Data Analysis*, 14:464–483, 2008.

[346] T.H. Scheike and M.J. Zhang. Analyzing competing risk data using the R timereg package. *Journal of Statistical Software*, 38:pii:i02, 2011.

[347] Y. Schen and S.C. Cheng. Confidence bands for cumulative incidence curves under the additive risk model. *Biometrika*, 55:1093–1100, 1999.

[348] C. Schmoor and M. Schumacher. Effects of covariate omission and categorization when analysing randomised trials with the Cox model. *Statistics in Medicine*, 16:225–237, 1997.

[349] G. Schulgen, M. Olschewski, V. Krane, C. Wanner, and G. Ruf. Sample sizes for clinical trials with time-to-event endpoints and competing risks. *Contemporary Clinical Trials*, 26:386–396, 2005.

[350] M. Schumacher, M. Olschewski, and C. Schmoor. The impact of heterogeneiy on the comparison of survival times. *Statistics in Medicine*, 6:773–784, 1987.

[351] S. Scolas, A. El Ghouch, and C. Legrand. Variable selection in a flexible parametric mixture cure model with interval-censored data. *Statistics in Medicine*, 35:1210–1225, 2016.

[352] S. Scolas, C. Legrand, , A. Oulhaj, and A. El Ghouch. Diagnostic checks in mixture cure models with interval-censoring. *Statistical Methods in Medical Research*, 27:2114–2131, 2018.

[353] K. Seppa, T. Hakulinen, H.J. Kim, and E. Laara. Cure fraction model with random effects for regional variation in cancer survival. *Statistics in Medicine*, 29:2781–2793, 2008.

[354] B.W. Silverman. Some aspects of the spline smoothing approach to non-parametric regression curve fitting. *Journal of the Royal Statistical Society, Series B*, 47:1–52, 1985.

[355] Y. So, G. Lin, and G Johnston. Using the phreg procedure to analysze competing risks data. 2015.

[356] C. Sofeu and V. Rondeau. How t use frailtypack for validating failure-time surrogate endpoints using individual ptient data from meta-analyses of randomized controlled trials. *Plos One*, 15, 2020.

[357] H. Song, Y. Peng, and D. Tu. A new approach for joint modeling of longitudinal measurements and survival times with a cure fraction. *Canadian Journal of Statistics*, 40:207–224, 2012.

[358] D.J. Spiegelhalter, A. Thomas, N.G. Best, and D. Lunn. WinBUGS Version 1.4 User Manual. 2003.

[359] C.F. Spiekerman and D.Y. Lin. Marginal regression models for multivariate failure time data. *Journal of the American Statistical Asociation*, 93:1164–1175, 1998.

[360] R. Sposto. Cure model analysis in cancer: an application to data from the childrens cancer group. *Statistics in Medicine*, 21:293–312, 2002.

[361] M. Stephens. Dealing with label switching in mixture models. *Journal of the Royal Statistical Society Series B*, 62:795–809, 2000.

[362] E. Steyerberg. *Clinical Prediction Models: A Practical Approach to Development, Validation and Updating.* Springer, New York 2009.

[363] W.W. Stroup. *Generalized Linear Mixed Models. Modern Concepts, Methods and Applications.* CRC Press, Boca Raton 2012.

[364] W.W. Stroup, G.A Miliken, E.A. Claassen, and R.D Wolfinger. *SAS for Mixed Models. Introduction and Basic Applications.* Cary, NC: SAS Institute, Inc., 2018.

[365] C.A. Struthers and J.D. Kalbfleisch. Misspecified proportional hazard models. *Biometrika*, 73:363–369, 2000.

[366] J. Sun. *The Statistical Analysis of Interval-Censored Failure Time Data.* New York: Springer-Verlag, 2006.

[367] J. Sy and J. Taylor. Estimation of a Cox proportional hazards cure model. *Biometrics*, 56:227–236, 2000.

[368] M. Tableman and J.S. Kim. *Survival Analysis using S. Analysis of Time-to-Event Data*. Chapan & Hall/CRC, Boca Raton 2004.

[369] J. Taylor. Semi-parametric estimation in failure time mixture models. *Biometrics*, 51:899–907, 1995.

[370] J. Taylor and N. Liu. Statistical issues invovled with extending standards models. In *Advances in Statistical Modeling and Inference: Essays in Honor of Kjell A Doksum, series in biostatistics*. Eds V. Nair. World Scieentific, Singapore, 2007.

[371] R Core Team. R: A language and environment for statistical computing, 2017. Vienna, Austria: R Foundation for Statistical Computing.

[372] T. Therneau and P. Grambsch. *Modeling Survival Data: Extending the Cox Model*. New York: Springer-Verlag, 2000.

[373] T.M. Therneau. *Coxme: Mixed effects Cox models*, 2015. version 2.2-5.

[374] T.M. Therneau. *Survival: Survival Analysis*, 2020. version 3.2-3.

[375] T.M. Therneau, P.M. Grambsch, and T.R. Fleming. Martingale-based residuals for survival models. *Biometrika*, 77:147–160, 1990.

[376] T.M. Therneau, P.M. Grambsch, and V. Shane Pankratz. Penalized survival models and frailty. *Journal of Computational and Graphical Statistics*, 12:156–175, 2003.

[377] M. Tournoud and R. Ecochard. Promotion time models with time-dependent exposure and heterogeneity: Application to infection disease. *Biometrical Journal*, 50:395–407, 2008.

[378] L. Trinquart, J. Jacot, S.C. Conner, and R. Porcher. Comparison of treatment effects measured by the hazard ratio and by the restricted mean survival times in oncology randomized controlled trials. *Journal of Clinical Oncology*, 34:1813–1819, 2016.

[379] A. Tsiatis and M. Davidian. Joint modeling of longitudinal and time-to-event data: an overview. *Statistica Sinica*, 14:809–834, 2004.

[380] A.A. Tsiatis. A nonidentifiability aspect of the problem of competing risks. In *Proceedings of the National Academy of Sciences of the United States of America*, volume 72, pages 20–22, 1975.

[381] A.A. Tsiatis. A nonidentifiability aspect of the problem of competing risks. *Proceedings of the National Academy of Sciences of the United States of America*, 72:20–22, 1975.

[382] A.A. Tsiatis. *Competing Risk*. New York: Wiley, 1999.

[383] A. Tsodikov. Asymptotic efficiency of a proportional hazards model with cure. *Statistics and Probability Letters*, 39:237–244, 1998.

[384] A. Tsodikov. A proportional hazards model taking account of long-term survivors. *Biometrics*, 54:1508–1516, 1998.

[385] A. Tsodikov. Estimation of survival based on proportional hazards when cure is a possibility. *Mathematical and Computer Modelling*, 33:1227–1236, 2001.

[386] A. Tsodikov. Semi-parametric models of long- and short-term survival: an application to the analysis of breast cancer survival in utah by age and stage. *Statistics in Medicine*, 21:895–920, 2002.

[387] A.D. Tsodikov. Semiparametric models: a generalized self-consistency approach. *Journal of the Royal Statistical Society, Series B*, 65:759–774, 2003.

[388] A.D. Tsodikov, J.G. Ibrahim, and A.Y. Yakovlev. Estimating cure rates from survival data: an alternative to two-components mixture models. *Journal of the American Statistical Association*, 98:1063–1078, 2003.

[389] C. Tudur-Smith, P.R. Williamson, and A.G. Marson. Investigating heterogeneity in an individual patient data meta-analysis of time to event outcomes. *Statistics in Medicine*, 24:1307–1319, 2005.

[390] M. Tweedy. An index which distinguishes between some important exponential families. Statistics: applications and new directions. In *Proceedings of the Indian Statistical Institute Golden Jubilee International Conference*. Eds. J. Ghosh and J. Roy, 1984.

[391] H. Uno, B. Claggett, L. Tian, E. Inoue, P. Gallo, T. Miyata, D. Schrag, M. Takeuchi, Y. Uyama, L. Zhao, H. Skali, S. Solomon, S. Jacobus, M. Hughes, M. Packer, and L.J. Wei. Moving beyond the hazard ratio in quantifying the between-group difference in survival analysis. *Journal of Clinical Oncology*, 32:2380–2385, 2014.

[392] F. Vaida and R. Xu. Proportional hazards model with random effects. *Statistics in Medicine*, 19:3309–3324, 2000.

[393] H. van Houwelingen and H. Putter. *Dynamic Prediction in Clinical Survival Analysis*. Chapman & Hall/CRC Press, Boca Raton 2011.

[394] I. Van Keilegom, M. Akritas, and N. Veraverbeke. Estimation of the conditional distribution in regression with censored data: a comparative study. *Computational Statistics and Data Analysis*, 35:487–500, 2001.

[395] R. Van Oirbeeck and E. Lesaffre. An application of harell's c-index to PH frailty models. *Statistics in Medicine*, 2010:3160–3171, 2010.

[396] B. Van Rompaye, S. Jaffar, and E. Goetghebeur. Estimation with Cox models: cause-specific analysis with misclassified cause of failure. *Epidemiology*, 23:194–202, 2012.

[397] J.W. Vaupel, K.G. Manton, and E. Stallard. The impact of heterogeneity in individual frailty on the dynamics of mortality. *Demography*, 16:439–454, 1979.

[398] J.W. Vaupel and A.I. Yashin. Heterogeneity's ruses: Some surprising effects of selection on population dynamics. *The American Statistician*, 39:176–185, 1985.

[399] G. Verbeke and G. Molenberghs. *Linear Mixed Models for Longitudinal Data*. New York: Springer-Verlag, 2000.

[400] E. Vittinghoff, S.C. Shiboski, D.V. Glidden, and C.E McCulloch. *Regression Methods in Biostatistics. Linear, Logistic, Survival and Repeated Measures Models*. New York: Springer-Verlag, 2005.

[401] S. Viviani, M. Alfo, and D. Rizopoulos. Generalized linear mixed joint model for longitudinal and survival outcomes. *Statistics and Computing*, 24:417–427, 2014.

[402] S.T. Wang, J.P. Klein, and M.L. Moeaschberger. Semi-parametric estimation of covariate effects using the positive stable frailty model. *Applied Stochastic Models and Data Analysis*, 11:121–133, 1995.

[403] L.J. Wei. The accelerated failure time model: A useful alternative to the Cox regression model in survival analysis. *Statistics in Medicine*, 11:1871–1879, 1992.

[404] R.E. Weiss. *Modeling Longitudinal Data*. Springer, New York 2005.

[405] H. White. Maximum likelihood estimation of misspecified models. *Econometrica*, 50:1–25, 1982.

[406] A. Wienke. *Frailty Models in Survival Analysis*. Chapman & Hall/CRC Press, New York 2010.

[407] E. Wileyto, Y. Li, and J.H.D. Chen. Assessing the fit of the parametric cure models. *Biostatistics*, 14:340–350, 2013.

[408] P.R. Williamson, R. Kolamunnage-Dona, P. Philipson, and A.G. Marson. Joint modelling of longitudinal and competing risks data. *Statistics in Medicine*, 27:6426–6438, 2008.

[409] P.R. Williamson, R. Kolamunnage-Dona, and C. Tudur-Smith. The influence of competing-risks setting on the choice of the hypothesis test for treatment effect. *Biostatistics*, 8:689–694, 2007.

[410] C.M.A. Wintrebert, H. Putter, A.H. Zwinderman, and H.C. van Houwelingen. Centre-effect on survival after bone marrow transplantation: Application of time-dependent frailty models. *Biometrical Journal*, 46:512–525, 2004.

[411] M.S. Wulfsohn and A.A. Tsiatis. A joint model for survival and longitudinal data measured with error. *Biometrics*, 53:330–339, 1997.

[412] J. Xu and Y. Peng. Nonparametric cure rate estimation with covariates. *Canadian Journal of Statistics*, 42:1–17, 2014.

[413] X. Xu and R. Brookmeyer. Bivariate frailty models for the analysis of multivariate survival time. *Lifetime Data Analysis*, 2:277–289, 1996.

[414] A. Yakovlev, B. Asselain, V. Bardou, A. Fouquet, and T. Hoang. A simple stochastic model of tumor recurrence and its application to data on premenopausal breast cancer. In *Biométrie et Analyse de Données Spatio-Temporelles*, pages 66–83, 1993.

[415] A. Yakovlev, A.D. Tsodikov, B. Asselain. Stochastic Models of Tumor Latency and Their Biostatistical Applications. Singapore; New Jersay: World Scientific, 1996.

[416] K. Yamaguchi. Accelerated failure-time regression models with a regression model of surviving fraction: an application to the analysis of permanent employment in Japan. *Journalof the American Statistical Assocation*, 87:284–292, 2013.

[417] Q. Yang, W.K. Fung, and G. Li. Sample size determination for jointly testing a cause-specific hazard and the all-cause hazard in the presence of competing risks. *Statistics in Medicine*, 37:1389–1401, 2018.

[418] A.I. Yashin and I.A. Iachine. Genetic analysis of durations: correlated fralty model applied to survival of Danish twins. *Genetic Epidemiology*, 12:529–538, 1995.

[419] A.I. Yashin, J.W. Vaupel, and I.A. Iachine. Correlated individual frailty: an advantageous approach to survival analysis of bivariate data. *Mathematical Population Studies*, 5:145–159, 1995.

[420] K.K.W. Yau and C.A. McGilchrist. ML and REML estimation in survival analysis with time dependent correlated frailty. *Statistics in Medicine*, 17:1201–1213, 1998.

[421] K.K.W. Yau and A.S.K Ng. Long-term survivor mixture model with random effects: application to a multi-centre clinical trial of carcinoma. *Statistics in Medicine*, 20:1591–1607, 2001.

[422] Y. Yilmaz, J.F. Lawless, I.L. Andrulis, and S.B. Bull. Insight from mixture cire modeling of molecular markers for prognosis in breast cancer. *Journal of Clinical Oncology*, 31:2047–2054, 2013.

[423] G. Yin. Bayesian cure rate frailty models with application to a root canal therapy study. *Biometrics*, 61:552–558, 2005.

[424] G. Yin and J. Ibrahim. A class of Bayesian shared gamma frailty models with multivariate failure time data. *Biometrics*, 61:208–216, 2005.

[425] G. Yin and J. Ibrahim. Cure rate model: a unified approach. *Canadian Journal of Statistics*, 33:559–570, 2005.

[426] B. Yu and R. Tiwari. A Bayesian approach to mixture cure models with spatial frailties for population-based cancer relative to survival data. *Canadian Journal of Statistics*, 40:40–54, 2012.

[427] D. Zeng and J. Cai. Simultaneous modelling of survival and longitudinal data with an application to repeated quality of life measures. *Lifetime Data Analysis*, 11:151–174, 2005.

[428] D. Zeng, G. Yin, and J. Ibrahim. Semiparametric transformation for survival data with a cure fraction. *Journal of the American Statistical Association*, 101:670–684, 2006.

[429] J. Zhang and Y. Peng. A new estimation method for the semiparametric accelerated failure time mixture cure model. *Statistics in Medicine*, 26:3157–3171, 2007.

[430] J. Zhang and Y. Peng. Accelerated hazards mixture cure model. *Lifetime Data Analysis*, 15:455–467, 2009.

[431] M.J. Zhang and J.P. Fine. Summarizing differences in cumulative incidence functions. *Statistics in Medicine*, 27:4939–4949, 2008.

[432] L. Zhao, B. Claggett, L. Tian, H. Uno, M.A. Pfeffer, S.D. Solomon, Trippa L., and L.J. Wei. On the Restricted Mean Survival Time Curve in Survival Analysis. *Biometrics*, 72:215–221, 2016.

[433] Y. Zhao, A. Lee, K. Yau, V. Burke, and G. McLachlan. A score test for assessing the cured proportion in long-term survivor mixture model. *Statistics in Medicine*, 28:3454–3466, 2009.

[434] B. Zhou, J. Fine, A. Latouche, and M. Labopin. Competing risks regression for clustered data. *Biostatistics*, 13:371–383, 2012.

[435] D. Zhuang, N. Schenker, J.M.G. Taylor, V. Mosseri, and B. Dubray. Analysing the effects of anemia on local recurrence of head and neck cancer when covariates values are missing. *Statistics in Medicine*, 19:1237–1249, 2016.

Index

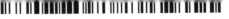

Printed in the United States
by Baker & Taylor Publisher Services